SCIENTIFIC CRITERIA TO ENSURE SAFE FOOD

Committee on the Review of the Use of Scientific Criteria
and Performance Standards for Safe Food
Food and Nutrition Board
Board on Agriculture and Natural Resources

INSTITUTE OF MEDICINE
NATIONAL RESEARCH COUNCIL
OF THE NATIONAL ACADEMIES

THE NATIONAL ACADEMIES PRESS
Washington, D.C.
www.nap.edu

THE NATIONAL ACADEMIES PRESS 500 Fifth Street, N.W. Washington, DC 20001

NOTICE: The project that is the subject of this report was approved by the Governing Board of the National Research Council, whose members are drawn from the councils of the National Academy of Sciences, the National Academy of Engineering, and the Institute of Medicine. The members of the committee responsible for the report were chosen for their special competences and with regard for appropriate balance.

Support for this project was provided by U.S. Department of Health and Human Services, Food and Drug Administration, under contract number 223-01-2460, Task Order 6, and the U.S. Department of Agriculture, Food Safety and Inspection Service, under contract number FSIS-27-B-01. The views presented in this report are those of the Committee on the Review of the Use of Scientific Criteria and Performance Standards for Safe Food and are not necessarily those of the funding agencies.

Library of Congress Cataloging-in-Publication Data

Committee on the Review of the Use of Scientific Criteria and Performance Standards for Safe Food.

Scientific criteria to ensure safe food / Committee on the Review of the Use of Scientific Criteria and Performance Standards for Safe Food, Food and Nutrition Board, Board on Agriculture and Natural Resources.

p. ; cm.

Includes bibliographical references.

ISBN 0-309-08928-X (hardcover), ISBN 0-309-50920-3 (PDF)

ISBN-13: 978-0-309-08928-9

1. Food—Safety measures 2. Food adulteration and inspection.

[DNLM: 1. Food Contamination—prevention & control. 2. Food Microbiology. 3. Food Supply—standards. WA 701 S416 2003] I. Title.

TX531.C586 2003

363.19′26—dc22

2003015501

Additional copies of this report are available from the National Academies Press, 500 Fifth Street, N.W., Lockbox 285, Washington, DC 20055; (800) 624-6242 or (202) 334-3313 (in the Washington metropolitan area); Internet, http://www.nap.edu.

For more information about the Institute of Medicine, visit the IOM home page at: **www.iom.edu.**

Printed in the United States of America.

THE NATIONAL ACADEMIES

Advisers to the Nation on Science, Engineering, and Medicine

The **National Academy of Sciences** is a private, nonprofit, self-perpetuating society of distinguished scholars engaged in scientific and engineering research, dedicated to the furtherance of science and technology and to their use for the general welfare. Upon the authority of the charter granted to it by the Congress in 1863, the Academy has a mandate that requires it to advise the federal government on scientific and technical matters. Dr. Bruce M. Alberts is president of the National Academy of Sciences.

The **National Academy of Engineering** was established in 1964, under the charter of the National Academy of Sciences, as a parallel organization of outstanding engineers. It is autonomous in its administration and in the selection of its members, sharing with the National Academy of Sciences the responsibility for advising the federal government. The National Academy of Engineering also sponsors engineering programs aimed at meeting national needs, encourages education and research, and recognizes the superior achievements of engineers. Dr. Wm. A. Wulf is president of the National Academy of Engineering.

The **Institute of Medicine** was established in 1970 by the National Academy of Sciences to secure the services of eminent members of appropriate professions in the examination of policy matters pertaining to the health of the public. The Institute acts under the responsibility given to the National Academy of Sciences by its congressional charter to be an adviser to the federal government and, upon its own initiative, to identify issues of medical care, research, and education. Dr. Harvey V. Fineberg is president of the Institute of Medicine.

The **National Research Council** was organized by the National Academy of Sciences in 1916 to associate the broad community of science and technology with the Academy's purposes of furthering knowledge and advising the federal government. Functioning in accordance with general policies determined by the Academy, the Council has become the principal operating agency of both the National Academy of Sciences and the National Academy of Engineering in providing services to the government, the public, and the scientific and engineering communities. The Council is administered jointly by both Academies and the Institute of Medicine. Dr. Bruce M. Alberts and Dr. Wm. A. Wulf are chair and vice chair, respectively, of the National Research Council.

www.national-academies.org

COMMITTEE ON THE REVIEW OF THE USE OF SCIENTIFIC CRITERIA AND PERFORMANCE STANDARDS FOR SAFE FOOD

CLAUDE EARL FOX *(Co-chair)*, Urban Health Institute, Johns Hopkins University, Baltimore, Maryland

CAMERON HACKNEY *(Co-chair)*, Davis College of Agriculture, Forestry and Consumer Sciences, West Virginia University, Morgantown

KATHRYN J. BOOR, Department of Food Science, Cornell University, Ithaca, New York

ELIZABETH BOYLE, Department of Animal Sciences and Industry, Kansas State University, Manhattan

MARSHA N. COHEN, Hastings College of the Law, University of California, San Francisco

JAMES S. DICKSON, Department of Microbiology, Iowa State University, Ames

DARRELL W. DONAHUE, Department of Chemical and Biological Engineering, University of Maine, Orono

JEFFREY M. FARBER, Bureau of Microbial Hazards, Health Products and Food Branch, Food Directorate, Health Canada, Ottawa, Ontario

ROBERT GRAVANI, Department of Food Science, Cornell University, Ithaca, New York

RICHARD L. GUERRANT, Division of Geographic and International Medicine, Health Sciences Center, University of Virginia, Charlottesville

NEAL H. HOOKER, Department of Agricultural, Environmental and Development Economics, The Ohio State University, Columbus

JOHN A. MARCY, Center of Excellence for Poultry Science, University of Arkansas, Fayetteville

DONALD W. SCHAFFNER, Department of Food Science, Rutgers University, New Brunswick, New Jersey

DONN R. WARD, Department of Food Science, North Carolina State University, Raleigh

Consultants

THOMAS P. GRUMBLY, Keystone Center, Keystone, Colorado

J. GLENN MORRIS, JR., Department of Epidemiology and Preventative Medicine, University of Maryland School of Medicine, Baltimore

ROBERT V. TAUXE, National Center for Infectious Diseases, Centers for Disease Control and Prevention, Atlanta, Georgia

SUBCOMMITTEE ON MEAT AND POULTRY

JAMES S. DICKSON *(Chair)*, Department of Microbiology, Iowa State University, Ames
ELIZABETH BOYLE, Department of Animal Sciences and Industry, Kansas State University, Manhattan
NEAL H. HOOKER, Department of Agricultural, Environmental and Development Economics, The Ohio State University, Columbus
JOHN A. MARCY, Center of Excellence for Poultry Science, University of Arkansas, Fayetteville
JIM E. RIVIERE, Center for Chemical Toxicology Research and Pharmacokinetics, College of Veterinary Medicine, North Carolina State University, Raleigh
JOHN G. SURAK, Department of Food Science and Nutrition, Clemson University, Clemson, South Carolina
TERRI WENGER, Trade and Consumer Protection, Wisconsin Department of Agriculture, Madison

SUBCOMMITTEE ON PRODUCE AND RELATED PRODUCTS, SEAFOOD, AND DAIRY PRODUCTS

ROBERT GRAVANI *(Chair)*, Department of Food Science, Cornell University, Ithaca, New York
KATHRYN J. BOOR, Department of Food Science, Cornell University, Ithaca, New York
DARRELL DONAHUE, Department of Chemical and Biological Engineering, University of Maine, Orono
LINDA J. HARRIS, Department of Food Science and Technology, University of California-Davis
CRAIG HEDBERG, Division of Environmental and Occupational Health, University of Minnesota, Minneapolis
W. STEVEN OTWELL, Department of Food Science and Human Nutrition, University of Florida, Gainesville
DONN R. WARD, Department of Food Science, North Carolina State University, Raleigh

Staff

RICARDO MOLINS, Study Director
MARIA ORIA, Program Officer
TAZIMA A. DAVIS, Research Assistant
SANAIT TESFAGIORGIS, Senior Project Assistant
GAIL E. SPEARS, Staff Editor
GARY WALKER, Financial Associate

FOOD AND NUTRITION BOARD

BOARD ON AGRICULTURE AND NATURAL RESOURCES

Staff

CHARLOTTE KIRK BAER, Director
DONNA LEE JAMEISON, Administrative Assistant

Preface

Protecting public health by promoting food safety has long been recognized as a state and federal responsibility. It has evolved through a series of legislative acts that responded to the fact that a significant proportion of human illness and deaths often have their genesis in the food supply. The U.S. Congress, concerned about recurrent controversy regarding the scientific basis of food safety criteria in regulating meat and poultry processing, commissioned the National Academies, through the Food Safety Inspection Service of the U.S. Department of Agriculture (USDA), to conduct the study that has resulted in this report. The study was to emphasize, but not be limited to, microbiological criteria currently in use in the meat and poultry industries.

Recognizing that the issues surrounding food safety criteria are common to all sectors of the food industry, the National Academies invited the Food and Drug Administration (FDA) to cosponsor the study. As a result, the scope of the study includes food safety criteria currently in use in the processing of seafood, produce and related products, and dairy products. An ad hoc committee appointed by the National Academies to examine the relevant general issues of interest to the USDA and FDA was charged with developing two reports, assisted by two subcommittees, one on meat and poultry and a second one on seafood, produce and related products, and dairy products. However, it was later agreed with the sponsors than only one report would be produced. The committee was asked to develop definitions for the terms "performance standard" and "criteria" and to (1) evaluate the scientific basis for existing criteria, particularly microbiological performance standards, applicable to the selected food groups, and the extent to which these standards are appropriate means of ensuring the safety of such foods within a Hazard Analysis and Critical Control Point (HACCP)-based system; (2) define the science-based process to establish food safety criteria and recommend guidelines as to what data are adequate and appropriate for use in developing new, or modifying existing, criteria; (3) examine whether current criteria accomplish what they purport to accomplish and the need to relate science-based criteria to public health objectives; (4) review the need for performance standards as measures of process control and the way such criteria are used under HACCP; and (5) recommend changes for improvement. During its deliberations, the committee and subcommittees heard from consumer, industry, and government representatives, and from interested individuals.

The National Academies appointed a committee comprised of 14 members with expertise and background in HACCP, public health, epidemiology of foodborne diseases, food regulatory processes, law, consumer perspective, food science, food microbiology, statistics of process control, process engineering, risk assessment of food contaminants, and microbial growth modeling. The composition and size of this committee changed after the first meeting; representation from the public health and regulatory areas was augmented. Several committee members participated also in one of the two subcommittees, each composed of seven members with expertise in processing of the food groups under study. The subcommittee chairs worked closely with the committee co-chairs and, in a real sense, the overall committee had four co-chairs. Despite the diversity of disciplines and backgrounds represented, very lively and often intense discussions gave way to committee consensus quickly and readily.

To supplement its expertise and to gather information on specific issues relevant to its charge, the committee conducted a workshop and held three open sessions as part of three of the committee's six meetings. The committee is grateful to the participants in the expert panel, Jorgen Schlundt, World Health Organization; Robert Tauxe, Centers for Disease Control and Prevention; Carol Tucker Foreman, Consumer Federation of America; Don L. Zink; Kaye Wachsmuth, Food Safety Inspection Service (retired); Michael Taylor, Resources for the Future; and Frank Busta, University of Minnesota. The committee's appreciation is also extended to the USDA and FDA staff that contributed information, particularly Robert Buchanan (FDA), Philip Derfler (USDA), Daniel Englejohn (USDA), Elise Golan (USDA), and William Garthright (FDA). In addition, the committee is grateful to Bruce Tompkin, International Commission on Microbiological Specifications for Foods, for his presentation to the committee. Special recognition is extended to the representatives of consumer groups, trade organizations, and the general public who contributed valuable information or views that greatly enhanced the committee's knowledge and perspective on the issues under consideration.

The Executive Summary presents the recommendations and the principal findings of the committee, as well as some of the main definitions developed or adopted by the committee in response to the charge. Chapter 1 describes the historical development of food safety regulatory approaches in the United States; Chapter 2 highlights the importance of foodborne disease surveillance and monitoring of microbial contaminants of food, both from a public health standpoint and as measures of the effectiveness of food safety criteria; Chapter 3 describes a science-based strategy for developing food safety criteria, including performance standards, and the procedures for obtaining the best data to support this process. It also discusses various food safety tools available to the regulatory agencies in developing and implementing science-based food safety criteria, including concepts for addressing the magnitude of the risk of foodborne illness and identifying factors that control that risk, a novel approach to relate performance standards to public health objectives, and the economics of food safety criteria, and provides recommendations for improvement. The discussion of each "tool" in the report is limited by design to that which is relevant to food safety, recognizing that some, such as statistical process control and the economic aspects of criteria, not only may be foreign to many food processors and food safety regulators, but are also methodologies that only recently are being brought into play in food safety. The subcommittees, in turn, contributed sector-oriented perspectives to the overall effort of the committee, examined relevant issues and criteria, and made recommendations for improvement specific to the food groups under consideration (Chapters 4 through 7). The final chapter (Chapter 8) summarizes the committee's findings and recommendations.

As the study progressed, several members left the committee for various reasons. The committee thanks Emilio Esteban, who contributed his knowledge and enthusiasm to this report, and to George Hardy, who was appointed to the committee but could not join it. Similarly, the committee thanks Glenn Morris and Thomas Grumbly, who changed their status from members to committee consultants.

This report has been reviewed in draft form by individuals chosen for their diverse perspectives and technical expertise, in accordance with procedures approved by the National Research Council's Report Review Committee. The purpose of this independent review is to provide candid and critical comments that will assist the institution in making its published report as sound as possible and to ensure that the report meets institutional standards for objectivity, evidence, and responsiveness to the study charge. The review comments and draft manuscript remain confidential to protect the integrity of the deliberative process. We wish to thank the following individuals for their review of this report:

Bill Aimutis, Cargill, Inc.; Christopher G. Atchison, The University of Iowa; Mindy Brashears, Texas Tech University; Dean O. Cliver, University of California, Davis; Donald E. Conner, Auburn University; P. Michael Davidson, The University of Tennessee; Jeff Farrar, California Department of Health Services; George J. Flick, Jr., Virginia Polytechnic Institute and State University; John Floros, Pennsylvania State University; Carol Tucker Foreman, The Food Policy

Institute, Consumer Federation of America; Linda Golodner, National Consumers League; Richard L. Hall, Independent Consultant, Food Industry; Myron M. Levine, The University of Maryland; Joseph M. Madden, Neogen Corporation; Nancy J. Rachman, Food and Chemical Practice Exponents, Inc.; Joan Rose, The University of South Florida; Robert E. Smith, R.E. Smith Consulting, Inc.; John Sofos, Colorado State University; Ewen C.D. Todd, Michigan State University; Bruce R. Tompkin, Conagra Refrigerated Prepared Foods; Laurian Unnevehr, The University of Illinois; and Kaye Wachsmuth, Independent Consultant, Public Health Microbiology.

Although the reviewers listed above have provided many constructive comments and suggestions, they were not asked to endorse the conclusions or recommendations nor did they see the final draft of the report before its release. The review of this report was overseen by Michael Doyle, University of Georgia, and Ronald W. Estabrook, University of Texas Southwestern Medical Center. Appointed by the National Research Council and Institute of Medicine, they were responsible for making certain that an independent examination of this report was carried out in accordance with institutional procedures and that all review comments were carefully considered. Responsibility for the final content of this report rests entirely with the authoring committee and the institution.

The co-chairs of the main committee and the chairs of the subcommittee, on behalf of the full committee, commend the staff for their excellence in support, editing, and contributions. Ricardo Molins, study director, was an invaluable resource to the committee members, bringing both a national and international perspective to the process in addition to assisting in building consensus among the committee members. The chairs also thank Maria Oria, program officer, for helping the committee focus on the issues of concern and for her valuable suggestions throughout the process. The committee is grateful to Tazima Davis, research assistant, and Sanait Tesfagiorgis, senior project assistant, for their support and dedication. The chairs would also like to acknowledge the helpful contributions of Allison Yates, director of the Food and Nutrition Board, whose leadership gave the committee the tools to build consensus on the issues, and of Charlotte Kirk Baer, director of the Board on Agriculture and Natural Resources. This report would not be possible were it not for the contributions of the staff and they have our deepest appreciation.

It is with great satisfaction that we thank the committee, subcommittees, and consultants for sharing with us their knowledge and efforts in accomplishing the heavy task entrusted to us in a relatively short time and with an admirable display of teamwork.

Claude Earl Fox, Cameron Hackney
Co-Chairs, Committee on the Review of the Use of Scientific Criteria and Performance Standards for Safe Food

Contents

Acronyms

ALOP	Appropriate level of protection
AMS	Agricultural Marketing Service
APC	Aerobic plate count
APHIS	Animal and Plant Health Inspection Service
BRFSS	Behavioral Risk Factor Surveillance System
BSE	Bovine spongiform encephalopathy
CAC	Codex Alimentarius Commission
CCP	Critical Control Point
CDC	Centers for Disease Control and Prevention
CFR	*Code of Federal Regulations*
CSPI	Center for Science in the Public Interest
CVM	Center for Veterinary Medicine
DMC	Direct microscopic count
DNA	Deoxyribonucleic acid
EPA	U.S. Environmental Protection Agency
ETEC	Enterotoxigenic *Escherichia coli*
FAO	Food and Agriculture Organization of the United Nations
FarmSO	Farm Safety Objective
FDA	Food and Drug Administration

FSO	Food Safety Objective
FSIS	Food Safety and Inspection Service
GAO	U.S. General Accounting Office
GAP	Good Agricultural Practice
GHP	Good Hygienic Practice
GLP	Good Laboratory Practice
GMP	Good Manufacturing Practice
HACCP	Hazard Analysis and Critical Control Point
HIMP	HACCP-based Inspection Model Project
ICMSF	International Commission on Microbiological Specifications for Foods
IFPA	International Fresh-cut Produce Association
ISO	International Organization for Standardization
ISSC	Interstate Shellfish Sanitation Conference
JECFA	FAO/WHO Joint Expert Committee on Food Additives
MPN	Most probable number
mRNA	Messenger ribonucleic acid
NACMCF	National Advisory Committee on Microbiological Criteria for Foods
NAHMS	National Animal Health Monitoring System
NARMS	National Antimicrobial Resistance Monitoring System
NASA	National Aeronautics and Space Administration
NFSS	National Food Safety System
NOAEL	No-observed-adverse-effect level
NRC	National Research Council
OCP	Other consumer protection
PCR	Polymerase chain reaction
PHS	Public Health Service
PMO	Grade A Pasteurized Milk Ordinance
PR/HACCP	Pathogen Reduction; Hazard Analysis and Critical Control Point Final Rule
PSO	Processing Safety Objective
QMRA	Quantitative microbial risk assessment

RA	Risk assessment
RTE	Ready-to-eat
RTI	Research Triangle Institute
SCC	Somatic cell count
SERA	*Salmonella* Enteritidis risk assessment
SPC	Statistical Process Control
TSRO	Transportation and Retail Safety Objective
USDA	U.S. Department of Agriculture
VTEC	Verotoxigenic *Escherichia coli*
WHO	World Health Organization
WTO	World Trade Organization

Executive Summary

GENERAL FINDINGS

The balance of progress in the reduction of certain human foodborne illnesses following implementation of the Hazard Analysis and Critical Control Point (HACCP) system in various areas of the food industry is decidedly favorable. The technical, financial, and educational efforts made by industry to implement HACCP and by the regulatory agencies to audit such implementation are commendable, but further improvements are warranted. The committee believes that the emphasis of food safety regulatory agencies must continue to be on prevention, reduction, or elimination of foodborne hazards along the food continuum.

In addition to specific issues related to each food group included in the study, several overarching issues were raised during the committee's deliberations. Despite improvements made in the area of food safety, the translation of science to practice is at best difficult in a regulatory environment. Because of the inherent deliberative nature of governmental bodies, scientific tools must be adopted and novel approaches to food safety must be sought. The need for regulatory control must be balanced with the need for regulatory flexibility and the expectation that an agency's actions reflect the most current and effective scientific methods available to protect the public health. However, the food safety community's understanding of science-based methodologies and concepts such as risk assessment or food safety objectives is limited, and much of the data needed to develop science-based strategies are often incomplete, nonexistent, or require extensive resources to generate. Furthermore, none of the scientific tools available to support the development of food safety criteria is a panacea; they all present limitations, such as gaps in research data, that need to be recognized and considered.

A second issue noted by the committee was the need to improve the management and use of food safety data to ensure that foodborne diseases are identified as early as feasible and that the origin of foodborne hazards and the most effective interventions to prevent, reduce, or eliminate them are identified. This leads the committee to conclude that there is also a need to better coordinate existing and emerging food safety information systems.

Third, the committee noted that the approach to developing, implementing, and enforcing food safety criteria, including performance standards, varies among regulatory agencies. Implementation problems, including questions about the authority of regulatory agencies to enforce performance standards, have contributed to diminishing the effectiveness of new regulatory measures aimed at controlling old and emergent foodborne hazards and have prompted many to question the effectiveness and appropriateness of the current system. As a result, implementation and enforcement activities need to be considered by regulators when developing food safety criteria.

Summary of Recommendations

Food safety regulatory agencies are applying a host of new control measures, from mandating the use of HACCP to increasing testing, with varying degrees of success, to ensure the safety of the food supply. A collective effort is needed to further improve the safety of food, and the following actions should be pursued:

- **Congress should require the development of a comprehensive national plan to harmonize the foodborne disease surveillance that is conducted by public health agencies with the monitoring of pathogens across the food production, processing, and distribution continuum that is conducted by food safety regulatory agencies.** Congress should allocate funds not only to develop and implement this plan, but also to enhance programs such as FoodNet, PulseNet, eLEXNET, foodborne outbreak reporting and data sharing, and other national foodborne disease surveillance systems conducted by public health authorities.
- **Congress should grant the regulatory agencies clear authority to establish, implement, and enforce food safety criteria, including performance standards, and the flexibility needed within the administrative process to update these criteria;** it should allocate funds to enable the regulatory agencies to undertake pilot studies and develop and maintain databases to support the development and updating of food safety criteria.

- **Food safety regulatory agencies should adopt science-based, transparent strategies to develop food safety criteria that**
  - **Clearly document the public health objective and the appropriate level of protection.**
  - **Obtain or generate the best scientific knowledge through the use of laboratory or field studies, risk assessments, and similar food safety tools.**
  - **Minimize knowledge gaps by conducting pilot programs of the proposed performance standard, by maintaining databases of critical information, or by conducting risk assessments that can be used to develop performance standards, using science-based expertise as needed.**
  - **Explicitly state the nature, limits, and extent of the scientific uncertainties.**
  - **Explicitly identify the assumptions, criteria, and expertise used to address the uncertainties in formulating the performance standard.**

- **The U.S. Department of Agriculture should take the following specific measures regarding scientific criteria, collecting data, and improving the safety of meat and poultry products:**
  - Periodically conduct baseline surveys to evaluate the microbiological status of carcass, trim, ground products, and ready-to-eat products, at processing and at retail.
  - Implement criteria for generic *Escherichia coli* levels for ground beef using the current generic *E. coli* criteria for carcasses as the model, and handle the resulting data from carcasses and ground beef through a national, anonymous database.
  - Develop a *Salmonella* performance standard for beef trim intended for grinding and reevaluate the current *Salmonella* performance standard for ground beef. Require that all beef trim for grinding be exposed to some verified pathogen reduction intervention.
  - Expand testing of *E. coli* O157:H7 to include trim destined for grinding so that contaminated trim can be diverted to further processing with verified interventions.
  - Urgently undertake research on the ecology of *E. coli* O157:H7 and other closely related serotypes in beef, from the farm through the trim, to identify appropriate control points.

— Until information on the ecology and mode of transmission of *E. coli* O157:H7 is available, and other effective preventive or corrective controls can be applied, only cooking to a high enough temperature or sufficient irradiation can ensure the safety of ground beef. The irradiation process does not replace the need for proper cooking. The committee urges regulatory and health authorities to (1) advise those members of the public who would prefer to minimize the risk of this product to cook irradiated and nonirradiated ground beef products to the appropriate temperature, (2) require these products to be clearly labeled with a warning of the potential for harm if not properly cooked, and (3) expand educational efforts to the public and target commercial and noncommercial food service managers and workers.

— Establish a research focus on intervention trials at all stages of the meat and poultry production process, from farm to table.

- **The Food and Drug Administration (FDA) should take the following specific measures regarding scientific criteria, HACCP, imported foods, and improving the safety of seafood, produce, and dairy products:**

— Include a process validation protocol in the *Fish and Fisheries Products Hazards and Control Guide* and appoint an advisory committee to periodically update this guide.

— Develop strategies to ensure the safety of imported seafood and produce by focusing on pathogen intervention strategies prior to shipment and on international harmonization of standards.

— Expand research on risks associated with many specific practices in the fresh produce sector, and on the potential for and significance of internalization of pathogens into fresh produce.

— Implement targeted educational programs to inform the public about the risks of consuming raw milk and raw milk products.

— Work with industry to conduct research to assess the pathogen reduction efficacy of cheese manufacturing conditions and to develop science-based performance standards for reduction of targeted pathogens in finished cheese products.

— Along with state authorities, consider requiring clear and concise labeling to identify cheeses manufactured from unpasteurized milk.

- **State health authorities should ban the sale of raw milk, as has already been done by FDA in interstate commerce.**

To assist the regulatory agencies in harmonizing the language in future food safety regulations, the committee developed or adopted definitions for several key terms as presented in Box ES-1.

BOX ES-1 Definitions

Public health objective: A measurable population-based target for maintaining or improving health.

Food safety objective: A statement of the maximum frequency and/or concentration of a hazard in a food at the time of consumption that is considered tolerable for consumers.

Performance standard: The degree to which a step or combination of steps in the production, processing, distribution, and/or preparation of a food must operate to achieve the required level of control over a hazard.

Microbiological criterion: A criterion that defines the acceptability of a product or food lot, based on the absence or presence or number of microorganisms, including parasites, and/or the quantity of their toxins/metabolites, per unit of mass, volume, area, or lot.

Microbiological standard: A mandatory microbiological criterion that is incorporated into a law, regulation, or ordinance.

Microbiological guideline: An advisory microbiological criterion used to inform food operators of the microbiological content that can be expected in food when best practices are applied.

KEY ISSUES

Regulatory Authority and Flexibility to Enact, Enforce, and Update Food Safety Criteria

Legal challenges to actions taken by regulatory agencies in response to violations of established food safety criteria have cast doubts on the agencies' authority to enforce criteria. While the committee did not undertake an analysis of these challenges, this situation should be promptly addressed through Congressional action.

Moreover, the current administrative process to modify food safety criteria is too cumbersome to allow appropriate and timely updating of these regulations to keep up with scientific and technological progress. To remedy this lack of flexibility, Congress should enable regulatory agencies the ability to incorporate flexibility into the administrative process so that food safety criteria can be efficiently adjusted to meet future public health goals. This flexibility includes incorporating new processing or assessment techniques and allowing the agencies the ability to change a performance standard to align it with the best contemporary scientific knowledge.

Regulatory agencies, in turn, need to be consistent in auditing and enforcing compliance with established criteria. Furthermore, because of the rapid growth of food imports, it is essential that regulatory agencies properly monitor and enforce compliance with established performance standards and guidelines in imported foods.

Basing Food Safety Regulations on Science

A major step in advancing a science-based food safety system has been the implementation of HACCP in various sectors of the food industry. The efforts made by industry and regulators to this effect are commendable and should continue.

Regulatory agencies should follow a strategy that combines the best available data with the best expert judgment, as an appropriate, science-based means to establish food safety regulations. Scientific tools such as Microbiological Risk Assessment, Food Safety Objectives, and Statistical Process Control are available to regulators when developing and monitoring compliance with regulations. Good science-based policies should allow flexibility and encourage innovation with minimal regulatory revisions. This implies a regulatory framework that specifies results, but not the methods used to achieve these results. It also implies flexible criteria that can be efficiently changed in response to changing public health goals.

The Need to Link Food Safety Criteria to Public Health Objectives

Food safety criteria have the common objective of protecting or improving public health. Therefore, science-based food safety criteria must be clearly linked to the public health problem they are designed to address. This link, which is not always present in current regulations, would also provide a means to measure the effectiveness of new and existing regulations. To establish this link, data from foodborne disease surveillance programs and from monitoring pathogen contamination in foods must be made compatible and should be integrated.

Timely collection, analysis, and dissemination of surveillance data are essential to minimize the spread of foodborne disease outbreaks to a larger population, particularly in the light of concerns about potential intentional contamination of food. Internal sharing and comparison of compatible surveillance data, and collaboration with international surveillance systems, are also essential. However, current microbial monitoring of food in the United States is fragmented and often incompatible with foodborne disease surveillance; this reduces the effectiveness of much of the monitoring and surveillance. Efforts to standardize methodology and data reporting methods, such as PulseNet, are beginning to produce invaluable information, and their expansion is fundamental to an effective surveillance system.

Similarly, to collect data that can be compared to foodborne disease surveillance data, there is a need for periodic surveys of pathogen contamination, at various stages in the production/consumption continuum, of foods frequently associated with foodborne illness. These data are necessary to identify the optimal locations and means for effective interventions, through appropriate criteria, that will enhance the safety of foods.

SUMMARY FINDINGS

Tools and Procedures to Establish Science-Based Food Safety Criteria

- The emphasis of food safety regulatory agencies must continue to be on the prevention, reduction, or elimination of foodborne hazards along the food production, processing, and distribution continuum, rather than on inspection of the end product.
- There is a need to define "acceptable levels" of hazard reduction at critical control points linked to public health objectives. The Food Safety Objective concept can help establish this link and define these levels, and it can also provide a theoretical framework to relate performance standards to public health objectives.
- Failure to develop HACCP plans that are appropriately specific for a given processing plant, line, and product may contribute to failure of the plan.
- There are inconsistencies in the interpretation and enforcement of HACCP regulations between and within the regulatory agencies.
- Quantitative microbial risk assessment offers the scientific tools to define the most effective solutions for lowering consumer exposure to foodborne microbial hazards.
- Statistical Process Control linked to continuous improvement must be a part of food safety regulations. The concept of "continuous improvement" is central to food safety.
- Depending on the quality of available data, food safety regulatory agencies could use controlled studies, expert opinion, or a combination thereof to develop science-based food safety criteria. Because of common gaps in available data and scientific knowledge, the combination strategy is the optimal science-based procedure to develop food safety criteria.
- Efficient and cost-effective collection of appropriate data for scientific decision-making may be facilitated through ongoing, systematic development of databases and targeted pilot studies to address specific data gaps.
- Documenting the limitations of the data and the assumptions used, and making this information available to the public, provide essential transparency to the process of developing food safety criteria.
- When appropriate data are available, a performance standard may be developed by (1) assuming that all food-processing companies are producing food of an acceptable level and setting the performance standard at a level such that the lowest compliant processor will pass, while all of the

noncompliant plants will fail, or (2) setting the performance standard at a level where only a portion of the processing plants will pass, thus enabling future adjustments to the standard.

- When zero tolerance is used as a performance standard, unique methodology issues need to be considered.
- Performance standards must be linked to a public health goal and must incorporate a measure of effectiveness in meeting the public health goal.
- Regulatory agencies need flexibility in administrative procedures to update food safety criteria to align them with the best contemporary scientific knowledge.
- It is difficult to quantify the individual costs and benefits of performance standards implemented as part of a broad regulatory change. The thesis that flexibility allows innovation, borne out in the area of environmental regulations, may be amenable to extension into the food safety regulatory environment.

Foodborne Disease Surveillance and the Monitoring of Microbial Contaminants in Food

- Foodborne disease surveillance is essential for defining trends in foodborne disease, identifying outbreaks, allocating the burden of disease among food groups, and evaluating food safety programs.
- Compatible bacterial subtype and antimicrobial resistance surveillance data from humans, animals, farms, and food products should be linked among federal agencies and state laboratories.
- Systematic sampling of animals for pathogens preslaughter and at point of slaughter to obtain a clear understanding of contamination routes is lacking. Periodic, systematic, nonregulatory microbiological surveys of food-processing plants, with sampling at various points, should be conducted to provide a basis to revise baselines on the prevalence of pathogen and indicator microorganisms for foods frequently implicated in foodborne disease outbreaks.
- Monitoring microbial pathogens in produce and seafood (domestic and imported), live animals (on farm and preslaughter), and final products, and comparison with human isolates through compatible serotyping and subtyping, would provide data to develop and evaluate food safety interventions and regulations. Without such data, it is not possible to clearly establish the contribution of current food safety criteria to improvements in public health.
- Epidemiological and food monitoring data are essential when developing quantitative microbial risk assessments for use as a basis for food safety criteria.

Safety Criteria for Meat and Poultry

- The rationale for the process control performance criteria for fecal contamination is based on the frequency and levels of contamination of beef carcasses with *E. coli* and is appropriate. However, if populations of generic *E. coli* are extremely low, other testing approaches may be necessary.
- The *E. coli* data collected by industry are not in the public domain. Collection of such data should be extended to ground beef, and all data should be handled through a national, anonymous repository.
- The *Salmonella* performance standards for carcasses and ground meat are valid criteria to reduce the levels of salmonellae in or on meat. However, if the populations or incidence of salmonellae are extremely low, other testing approaches may be necessary.
- The *Salmonella* performance standard for ground beef products may not reflect the overall quality of the grinding operation. It may instead be a reflection of the quality of incoming raw materials.
- A *Salmonella* performance standard or other appropriate criterion is needed for beef trim intended for grinding.
- All meat intended for trim for ground products, especially ground beef, and including trim from heads, should be exposed to some form of verified pathogen reduction intervention.
- Based on public health data, the zero tolerance policy for *E. coli* O157:H7 in ground beef has been insufficient to reduce the rate of human illness attributable to this microorganism. It is important to emphasize the need for testing and interventions prior to the grinding operation.
- Information on the ecology and mode of transmission of *E. coli* O157:H7 and related serotypes is urgently needed to help develop preventive measures and effective interventions.
- Currently, only cooking to a high enough temperature or sufficient irradiation can ensure the safety of ground beef. The irradiation process does not replace the need for proper cooking.
- The guidelines requiring a specific lethality for *Salmonella* as a critical control point in HACCP plans for production of cooked beef and poultry and other related products are not well justified scientifically and have resulted in an excessively conservative performance standard.
- The scientific bases for the stabilization performance standards required in the production of cooked beef and poultry and other related products are not clear; the validity of the data and assumptions is difficult to determine. These standards do not include cured meat products and should not be applied to these products.
- Development of a standard using a safety margin based on a highly conservative worst-case scenario may lead to production of overprocessed products of inferior quality, as well as to undue economic burdens for the

processor. An inadequate safety margin may lead to production of unsafe products.

- Efforts to reduce the pathogenic contamination of animals preslaughter are a key part of a farm-to-table food safety strategy.
- Substantial declines since 1996 in several bacterial foodborne diseases in the United States indicate that the collective efforts to improve food safety are achieving improvements in public health. It is likely that the Pathogen Reduction/HACCP rule has contributed to the declines in infections caused by the meat-associated pathogens *Campylobacter*, *Listeria monocytogenes,* and *Yersinia enterocolitica;* it is also likely, however, that concurrent changes in distribution, retail, and consumer behavior also played a role.
- Measuring changes in consumer behavior, as well as subtyping microbial pathogen isolates from various food sources and comparing the results with isolates from human infections, could help define a cause-and-effect relationship between performance standards and improved public health.
- Emphasizing contamination prevention rather than end-product testing to ensure the safety of meat is justified. The conclusion of previous National Academies' reports that carcass-by-carcass inspection is an ineffective food safety strategy remains valid. Meat and poultry processors and regulators should use process control techniques to ensure that performance standards for meat and poultry are met.

Safety Criteria for Seafood

- Mandatory seafood HACCP has made positive contributions to seafood safety; further benefits will depend on continuing education and technical innovation. FDA's *Fish and Fisheries Products Hazards and Control Guide* (the Guide) is both innovative and useful.
- A structured protocol for process validation that addresses criteria for qualifying "processing authorities" and for structuring sampling plans, experimental designs, and appropriate methodologies is lacking in the Guide. Similarly, a regulatory protocol is necessary to apply new, rapid analytical methodologies to process validation and routine verification.
- Appropriate control of some chemical hazards in seafood is satisfactorily achieved through restrictions on harvesting sites or by using vessel and plant records. End-product testing provides a useful verification tool for control of these hazards.
- The implementation of postharvest treatments to progressively reduce the average number of annual reported illnesses attributed to raw oysters required by the Model Ordinance is a unique, flexible approach to safety; it establishes a public health objective and requires adequate industry performance without mandating a specific process or performance standard.

- Screening limited quantities of imported seafood products at points of entry is not consistent with the preventive concept of HACCP. Prevention of safety hazards in imported seafood must place greater emphasis on pathogen intervention strategies prior to shipment. Application of the Guide to increase seafood safety in international commerce requires immediate attention.

Safety Criteria for Produce and Related Products

- Fresh produce safety is of concern because microbial pathogens introduced on fresh produce at any point may be present at the point of consumption.
- Data on risks associated with many specific practices in the fresh produce sector are lacking. Research is needed on the likelihood of internalization of pathogens into fresh produce and its underlying mechanisms.
- There are concerns about the harmonization of food safety practices for imported produce. Imported produce should follow the same or equivalent Good Agricultural Practices that are required in domestic production.
- Because the use of a D-value concept to calculate thermal processes is being challenged, the appropriateness of the 12-D process for canning low-acid foods should be scientifically reevaluated.
- Reflecting the array of products and scenarios, FDA has developed guidance documents or required standards to address produce safety. Some managing strategies that have been implemented are:
  - — Good Agricultural Practices in the field and packing houses; required Good Manufacturing Practices in fresh-cut operations.
  - — Implementation of HACCP in fruit and vegetable juice production. The derivation of the sampling program for generic *E. coli* in fruit juices involving surface treatment of whole fruit is an excellent example of using the combination strategy to develop a performance standard and could be used as a model when developing future food safety criteria. In contrast, the justification of the 5-D pathogen reduction process for juices lacks transparency.
  - — An appropriate action level of 50 mg/kg for patulin in apple juice, apple juice concentrates, and apple juice products.
  - — Issuing guidance documents on practices to be followed by sprout producers.
  - — Establishing appropriate pesticide tolerances in produce.

Safety Criteria for Dairy Products

- The application of regulations within the evolving Grade A Pasteurized Milk Ordinance can be directly credited with reducing the incidence of milk-borne disease. The development, implementation, and enforcement of the Ordinance provide a good model for an integrated strategy for food safety assurance. It involves all stakeholders, is based on science, and is appropriately transparent. This model also provides a specific structure and mechanism for a biennial review of existing regulations, which could be used in other sectors of the food industry.

- A scientifically appropriate performance standard for the reduction of a targeted pathogen in finished cheese products is needed.
- Research is needed on pathogen survival in cheese made from sub-pasteurized milk, and educational programs that illustrate the hazards of raw milk and raw milk-product consumption are warranted. Cheeses manufactured from subpasteurized milk should be clearly and prominently labeled as such at the point of purchase.
- State authorities should ban the sale of unpasteurized milk because of its inherent risks. Targeted educational programs that illustrate the hazards of raw milk consumption are also warranted.

1

Historical Perspective on the Use of Food Safety Criteria and Performance Standards

The public health system in the United States traces its origins to the latter part of the nineteenth and early twentieth centuries, with its development paralleling the shift of the U.S. population from rural to urban settings. In the mid-nineteenth century there were concerns that life expectancy was decreasing in the rapidly growing cities (Hutt and Merrill, 1991), leading to demands for government intervention to control epidemics of disease and to assure that the food and water provided by others was safe (Hutt and Merrill, 1991). Before the 1870s, except for a few staples such as flour, almost all of the food consumed in the United States was either made in the home or purchased from neighbors; gradually, however, more and more food came from factories or was shipped long distances to market, so that consumers were unaware of the source of the food, the ways in which it had been processed and handled, or even what it contained (Alsberg, 1970; Roe, 1956). At the same time, "competition in sales and in the development of products created incentives for illegal profits through the debasement of manufactured foods and the mislabeling of those products" (Roe, 1956).

In the late eighteenth and nineteenth centuries, medical science equated dirt with disease, and consequently early public health regulatory efforts placed a strong emphasis on sanitation and elimination of "filth" (Chapin, 1970). This was reflected in the Massachusetts Health Act of 1797, in which towns were instructed to establish a health committee and appoint a health officer whose sole prescribed duty was "to remove all filth of any kind whatever . . . whenever such filth shall, in their judgment, endanger the lives or the health of the inhabitants thereof" (Chapin, 1970).

By the end of the nineteenth century, there was increasing recognition that infectious diseases resulted from the action of microorganisms. Sternberg, in 1880, published the first American book on bacteriology, and during the next 30 to 40 years a series of landmark studies were conducted linking specific infectious agents to epidemics of disease and documenting routes by which these agents might be transmitted (Gorham, 1970). Among others, an outbreak of typhoid fever at Wesleyan University in Middletown, Connecticut, in 1894 provided the first clear evidence of transmission of typhoid fever in the United States by contamination of oysters (Clem, 1994). However, despite the explosion in microbiological knowledge, public health officials continued to focus much of their effort on elimination of "filth, foul odors, and the decomposition and fermentation of animal and vegetable matter" in keeping with the generally accepted concept that "disease breeds in filth" (Gorham, 1970).

It was in this social and scientific context that Upton Sinclair published *The Jungle*, a scathing commentary on the industrial society that portrayed numerous abuses in the slaughter industry. Responding to this book and associated public concerns, in 1906 Congress passed the Federal Meat Inspection Act, which provided for the inspection of slaughter facilities in order to prevent the introduction of dead, diseased, disabled, and dying animals into the food supply. In keeping with the prevailing public health views, the scientific basis for this act was firmly planted in the filth theory of disease; the act did not mention specific pathogens. Inspectors used their sight, touch, and smell (organoleptic inspection) to detect and exclude filth and dead and decaying animals from slaughter. As dead, diseased, disabled, and dying animals became increasingly less of a problem, prevention of fecal contamination became a major focus of the inspection system. This was accompanied by increasing government regimentation of the entire slaughter process to optimize the opportunities for inspectors to detect filth, fecal contamination, or evidence of disease in slaughtered animals.

In this same time period, there was also increasing federal attention given to issues of food adulteration and mislabeling. As summarized by Roe (1956), Professor E.F. Ladd, then Food Commissioner of North Dakota, reported in a magazine article in 1905 that he "was unable to find any chicken or turkey in products designated as 'potted chicken' or 'potted turkey'." He noted a wide use of chemical preservatives, such as boric acid, and extensive use of coal-tar dyes in foods. He found that about 70 percent of the chocolate and cocoa on the market was adulterated with cocoa shell or other substitutes. Reported sales of "Vermont maple syrup" exceeded the production capacity of Vermont by about tenfold. Investigation of adulteration of food and drugs by the Division (then Bureau) of Chemistry of the U.S. Department of Agriculture (USDA) (the predecessor of today's Food and Drug Administration [FDA]), under the leadership of Dr. Harvey W. Wiley, led to widespread publicity about the adulteration of common foodstuffs. Wiley's so-called "poison squad" of 12 USDA employees used themselves as subjects to test the safety of widely-used food preservatives between 1902 and 1904, engendering significant public concern (Hutt and Merrill, 1991). These concerns culminated in 1906 with the passage of the Federal Food and Drugs Act, which contained prohibitions against misbranding and adulteration. As in meat and poultry inspection, the regulatory focus was on chemical contaminants and filth, rather than exclusion of specific pathogens. Even in the 1938 Food, Drug, and Cosmetic Act, which broadened and expanded the 1906 act, a food was defined as adulterated if it contained a poisonous or deleterious substance; if it consisted in whole or in part of any filthy, putrid, or decomposed substance; if it had been prepared, packed, or held under unsanitary conditions; if it was the product of a diseased animal or one dead before slaughter; or if its container was composed of any poisonous or deleterious substance (Slocum, 1956).

It was in shellfish, with their recognized association with typhoid fever, that microbiological criteria first began to play a major role in food protection (Clem, 1994). With an increasing appreciation of the linkage between typhoid fever, raw shellfish consumption, and fecal contamination of harvest waters, efforts were focused at an early point on development of bacteriological methods for defining contamination. In 1909 the American Public Health Association appointed a committee to develop a "standard" bacteriological technique for screening oysters and other shellfish, which recommended use of a tube dilution method for the presence of *Escherichia coli*. In an effort to gain data on levels of contamination, USDA's Bureau of Chemistry conducted an extensive bacteriological study along the Atlantic and Gulf coasts between 1908 and 1910. While individual states began to implement increasingly stringent shellfish sanitation programs in the decade that followed, it required a major, multi-state outbreak of typhoid fever in 1924 to mobilize public opinion and drive public health action at a national level. The Surgeon General of the United States called a conference of health officials on February 19, 1925, to deal with this issue. Among other resolutions, the conference recommended that "The product [raw oysters] must conform to an established bacterial standard and must meet Federal, State, and local laws and regulations relative to salinity, water content, and food proportion, and must conform to the pure food laws standard" (Clem, 1994). This recommendation generated a great deal of controversy based on concerns that ranged from the public health importance of bacteriological findings to technical issues related to appropriate cut-off levels for indicator organisms. However, the following two decades saw the development of increasing scientific consensus on appropriate scientific methods and criteria for bacteriological screening of harvest waters, a consensus that formed the basis for the bacteriological criteria currently used by the National Shellfish Sanitation Program for certification of shellfish and shellfish-growing waters.

The latter part of the twentieth century saw the establishment of another major regulatory agency, the U.S. Environmental Protection Agency (EPA), which is responsible for the licensing and registration of pesticides and sets limits on pesticide residues in food. It also oversees drinking water quality and safety. In contrast to FDA and USDA, and reflecting the time at which the agency was established, the basic EPA regulatory framework was constructed on a much more up-to-date science base, which recognized the existence of both chemical and microbiological contaminants. For certain pathogenic microorganisms, such as *Cryptosporidium* and *Giardia lamblia*, EPA has set a maximum contaminant level goal of zero, reflecting the fact that any amount of these pathogens in drinking water may pose a risk to health. EPA also sets enforceable regulatory limits in the form of required treatment techniques, maximum contaminant levels, or both. These regulatory standards are required by law to achieve levels as close as feasible to the maximum contaminant level goal, taking into account the best available treatment technology and costs of treatment (EPA, 2002a, 2002b).

While there are differences in the science base on which the regulatory structure is based, a common theme through all of these regulations is the recognition of the need for "performance standards" to provide clear articulation of what is and is not acceptable in the process or system being regulated. For the meat and poultry industry, it is exclusion of dead, diseased, disabled, and dying animals from the food supply; for processed foods, it is exclusion of adulterants and correct labeling; for oysters, it is the absence of high levels of fecal bacteria in harvest waters; while for EPA it is the presence of specific chemical or microbiological hazards. The need for such standards in the food industry goes to the heart of regulatory theory, which recognizes the necessity for the government to establish standards as a counterbalance to private economic incentives.

In the absence of government standards, companies willing to spend funds to assure protection of the public health are disadvantaged by the need to compete with companies unwilling to do so, because the latter could sell their products at a lower price. Some consumers might be willing to spend more on a "better" or "safer" product; poorer consumers, of course, would be unable to do so and would bear greater food safety risks than more affluent consumers. Price differentials for safer products would not be possible in many parts of the food marketplace, however, as most foodstuffs are sold as unbranded commodities at the beginning of the food chain, and often (as with most meat, poultry, and produce) at the retail level. Thus, even if society were willing to rely upon the market to encourage food safety, it is unlikely to be an effective producer of safety because of the commodity nature of most food transactions, as well as the difficulty of connecting foodborne illness with particular eating occasions or individual foods. For the same reasons, personal injury litigation provides only a weak incentive for food companies to improve their food safety efforts, because there is a low probability that they will be sued for foodborne illness, the damages they would pay are likely to be small, and there is a low probability that such litigation would have negative public relations consequences (Buzby and Frenzen, 1999).

Current food safety regulatory standards in the United States have developed over the last century through the accumulation of new food safety legislation and the standard-setting activities of the regulatory agencies, including FDA, USDA, EPA, and the National Marine Fisheries Service. By legislation, Congress has set generic standards for naturally occurring toxins (deemed unlawful if "ordinarily injurious"), added "poisonous or deleterious" substances (deemed unlawful if they "may render" the food injurious), and intentional food additives, animal drugs, and pesticide residues (deemed safe if there is a "reasonable certainty of no harm"). While applying these and other generic food safety standards, the regulatory agencies have set more specific food safety standards. These include tolerances (which set legal limits) on the presence of chemicals in food, prohibitions on specific microbial pathogens in specific foods, standards for process control, and standards defining the acceptable outcome of a food process for reducing pathogenic contamination. All of these are performance standards in the sense that they define what must be achieved in controlling risk factors for food safety. They have been set over a period of years and under diverse circumstances by USDA, FDA, and EPA based on a host of scientific, legal, and practical constraints.

THE IMPACT OF CHANGING SCIENTIFIC AND SOCIETAL CONDITIONS ON STANDARDS

The U.S. food regulatory system is a patchwork of standards developed across a century that has seen dramatic changes in society and science. While the standards established in the early part of the twentieth century were highly successful in accomplishing the objectives to which they were targeted, their success, and our increasing scientific sophistication, has led to the recognition of new problems that cannot be adequately addressed using existing standards. This is highlighted by two examples:

1. *Use of fecal coliform indicators for shellfish.* As discussed earlier, fecal coliform standards for shellfish harvest waters were implemented as a response to public health concerns about the spread of typhoid fever through raw molluscan shellfish. These standards have been successful in minimizing the risk of illness due to pathogens present in fecal material, and their original intent—to prevent recurrent outbreaks of oyster-associated typhoid fever—has clearly been achieved. At this time, the leading causes of shellfish-associated illness and death in this country are bacteria of the *Vibrio* species, which can cause diarrheal disease and potentially fatal bloodstream infections in susceptible hosts (Altekruse et al., 2000; Hlady and Klontz, 1996; IOM, 1991). *Vibrionaceae* are free-living marine bacteria; in one study of the Chesapeake Bay, *V. vulnificus* (the species responsible for most oyster-associated deaths annually) alone accounted for 8 percent of the total culturable heterotrophic bacteria in the samples (Wright et al., 1996). Because of their free-living status, *Vibrionaceae* are not associated with fecal contamination, and, consequently, the fecal coliform microbial performance standard has not been effective in reducing the rate of *Vibrio*-associated illness.

2. *Use of organoleptic inspection for poultry.* As noted earlier, organoleptic inspection was initiated to prevent the introduction of dead, diseased, disabled, or dying animals into the food supply. In this sense, it has been highly effective: flocks coming to slaughter tend to be highly homogeneous and free of disease, and animals that die before slaughter never make it into the slaughterhouses. Today *Campylobacter* is the leading cause of poultry-associated foodborne illness. *Campylobacter* species are part of the colonizing intestinal flora of normal, healthy chickens; exclusion of dead, diseased, disabled, and dying birds does not control this problem. Organoleptic inspection focuses on the identification of birds contaminated with feces; these birds are subsequently removed from the processing line for reprocessing. However, although visible fecal contamination is a relatively rare event, in some studies *Campylobacter* has been isolated from over 80 percent of chicken parts available at retail sale (NRC, 1987). As it is virtually impossible for organoleptic inspection techniques to identify products bearing "invisible" microbial contamination by a specific pathogen such as *Campylobacter*, it is unrealistic to expect that organoleptic standards will have an important impact on reducing the incidence of *Campylobacter* infections in humans.

FRAGMENTATION OF THE CURRENT REGULATORY SYSTEM

The report *Ensuring Safe Food from Production to Consumption* (IOM/NRC, 1998) adequately described the fragmentation of the current food safety regulatory system. At least a dozen federal agencies administer more than 35 statutes and are overseen by 28 congressional committees. Four federal agencies (FDA, part of the Department of Health and Human Services; the Food Safety and Inspection Service (FSIS), part of USDA; EPA; and the National Marine Fisheries Service, part of the U.S. Department of Commerce) play the major roles. State and local health departments play important roles as well; as at the federal level, many jurisdictions have multiple agencies involved in assuring food safety. Jurisdiction over a particular food, or a particular problem, depends not only upon geography, but also upon the type of food product involved and the level of the food chain at which the problem is found.

The regulatory system is fragmented because of the statutes that created the food safety agencies and authorize their activities. As noted earlier, the system arose in response to public concerns. The statutory framework for the federal food regulatory system has its antecedents in legislation written originally in 1906; major revisions created the Federal Food, Drug, and Cosmetic Act in 1938 and the Wholesome Meat Act in 1967. As early as 1949, a federal advisory committee recommended significant reorganization of the food safety system (IOM/NRC, 1998), but no significant structural reform has ever occurred. This statutory framework for government food safety regulation poses a significant set of challenges and has had a clear negative impact on implementation and enforcement of modern, science-based performance standards by the regulatory agencies.

For example, in the case of *Supreme Beef Processors v. USDA* 275 F. 3d 432 (5th Cir. 2001), a federal appeals court decided that USDA did not have statutory authority to withdraw its inspectors from a meat processing and grinding plant—an action that would shut it down—even though the plant had failed to meet the *Salmonella* performance standard on three consecutive occasions. Because *Salmonella* is present in a substantial percentage of raw meat and poultry products, it is not considered an adulterant. Its presence in raw meat, therefore, does not prevent the meat from passing inspection and being marked by USDA as "inspected and passed." Nor is the presence of *Salmonella* deemed to render a product "injurious to health," because normal cooking will destroy the pathogen (275 F. 3d at 439). The relevant statute, the Federal Meat Inspection Act, provides that a meat product is adulterated if it has been prepared, packed, or held under unsanitary conditions whereby it may have become contaminated with filth or whereby it may have been rendered injurious to health (21 U.S.C. §601(m)(4)). As noted earlier, this language reflects the prevailing scientific theories from 100 years ago, which equated filth with disease. This contrasts with our current understanding that infectious diseases are caused by specific pathogenic microorganisms (such as *Salmonella*) that may be transferred to, and multiply in, a product as it moves through the continuum of slaughter and processing. It also fails to reflect our understanding that such microorganisms can be readily transferred from a raw product to other foods in a kitchen, thereby serving as a cause of foodborne illness even if the product that introduced the microorganism into the kitchen is subsequently cooked. USDA's performance standard for *Salmonella* in beef was set to provide a proxy for the presence or absence of other pathogens. USDA has authority to shut down a plant for insanitation, but USDA did not allege unsanitary conditions at the Supreme Beef plant. Rather, it challenged the *Salmonella* level in the ground beef that the plant produced. The court concluded that USDA's statute cannot be used "to regulate characteristics of the raw materials that exist" before the meat product is brought into the inspected plant: "The performance standard is invalid because it regulates the procurement of raw materials" (275 F. 3d at 441).

From the perspective of the consumer, it is irrelevant when or how a pathogen gets into the food supply. The fact that *Salmonella* (or *E. coli* O157:H7 or other pathogens) is introduced into a product at slaughter rather than during grinding does not negate its public health impact. The *Ensuring Safe Food from Production to Consumption* (IOM/NRC, 1998) report recommends modifying the federal statutory framework for food safety to eliminate fragmentation and enable the creation and enforcement of science-based standards.

DEVELOPMENT OF NEW REGULATORY APPROACHES

The need for new types of inspection approaches and new performance standards to deal with current food safety problems has been emphasized in a series of reports by government and private organizations. The key reports include:

- *Meat and Poultry Inspection: The Scientific Basis of the Nation's Program* (NRC, 1985b). This report recommended that FSIS focus on pathogenic organisms and that all official establishments adopt Hazard Analysis and Critical Control Point (HACCP) systems to control pathogens and other hazards.
- *An Evaluation of the Role of Microbiological Criteria for Foods and Food Ingredients* (NRC, 1985a). This report recommended the implementation of microbiological guidance as part of HACCP systems, although criteria containing specific limits for pathogens were considered impractical in some instances.
- *Poultry Inspection: The Basis for a Risk-Assessment Approach* (NRC, 1987). This report looked specifically at poultry slaughter and processing. It highlighted the lack of efficacy of the current organoleptic inspection system in reducing foodborne illness and recommended implementation of a HACCP-based regulatory system.
- *Cattle Inspection* (IOM, 1990). This report also emphasized the lack of a scientific basis for organoleptic inspection and proposed implementation of a HACCP-based system.
- *Seafood Safety* (IOM, 1991). This report summarized current problems and regulatory approaches for control of seafood-associated illness. Again, a HACCP-based approach was recommended as a possible basis for regulatory intervention.
- *"Food Safety: Risk-Based Inspections and Microbial Monitoring Needed for Meat and Poultry"* (Harman, 1994). In his testimony before a House subcommittee, Harman, speaking for the General Accounting Office, stated that "A HACCP system is generally considered the best approach currently available to ensure safe foods because it focuses on preventing contamination rather than detecting contamination once it has occurred."
- *Hazard Analysis and Critical Control Point System and Guidelines for its Application* (CAC, 1997). This report recommended that countries incorporate HACCP principles into their food industries.
- "Hazard Analysis and Critical Control Point Principles and Application Guidelines" (NACMCF, 1998). These principles endorsed the HACCP system as an effective and rational approach to the assurance of food safety.

A consistent theme in these reports is the importance of encouraging industry to move toward the adoption of a HACCP system. HACCP is a preventive system for food safety process control that was originally developed as a contract specification by the National Aeronautics and Space Administration (NASA) in cooperation with the U.S. Army's Natick Laboratory, and subsequently implemented by Pillsbury as HACCP under the direction of Dr. Howard Bauman (Lachance, 1997). The initial purpose of the concept was to minimize the risk of foodborne disease during space flights, but it has subsequently been adopted in many industries. The HACCP method addressed NASA's need for absolute freedom from potentially catastrophic disease-producing bacteria and toxins in food delivered to astronauts. Since the 1980s, the HACCP method has been adopted by other agencies in the United States and abroad. HACCP involves seven principles (see Chapter 3) that must be backed by sound scientific knowledge (e.g., published microbiological studies on time and temperature factors for controlling foodborne pathogens).

As noted repeatedly in the reports cited above, HACCP provides an attractive framework by which companies can minimize the risk of illness associated with their products. The problem comes, however, in integrating HACCP concepts into a regulatory system. The food safety standards of an earlier age were "command and control" in nature; for example, no fecal contamination of carcasses and inspectors standing in each plant with a rulebook written by the government to enforce the regulation. The past decade has seen development of a variety of creative approaches to integrate regulatory controls with HACCP. Within this process, however, there have been several problem areas:

- The need to match the inherent flexibility of HACCP with a similarly flexible regulatory system that encourages plants to analyze and monitor their own hazard profile and respond accordingly. That is, it must be determined how to move away from the old command and control approach while maintaining sufficient regulatory control to protect the public health.
- How to deal with the recognized fact that science is constantly changing. Plans and regulatory approaches that are based on the best available science one year may be totally outdated by the following decade (or the following year); both HACCP and the associated regulatory controls must have the flexibility to deal with these changes. Many small- and medium-sized food-processing facilities lack the level of scientific expertise that would allow them not only to stay abreast of changes, but also to apply the implications of the changes to industrial operations. These facilities have difficulty applying the concepts of HACCP without significant guidance. A certain amount of structure is required and often desired by these companies; however, by providing this structure, some of the flexibility theoretically afforded by these concepts is lost. Finding a balance that allows

for flexibility but acknowledges the scientific limitations of many food processors will continue to be a challenge.
- The lack of a generally accepted approach to setting regulatory controls and performance standards that result in a reduction of human disease.

Subsequent sections highlight the status of current regulatory approaches and the ways in which regulatory standards have been and are being established today in the context of an increasing emphasis on the use of HACCP as a means of minimizing risk of foodborne illness. The key elements in the development of one such regulatory system, the USDA Pathogen Reduction (PR)/HACCP Final Rule, are provided in detail below.

Example of the Development of a New Regulatory Approach

In 1994 FSIS began a review and revision of existing food safety regulations for meat and poultry that led to the publication of the PR/HACCP rule (FSIS, 1996). While numerous National Academies' and other expert committees and groups had recommended changes in the regulatory system, an outbreak—this time, the *E. coli* O157:H7 outbreak from hamburgers in restaurants in the western United States—was again the major driving force for regulatory change. The primary objective of the new regulation was to reduce meat- and poultry-associated foodborne illness. In keeping with the prior National Academies' and other expert reports, HACCP served as the core of the new regulatory structure.

In brief, the PR/HACCP rule requires all meat and poultry slaughter and processing establishments to design and implement a HACCP system, with the schedule of implementation dependent on plant size. The exact elements of the HACCP plan are not specified in order to: encourage companies to carefully evaluate the particular public health hazards associated with each specific product line and plant; provide companies with the freedom to develop innovative methods for control of these hazards; and provide companies with the flexibility to identify Critical Control Points that would have maximal utility in the control of potential hazards in their products.

It was fully anticipated that generic HACCP plans would rapidly emerge; however, it was also hoped that, in even the smallest plants, generic plans would be carefully evaluated, and plant owners would take advantage of the flexibility inherent in the system to develop new and creative approaches to control foodborne pathogens. To encourage such innovation, implementation of the PR/HACCP rule was accompanied by ongoing efforts to reduce the regulatory control that FSIS had previously maintained on all aspects of slaughter and processing, including the traditional tight control over any change in plant design or operation. There was also recognition that many of the major foodborne pathogens were colonizers of the animal intestinal tract, and, consequently, there was value in monitoring (and minimizing) fecal contamination of carcasses. As such, the PR/HACCP rule required that, as part of their HACCP program, plants implement a microbiological monitoring program for generic *E. coli* as a marker for fecal contamination in carcasses at slaughter operations (FSIS, 1996).

While efforts were being made to encourage flexibility and innovation through implementation of HACCP, there was also recognition that there had to be some type of regulatory "floor" to clearly define minimal acceptable levels of performance. As the goal of these regulatory changes was to reduce the incidence of meat- and poultry-associated foodborne illness, it was felt that such standards should focus on the effectiveness of a plant's HACCP program in reducing contamination of product with specific, known pathogens. At the time the PR/HACCP rule was being prepared, *Salmonella* species were recognized as having the greatest economic impact among the known bacterial foodborne pathogens. *Salmonella* was also present in all product classes that were being regulated, and it could be readily isolated using a well-established laboratory methodology available for its identification. Based on these considerations, the decision was made to establish a *Salmonella* performance standard.

Given the low levels and uneven nature of contamination on a carcass and the ability of pathogenic microorganisms to rapidly multiply at the appropriate temperatures, and recognizing some of the technical issues involved in trying to quantify *Salmonella* on a single carcass, the percentage of carcasses contaminated was used as the basis for the standard. The decision was made to set the initial standard at a level equal to the current national mean for that product class (e.g., in studies conducted in the early 1990s, 25 percent of broiler chickens were found to be contaminated with *Salmonella*; consequently, the *Salmonella* performance standard for plants was set at 25 percent contamination). The concept was that the new standards would create accountability for all slaughter plants to target and control *Salmonella* and require plants performing worse than the national mean to at least bring their incidence of contamination down to that level. USDA intended that, as the incidence of contamination and the national mean declined, the *Salmonella* performance standard would be reduced accordingly, thereby inducing further reductions in *Salmonella* within the demonstrated capability of the industry, as reflected in the new national mean.

In addition to monitoring *Salmonella* contamination at individual plants (and in keeping with recommendations in prior National Academies reports), the Centers for Disease Control and Prevention, working with FSIS and FDA, set up a national sentinel surveillance system for foodborne illnesses to provide data to assess the effectiveness of the PR/HACCP rule in reducing the national incidence of foodborne illness (see Chapter 2). As described in subsequent chapters, this system, later named FoodNet, has served as a key element in monitoring foodborne disease incidence in the United States.

Significance of Zero Tolerance

Regulators often confront the notion that they should have "zero tolerance" for anything (such as pathogens in the food supply) that is deemed to pose a risk to public health or safety. The term zero tolerance resonates with the public, which is appropriately seeking assurance of the safety of the products it consumes. Sometimes regulators use the term zero tolerance in reference to a pathogen or environmental contaminant to indicate that whenever a particular problem is found, strict regulatory action will be taken.

The term zero tolerance is commonly used in the media in respect to issues of science, including food safety, but also in many other contexts. For example, zero tolerance has been used to comment about drug-law enforcement, drug-testing policies in sports (Goldberg, 2000; Mann, 2000), crime (Gembrowski, 2000), and security violations (Pincus, 2000). Businesses frequently note their zero tolerance of offensive behavior (for example, eBay has zero tolerance for illegal items auctioned on its site [Harmon, 1999], and AOL has a policy of zero tolerance for hate messages in its chat rooms and message boards [Farhi, 2001]). Zero tolerance is a powerful term, with the intended connotation of the complete absence of the hazard or inappropriate behavior at issue, and it is popularly perceived as assurance of protection against—or at least official intolerance of—that hazard or behavior.

Laws and regulations, in contrast, use the term zero tolerance (or a tolerance of zero) sparingly. It does not appear in either Title 7 (Agriculture) or Title 21 (Food and Drugs) of the U.S. Code. It appears in the U.S. Code only in reference to binge drinking on college campuses in 20 U.S.C. §1011h(b)(3), and behavioral guidelines for members of the Job Corps in 29 U.S.C. §§2892(b)(2), 2899(d)(7). It appears in sections of the Code of Federal Regulations that concern food and drugs only in respect to new animal drugs used in animal feed for which no residue (zero tolerance) is allowed to be found in the animal after slaughter (21 C.F.R. §558.3, general rule; see, e.g., 21 C.F.R. §§ 172.820, 556.110, 556.120, 556.140). That is, if any residue of these drugs is found, the user is in violation. In addition, there are some food safety regulations that use zero as a standard (e.g., zero percent prevalence of cattle affected with bovine tuberculosis), without including the zero tolerance phrase.

Nevertheless, zero tolerance appears in *Federal Register* discussions of regulatory policies by both USDA and FDA. Sometimes zero tolerance is rejected because, for example, there can be no zero tolerance policy for genetic contamination in organic foods because it would be "impossible to achieve" (AMS, 2000) or because zero tolerance for ingesta in poultry is too costly to achieve (USDA, 2002). In other situations it is determined to be the appropriate policy: zero tolerance, defined as "no detectable level of viable pathogens," for *Listeria monocytogenes* in ready-to-eat products (FSIS, 2001) or zero tolerance for visible fecal material (FSIS, 2000).

Scientists are often dismayed by the use of this term because they recognize the inability to ensure, in most situations, the complete absence of pathogens and contaminants and the limitations of any feasible sampling plan to check for their total absence. The issue is not a new one; the National Academy of Sciences issued a report in November 1965 (NRC, 1965) on no residue and zero tolerance as they relate to the registration of pesticides, the setting of tolerances for pesticides, and FDA enforcement of pesticide residues in foods. This report considered the development of increasingly sensitive analytical methods for residue detection, the problem of background levels of pesticide residues not related to immediate applications to food products, and the scientific and administrative barriers to employing zero tolerance for pesticide regulation. However, scientists do recognize that a preference for zero "is influenced by the wish to emphasize that absence is the desired objective (although it cannot be guaranteed) and by the knowledge that once pathogens are found, the finding cannot be ignored" (ICMSF, 2002). The various uses of and limits for this term, therefore, must be properly analyzed.

The committee has adopted for its purposes the following definition of zero tolerance:

> Lay audience perception of the absence of a hazard that cannot be scientifically assured, but is operationally defined as the absence of a hazard in a specified amount of food as determined by a specific method.

This definition reflects two points that may seem to be in conflict, but are actually reconcilable:

1. Some people perceive zero tolerance as meaning the absence of a hazard.
2. The absence of a hazard cannot be scientifically assured. However, in regulatory practice the concept requires the absence of the hazard in a specified amount of food as determined by a specific method and sampling protocol. If the hazard is found, regulators will take action.

With agreement that zero tolerance is a regulatory and lay concept that specifies an ideal, but that science can strive for but never meet that ideal, disagreements over the use of the term should be minimized.

REFERENCES

Alsberg CL. 1970. Progress in federal food control. In: Ravenel MP, ed. *A Half Century of Health.* New York: Arno Press and the New York Times. Pp. 211–220.

Altekruse SF, Bishop RD, Baldy LM, Thompson SG, Wilson SA, Ray BJ, Griffin PM. 2000. *Vibrio* gastroenteritis in the U.S. Gulf of Mexico region: The role of raw oysters. *Epidemiol Infect* 124:489–495.

AMS (Agricultural Marketing Service). 2000. National organic program; Final rule. *Fed Regist* 65:80547–80596.

Buzby JC, Frenzen PD. 1999. Food safety and product liability. *Food Policy* 24:637–651.

CAC (Codex Alimentarius Commission). 1997. *Hazard Analysis and Critical Control Point System and Guidelines for Its Application.* Annex to CAC/RCP 1-1969, Rev. 3-1997. Rome: Food and Agriculture Organization of the United Nations.

Chapin CV. 1970. History of state and municipal control of disease. In: Ravenel MP, ed. *A Half Century of Health.* New York: Arno Press and the New York Times. Pp. 133–160.

Clem JD. 1994. Historical overview. In: Hackney CR, Pierson MD. *Environmental Indicators and Shellfish Safety.* New York: Chapman & Hall. Pp. 1–29.

EPA (U.S. Environmental Protection Agency). 2002a. *Current Drinking Water Standards.* Online. Available at http://www.epa.gov/safewater/mcl.html. Accessed January 23, 2002.

EPA. 2002b. *Setting Standards for Safe Drinking Water.* Online. Available at http://www.epa.gov/safewater/standard/setting.html. Accessed January 23, 2002.

Farhi P. 2001, Sept. 8. Sticky web: Threats on ACLU site pose free-speech dilemma. *The Washington Post.* P. C01.

FSIS (Food Safety and Inspection Service). 1996. Pathogen reduction; hazard analysis and critical control point (HACCP) systems; Final rule. *Fed Regist* 61:38805–38855.

FSIS. 2000. Announcement of and request for comment regarding industry petition on hazard analysis and critical control point (HACCP) inspection. *Fed Regist* 65:30952–30956.

FSIS. 2001. Performance standards for the production of processed meat and poultry products; Proposed rule. *Fed Regist* 66:12589–12636.

Gembrowski S. 2000, June 23. Schools cannot eliminate violence, panel says. *The San Diego Union-Tribune.* P. B2.

Goldberg J. 2000, Sept 29. Olympic dreams. Op-ed. *The Washington Post.* P. A32

Gorham FP. 1970. The history of bacteriology and its contribution to public health work. In: Ravenel MP, ed. *A Half Century of Health.* New York: Arno Press & the New York Times. Pp. 66–93.

Harman JW. 1994. *Food Safety: Risk-Based Inspection and Microbial Monitoring Needed for Meat and Poultry.* Testimony, 04/19/94, GAO/T-RCED-94-189. Washington, DC: General Accounting Office.

Harmon A. 1999, Sept. 3. Auction for a kidney pops up on eBay's site. *New York Times.* P. A13.

Hlady WG, Klontz KC. 1996. The epidemiology of *Vibrio* infections in Florida, 1981–93. *J Infect Dis* 173:1176–1183.

Hutt PB, Merrill RA. 1991. *Food and Drug Law: Cases and Materials*, 2nd ed. Westbury, NY: Foundation Press. Pp. 8–9.

ICMSF (International Commission on Microbiological Specifications for Foods). 2002. *Microorganisms in Foods 7. Microbiological Testing in Food Safety Management.* New York: Kluwer Academic/Plenum Publishers.

IOM (Institute of Medicine). 1990. *Cattle Inspection.* Washington, DC: National Academy Press.

IOM. 1991. *Seafood Safety.* Washington, DC: National Academy Press.

IOM/NRC (National Research Council). 1998. *Ensuring Safe Food from Production to Consumption.* Washington, DC: National Academy Press.

Lachance PA. 1997. How HACCP started. *Food Technol* 51:35.

Mann J. 2000, Nov. 15. Voters getting wise to the war on drugs. *The Washington Post.* P. C13.

NACMCF (National Advisory Committee on Microbiological Criteria for Foods). 1998. Hazard analysis and critical control point principles and application guidelines. *J Food Prot* 61:1246–1259.

NRC (National Research Council). 1965. *Report on 'No Residue' and 'Zero Tolerance'.* Washington, DC: National Academy of Sciences.

NRC. 1985a. *An Evaluation of the Role of Microbiological Criteria for Foods and Food Ingredients.* Washington, DC: National Academy Press.

NRC. 1985b. *Meat and Poultry Inspection: The Scientific Basis of the Nation's Program.* Washington, DC: National Academy Press.

NRC. 1987. *Poultry Inspection: The Basis for a Risk-Assessment Approach.* Washington, DC: National Academy Press.

Pincus W. 2000, Sept. 25. Lab crackdown criticized: Report says changes could actually harm security. *The Washington Post.* P. A02.

Roe RS. 1956. The Food and Drugs Act—Past, present, and future. In: Welch H, Marti-Ibanez F, eds. *The Impact of the Food and Drug Administration on our Society.* New York: MD Publications. Pp.15–17.

Slocum GG. 1956. Prevention and control of food poisoning. In: Welch H, Marti-Ibanez F, eds. *The Impact of the Food and Drug Administration on our Society.* New York: MD Publications. Pp. 83–84.

USDA (U.S. Department of Agriculture). 2002. Semiannual regulatory agenda, spring 2002. *Fed Regist* 67:32826–32909.

Wright AC, Hill RT, Johnson JA, Roghman M-C, Colwell RR, Morris JG Jr. 1996. Distribution of *Vibrio vulnificus* in the Chesapeake Bay. *Appl Environ Microbiol* 62:717–724.

2

The Science of Public Health Surveillance

THE TOOLS OF PUBLIC HEALTH SURVEILLANCE

Public health surveillance is the ongoing, systematic collection, analysis, interpretation, and dissemination of health outcome-specific data for use by the public health sector to reduce morbidity and mortality and to improve health (Thacker and Berkelman, 1988). Surveillance of many infections and intoxications, including those that are foodborne, has been a fundamental public health activity for many years. Human foodborne disease surveillance is conducted for three principal reasons: (1) to identify, control, and prevent outbreaks of foodborne disease, (2) to monitor trends and determine the targets and efficacy of control measures, and (3) to determine the burden of specific diseases on public health (Potter et al., 2000).

By detecting outbreaks and their sources quickly, surveillance can lead to control of an acute health hazard, for example, by removing a contaminated product from the market or by temporarily closing a hazardous kitchen. Outbreak investigations can also identify critical gaps in knowledge, leading to applied research and ultimately to better long-term prevention as unsafe food handling processes are corrected or new food hazards are identified and controlled.

The information gathered through surveillance and subsequent investigations of outbreaks and of sporadic cases can reveal the magnitude and trends of foodborne diseases, which helps policy makers target prevention strategies. This information is also critical to the design and evaluation of risk assessments. Improved understanding of foodborne diseases, in turn, can help researchers recognize new problems, such as entirely new hazards (e.g., microbes or toxins)

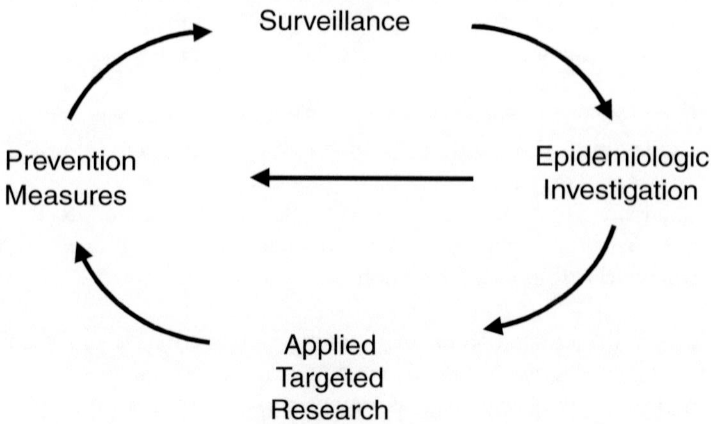

FIGURE 2.1 The cycle of public health prevention.

or known hazards that may appear in foods not previously associated with them. Most foodborne pathogens were discovered during outbreak investigations, and much of the knowledge we have about specific hazards and how they enter the food supply also was gained during the course of investigations. As new foodborne disease sources and agents emerge, the efforts to control them through application of the Hazard Analysis and Critical Control Point (HACCP) system and other control strategies must constantly evolve. Surveillance is a keystone in the effort to define, control, and prevent foodborne diseases (Figure 2.1).

In the United States, foodborne disease surveillance is primarily conducted by local and state public health agencies. In fact, local surveillance for diseases of public health concern has been conducted for centuries. In the nineteenth century, fear of cholera led to the establishment of permanent municipal health departments and disease surveillance, even before the microbe that caused it was identified (Rosenberg, 1987). Reporting of typhoid fever cases and deaths drove many improvements in water and food safety at the beginning of the twentieth century. Increased concern following the large *Escherichia coli* O157:H7 outbreak in 1993 associated with consumption of undercooked ground beef (Bell et al., 1994) stimulated enhancements in surveillance for foodborne infections (FSIS, 1998c).

Strategies in Public Health Surveillance

There are specific strategies to collect information that may serve as a basis for making food safety policy decisions. The surveillance strategies for outbreaks and sporadic cases of diseases that are often foodborne are:

1. Monitoring case reports of specific, notifiable infections
2. Investigating and reporting outbreaks of illnesses associated with events or establishments
3. Investigating and reporting unusual clusters of cases of specific infections
4. Vigilantly surveilling (termed sentinel site surveillance) for specific conditions that may or may not be notifiable
5. Laboratory subtyping of pathogens isolated from human infections
6. Surveying the population to measure trends in diarrheal illness, consumer behavior, and food consumption

One surveillance method may be more appropriate than another, and these methods may also be used alone or in combination, depending on the purpose. For example, subtyping of pathogens may be performed to confirm the source of an outbreak.

The specific surveillance strategies are conducted either nationwide or in several sentinel sites that represent the whole population. Surveillance conducted to detect outbreaks and protect the public should cover the whole population, should include conditions most likely to appear in outbreak form, and in some instances, should focus on settings where outbreaks are likely to occur. Some outbreaks are not tightly clustered in time and space, and thus are not evident in surveillance conducted in one location. To detect dispersed outbreaks, it can be critical to compare specific markers of the infecting organisms, such as genetic "fingerprints," across many jurisdictions (Swaminathan et al., 2001). Such comparison of subtypes may reveal an unusual clustering of infections with a single strain of a pathogen that can then be further investigated. Public health laboratories use subtyping methods and are linked in a national network to permit rapid comparison of results and to provide warning of dispersed outbreaks. For example, the network of state public health laboratories detected a multistate cluster of *Salmonella* Newport infections that had the same pulsed-field gel electrophoresis profile. As a result of the investigation of genetic profiles, 78 infections in 13 states were linked to consumption of imported mangoes (Sivapalasingam et al., 2000).

If the purpose of surveillance is to measure the public health burden of disease or track long-term trends in the nation as a whole, more detailed data collected from a representative sample of sites around the country is likely to provide more accurate information (Angulo and Swerdlow, 1999). This sentinel-site approach can provide data on important illnesses, such as *Campylobacter* or *Vibrio* infections, that are not well represented in national surveillance systems because they rarely appear in outbreak form and are not reportable in many jurisdictions.

For the purpose of determining the food source of infections, surveillance based on outbreak investigations provides answers for those illnesses that frequently appear in outbreak form. For illnesses that rarely appear as outbreaks, case studies can give a general answer as to the source of illnesses that are strongly tied to specific sources, and case-control studies can provide information if the sources are complex. As described later, the committee feels that to construct a detailed quantification of the contribution of specific animal or food sources to foodborne diseases, systematic monitoring of pathogens in food and animal reservoirs using molecular subtyping and comparison of strains with isolates from human infections are urgently needed.

The following sections describe how these strategies are utilized in both nationwide and sentinel site surveillance by public health agencies in the United States. Specialized surveys that relate the contribution of consumer behavior to the level of specific foodborne illness risk are described as well. Finally, several factors that limit the value of surveillance systems are discussed.

Nationwide Surveillance of Notifiable Diseases

Many counties and states have collected notifiable disease reports for more than a century, covering an ever-expanding list of illnesses. Since 1961, these reports have been voluntarily submitted to the Centers for Disease Control and Prevention (CDC), which publishes them as weekly and annual summaries (Thacker, 1994). At its annual meetings, the Council of State and Territorial Epidemiologists decides which specific illnesses should be nationally notifiable. This general umbrella of reporting covers all areas of the United States; provides information useful to local, state, and national authorities; and is relatively inexpensive. Most disease reporting is passive from the standpoint of the public health system, which means that clinicians and laboratories are asked to report cases on their own initiative. Basic case surveillance has been enhanced for some infections by further characterization of the infecting pathogen in public health laboratories. This voluntary case surveillance was first begun for *Salmonella*. Following large, multistate outbreaks of salmonellosis early in the 1960s, health department laboratories in states and large cities began to serotype strains of *Salmonella* isolated from humans; the results of this subtyping were shared with CDC as well in order to detect outbreaks affecting more than one state. Since 1962, national *Salmonella* surveillance has depended on this serotype-based reporting (Olsen et al., 2001). These data have been critical to the detection of many outbreaks of salmonellosis each year. Since 1990, these data have been relayed electronically from states to CDC via the Public Health Laboratory Information System (Bean et al., 1992). In addition, since 1995 these data have been routinely examined using an automated statistical outbreak detection algorithm that compares current reports with the preceding 5-year mean number of cases for the same geographic area and week of the year to look for unusual clusters of infection (Hutwagner et al., 1997). The usefulness of the outbreak algorithm is limited by the timeliness of reporting and the high background rates of reporting for common serotypes such as *S.* Typhimurium and *S.* Enteritidis. The greatest sensitivity for *Salmonella* serotyping to detect meaningful clusters is for the rare serotypes, whereas further differentiation is necessary for the most common serotypes.

The utility of serotyping as an international designation for *Salmonella* subtypes has led to its widespread adoption. In a recent survey, 61 countries reported that they used *Salmonella* serotyping for public health surveillance (Herikstad et al., 2002a). A new World Health Organization (WHO) website (WHO, 2002) collects and presents the results of this serotyping. This website is a new mechanism for the global surveillance of foodborne diseases.

Molecular subtyping is now expanding the power of surveillance to detect outbreaks that appear as sporadic cases and is improving the ability of public health authorities to investigate outbreaks by comparing the molecular "fingerprint" of bacterial strains associated with sporadic cases of a foodborne disease. These new techniques can define subtypes within a single species or serotype and provide useful strain differentiation for a growing number of pathogens (Swaminathan et al., 2001). State public health laboratories began using an assay standardized at CDC for *E. coli* O157:H7 after it proved useful in the 1993 West Coast outbreak associated with the consumption of undercooked ground beef; they have now expanded the use of this technique to common serotypes of *Salmonella* such as Typhimurium and Enteritidis, and to *Listeria monocytogenes* (Swaminathan et al., 2001). Developing this capacity at the state level also enhanced rapid detection of multicounty clusters within the state (Bender et al., 1997, 2001). Standardized subtyping protocols have now been developed for seven pathogens; next-generation, gene-based technologies are under development.

Recently, PulseNet, a national network formed by linking all state public health laboratories via the Internet, with a national database maintained by CDC, made it possible to rapidly identify and investigate multistate clusters. Once a cluster of infections caused by strains with the same fingerprint is identified, rapid epidemiological investigation can determine whether the cluster is a true outbreak with a common source. Laboratories at the Food and Drug Administration (FDA) and the U.S. Department of Agriculture (USDA) also participate in this network so that isolates from foods and animals can be compared within the system. It is noteworthy that Canada has already adopted a compatible system and that the European network for laboratory-based surveillance of foodborne infections, EnterNet, has similar plans. The participation of Canada, Europe, Asia, and other regions could make it possible to detect multiregional clusters of foodborne disease (Swaminathan et al., 2001).

Monitoring levels of antimicrobial resistance in foodborne pathogens is another form of subtype-based surveillance. Since 1996, the National Antimicrobial Resistance Monitoring System (NARMS) for enteric bacteria, a collaborative effort of CDC, USDA, and FDA, has been monitoring the prevalence of resistance in *Salmonella*, *Campylobacter*, and other foodborne bacterial pathogens isolated from humans, animals, and foods (Marano et al., 2000). This type of surveillance provides information about the trends in microbial resistance to specific drugs, identifies the emergence of new resistance threats, and permits the comparison of strains identified in various locations. This information is useful to public health officials who are involved in controlling highly resistant strains, to clinicians making treatment decisions, and to regulators who can better evaluate the association between antibiotics used in animals or the environment and resistance developed in human pathogens.

In summary, nationwide surveillance systems for cases of foodborne infection are valuable tools for defining trends, identifying outbreaks, and evaluating food safety programs. In some situations, serotyping and subtyping of pathogens, coupled with nationwide surveillance, provide an ideal system to link a cluster of cases.

Considering that state and local public health systems provide the only nationwide population-based surveillance for foodborne diseases, and that outbreak investigations are critical to identify new pathogens and new food safety hazards, the committee recommends that foodborne outbreak investigation and reporting by state and local health departments be enhanced. Training and personnel and laboratory support should be provided to enable rapid, thorough, and accurate investigation and reporting of foodborne outbreaks by local and state health departments, with performance evaluated through systematic review of outbreak reports. In addition, timely analysis and dissemination of results to regulators, industry, and the public is essential. Time series analysis (as discussed in Chapter 3) would also be a valuable analysis technique in this area.

Sentinel Site Surveillance

In contrast to the national umbrella of routine notifiable disease surveillance supplemented with public health laboratory subtyping, a different strategy, sentinel site surveillance, can provide more detailed information about specific illnesses that are likely to be foodborne. This strategy was first developed for monitoring cases of hepatitis, for which detailed laboratory and epidemiological data are crucial (Bell et al., 1998).

A more recent example of this type of surveillance is the Foodborne Disease Active Surveillance Network (FoodNet), a collaborative program of CDC, sentinel sites (currently nine sites), USDA, and FDA under the aegis of CDC's Emerging Infections Program (Angulo and Swerdlow, 1999). The establishment of FoodNet was stimulated by a request from USDA's Food Safety and Inspection System (FSIS) for a system to ascertain the public health impact of USDA's Pathogen Reduction; Hazard Analysis and Critical Control Point Final Rule (PR/HACCP rule). FoodNet began with an initial five-site area in 1996 and expanded to nine sites by 2001. The current surveillance area covers 37.8 million persons, or approximately 13 percent of the U.S. population (CDC, 2002a).

FoodNet conducts active case ascertainment for foodborne diseases, accompanied by epidemiological studies designed to help better understand the epidemiology of foodborne diseases in the United States. Active case ascertainment means that public health authorities regularly contact clinical laboratories to obtain case reports of diagnosed illnesses; therefore, the results do not depend on which infections are locally notifiable or on local resources available for surveillance. Thus, because reporting is more uniform and complete, active case ascertainment yields better data than passive reporting systems. However, it is also more expensive and limited in geographic scope. In addition to case ascertainment, FoodNet surveys laboratory, physician, and patient practices that cause an individual case to be diagnosed. Also, FoodNet has been a platform for conducting case-control studies of sporadic infections in order to identify general risk factors for infection that distinguish the persons who get ill from those who stay healthy. This information has been used to better define the burden of foodborne illness (Mead et al., 1999), to evaluate the risk factors for specific infections (e.g., in the *Campylobacter* case-control study [Friedman et al., 2000b]), and to track the trends in major foodborne infections (CDC, 2002a).

To provide real-time tracking of human case surveillance, the committee recommends that the capacity of the sentinel sites of FoodNet to rapidly interview (i.e., as soon as possible after the case is diagnosed, as opposed to two to three weeks later when active surveillance contacts with the laboratory detect the case, a cluster is identified, or some other event shows the need for follow-up) individual illness cases that are potentially foodborne, to track real-time interviews, and to collect and subtype *Listeria*, *E. coli* O157:H7, and *Salmonella* isolates from human infections, be enhanced as soon as feasible. (Although several subtyping schemes exist for *Campylobacter*, none has yet been shown to be useful and practical in the public health setting for routine testing of all isolates.) All cases of infection from pathogens covered by FoodNet surveillance should be interviewed. In addition, the committee believes that international collaboration and the sharing of methods and microbiological and illness surveillance data between the United States and other surveillance systems such as WHO's Global SalmSurv (WHO, 2002) and Europe's EnterNet must be strongly supported.

Foodborne Outbreak Reporting

A foodborne outbreak is a cluster of two or more similar infections that are shown by investigation to result from ingestion of the same food (Olsen et al., 2000). Local and state health departments conduct most foodborne outbreak investigations. Since 1967, CDC has collected reports of outbreaks of foodborne illnesses investigated by local, state, and national public health authorities (Olsen et al., 2000). Reports of outbreaks include the nature of the pathogen or toxin, the type of food that caused the outbreak, and some information about factors that contributed to the outbreak. Before 1998, these reports were collected on paper and slowly reviewed and compiled. The system is now being overhauled with an improved form, the active solicitation of reports from states, the introduction of Internet-based reporting (Electronic Foodborne Outbreak Reporting System), and the more rapid analysis and dissemination of results (FDDB, 2002a).

The foodborne outbreak surveillance system has provided useful information on long-term trends for many pathogens for which surveillance otherwise does not exist, as well as summaries of the outbreaks caused by a particular pathogen, hazard, or food (Bean and Griffin, 1990). In the future, it may provide more systematic detection of clusters of outbreaks, based on both laboratory testing and epidemiological assessment of the outbreak presentation (Hall et al., 2001). The committee considers the systematic analysis of information on outbreaks gathered through this system as an effective tool for allocating the burden of many infections and other hazards across broad food categories.

Specialized Surveys of Behavior

FoodNet and other surveillance efforts also provide systematic data on behavior of the population and exposure to specific risks. Studies conducted through the CDC Behavioral Risk Factor Surveillance System (BRFSS) documented the high frequency of risky food behavior (Yang et al., 1998). More recently, FoodNet population surveys have provided population-based data on the incidence of diarrheal illness and the likelihood of seeking medical care for a diarrheal illness; this information was critical to develop a general estimate of the burden of foodborne disease (Herikstad et al., 2002b; Mead et al., 1999). The surveys also provided general population-based data on the frequency of exposure to a wide variety of foods and other potential sources of intestinal infection (Consumer Studies Branch, 2002; FDDB, 2002b).

Another potential source of information is the complaint systems maintained by local and state health departments to which individuals can report illnesses or hazardous conditions they believe may be related to food (Samuel et al., 2001). While such systems are far less specific than systems built on diagnosed cases of illness, they may provide an early warning of problems.

Limitations of Surveillance

One limitation inherent in all surveillance systems is that many cases go unrecognized for a variety of reasons. For example, cases may not be detected because people who are ill do not seek medical care, physicians and laboratories may not make a specific diagnosis, diagnosed cases may not be reported to authorities, and authorities with limited resources may not investigate or report cases. This last factor becomes especially significant if the surveillance program is voluntary, as is the case with outbreak reporting by local and state agencies.

Data collected in this voluntary manner do not correspond to a nationally representative sample of the population because reporting depends on other variables, such as local resources or whether a particular disease is notifiable (CDC, 2001). Even in active surveillance programs, such as FoodNet, the number of cases is underestimated because people do not seek medical care or because cases are reported only when they are confirmed by a laboratory. Therefore, the actual number of cases that occurs is likely to be substantially greater than the number of cases reported. For example, it has been estimated that 38 cases of salmonellosis occur for every 1 that is reported (Voetsch et al., 1998). Many outbreaks are also likely to be unrecognized. A common-source outbreak in a restaurant may not be recognized because patrons were exposed in small groups that were unknown to each other. For some foodborne infections, the incubation period may be long enough to obscure the relationship with the meal unless persons attending a large gathering, such as a banquet or wedding reception, have some reason to compare their experiences afterwards.

A second limitation is the difficulty in attributing a specific case to a specific food. Many infections can be transmitted by a variety of foods and by routes other than food. In the sporadic case of illness, the person may have consumed many foods and may have had other potentially risky exposures in the days preceding illness, making it difficult to determine the source of the illness. In an outbreak setting, where careful comparison of food consumption patterns of a group of ill persons with those of a group who remained well can identify the immediate food vehicle, it is still difficult sometimes to determine which of the various ingredients was the source of the illness. However, many outbreak investigations are definitive, and comparison of patterns observed among groups of outbreaks can help define patterns.

Finally, surveillance can only count what is measurable and known. Because diagnosis of Norwalk-like virus (recently designated "Noroviruses") infections is not routinely performed in clinical laboratories, for example, this extremely common illness cannot be monitored with the same type of case-based surveillance that is conducted for infections caused by *Salmonella* or *Campylobacter*, for which routine diagnostic tests are available. The importance of Norwalk-like virus infections can be defined from outbreaks where the typical combination of signs, symptoms, incubation period, and duration of illness can be documented and where specimens reach specialized laboratories that can make the diagnosis (Bresee et al., 2002). Similarly, enterotoxigenic *E. coli*, the cause of much travelers' diarrhea, is increasingly recognized as a cause of outbreaks in the United States, but may also be an unrecognized common cause of sporadic cases because the specialized tests to detect it are rarely applied (Dalton et al., 1999; Guerrant et al., 1990). It is likely that there are many foodborne disease agents yet to be discovered which, consequently, are not currently tested for in any laboratory (Tauxe, 1997).

Similarly, behavioral risk-factor surveillance is subject to limitations. This type of surveillance depends on what people can and will report. People may overestimate how often they perform socially desirable behaviors such as hand washing. Questions about risk exposures also depend on what the consumer observes. People are not likely to know if the food they ate was cross-contaminated in the kitchen, even if they prepared it themselves. The observations individuals can make may be a less-than-perfect measure of risk. Although the FoodNet population survey used consumption of pink ground beef as an assessment of cooked meat doneness and safety, research has clearly demonstrated that cooked meat color is not an acceptable indicator for these parameters (Berry et al., 1998; FSIS, 1998a, 2000; Hunt et al., 1999). Premature browning and a persistent pink color are two conditions that can occur in ground beef patties, influencing internal beef patty color, whether or not a patty has been cooked to an internal temperature of 160°F (Hunt et al., 1999; Killinger et al., 2000). In a nationwide evaluation, Berry and coworkers (1998) found 47.4 percent of hamburgers cooked to 160°F retained some pink color, and 15.8 percent still retained some pink color when cooked to 175°F. In addition, more than 25 percent of fresh-cooked hamburgers (meat was never frozen) were brown or nearly brown internally although hamburgers were only cooked to 150°F.

RESULTS FROM PUBLIC HEALTH SURVEILLANCE

The Burden of Disease

An estimation of the burden of disease is very useful when regulatory agencies make decisions about the focus and allocation of resources. The burden of disease attributable to foods has only been estimated in a general way; if the estimate of this burden was specific for particular foodborne diseases and food groups, more informed decisions could be made by regulatory agencies.

Information from surveillance has recently been integrated into a general estimate of the overall burden of foodborne disease in the United States (Mead et al., 1999). This estimate included the number of cases, hospitalizations, and deaths that were attributed to specific pathogens and to the large number of illnesses that remain unaccounted for. These pathogen-based point estimates can provide a benchmark for assessing the economic impact of foodborne diseases, such as the $6.9 billion estimated cost to society from the diseases caused by the major foodborne bacterial pathogens (Buzby and Roberts, 1996). Some foodborne infections can also cause chronic complications in a small percentage of cases; for example, kidney failure related to *E. coli* O157:H7 has been reported in 4 to 8 percent of cases (Griffin et al., 2002), and Guillain Barré syndrome paralysis may complicate 1 in 1,000 *Campylobacter* infections (Nachamkin et al., 2000). There may be other complications of and sequelae from foodborne diseases. For example, it has recently been reported that people infected with multiresistant salmonellae are more likely to die in the 6 months following the infection than uninfected individuals (Helms et al., 2002). The full impact of illnesses includes acute morbidity and mortality, as well as the impact of subsequent complications and of long-term effects, such as life-long impairments from congenital toxoplasmosis or early childhood diarrheal illnesses in impoverished areas (Guerrant et al., 2002). With more information about the frequency, duration, and disability caused by these complications, the burden of foodborne illness could be reestimated on a basis such as Disability Adjusted Life Years, a measure used to characterize the burden of many other public health problems (Murray and Lopez, 1997).

Surveillance data can subdivide the burden of a specific infection. For example, the contribution of specific *Salmonella* serotypes to the overall burden of salmonellosis can be derived from their frequency. More specifically, the three most common serotypes of *Salmonella*, Typhimurium, Enteritidis, and Newport, together accounted for nearly half of all reported cases of salmonellosis in 2001, and thus of the burden of salmonellosis (Table 2.1).

The burden of reported foodborne outbreaks can also be measured. National foodborne outbreak reporting from 1998 through 2000 gave a combined annual incidence of 4.8 outbreaks per 1 million persons in the population (FDDB, 2002a). However, in addition to the limitations mentioned above, measuring the burden of disease due to outbreaks presents special challenges. For example, small outbreaks are particularly likely to go unrecognized and unreported, and it is likely that outbreak surveillance undercounts the true frequency of events for the reasons noted earlier. Moreover, a substantial fraction of outbreak investigations do not determine either the causative agent (the etiology) or the specific food that

TABLE 2.1 The Top Ten *Salmonella* Serotypes Reported from Humans in 2001

Rank	Serotype	Number of Reported Cases	Percentage of the Total
1	Typhimurium	6,999	22.1
2	Enteritidis	5,614	17.7
3	Newport	3,158	10.0
4	Heidelberg	1,884	5.9
5	Javiana	1,067	3.4
6	Montevideo	626	2.0
7	Oranienburg	595	1.9
8	Muenchen	583	1.8
9	Thompson	514	1.6
10	Saint Paul	469	1.5
Subtotal		21,509	67.9
Total		31,675	

SOURCE: FDDB (2002c).

was contaminated (the food vehicle), information that is critical in assigning the burden of disease and focusing resources on areas of most concern. Between 1993 and 1997, among the 2,751 foodborne outbreaks reported to CDC and included in a published summary, an etiology was reported for 838 (32 percent) and a food vehicle for 967 (35 percent) (Olsen et al., 2000). Clinical and epidemiological profiling of outbreaks with unconfirmed etiology indicates that many of these can still be put into meaningful categories (Hall et al., 2001). Among outbreaks investigated that affected at least ten persons in FoodNet sites in 1998 and 1999, 30 percent had a determined etiology and 57 percent had a reported vehicle (Jones et al., 2000).

One reason the etiology of many outbreaks goes unconfirmed is that appropriate clinical samples are not collected and tested (Garman et al., 2002). Thus, only large outbreaks are likely to be characterized. The committee believes that allocation of more resources for diagnostic testing and investigation could increase the proportion of foodborne disease outbreaks that are characterized.

Trends in Foodborne Disease

Standard case surveillance data, such as that collected from the national *Salmonella* surveillance program, provide nationwide data on the prevalence and trends of specific serotypes of *Salmonella*. However, unreported cases—due to not seeking medical attention or not performing the diagnostic—occur. The results over time show substantial variation in the incidence of specific serotypes as epidemics emerge and are controlled (Figure 2.2). The national incidence of *S.*

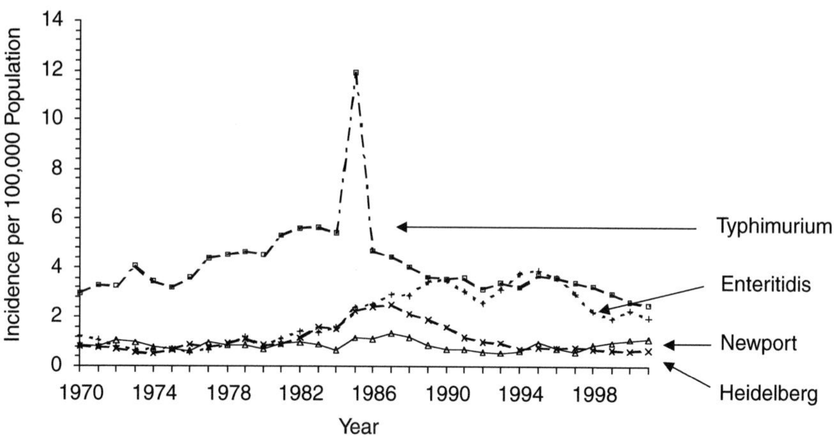

FIGURE 2.2 Trends in incidence of the top four *Salmonella* serotypes 1970–2001. SOURCE: CDC (2002b).

Enteritidis infections shows the progress of this primarily egg-associated epidemic. The epidemic began in the 1980s and reached a peak in 1995. Although the incidence of this serotype has decreased by approximately 48 percent since 1995, it remains well above the pre-epidemic baseline of 1 per 100,000 population, at par with *S.* Typhimurium as the most prevalent salmonellae serotypes. The increase and subsequent return to baseline in *S.* Heidelberg, a serotype usually associated with poultry, is also evident. In contrast, because significant variation has occurred since 1995 in the number of reported cases of *S.* Newport, a serotype usually associated with cattle, the trend is not so clear, but there are indications that it is on the increase and it is currently the third most common serotype (FDDB, 2002c). Systematic review of the *Salmonella* surveillance data through 1997 indicates that there have been important declines in several serotypes associated with swine and with poultry, and increases in serotypes associated with reptiles (such as pet turtles and snakes) (Olsen et al., 2001).

Another surveillance system that provides trends for the illnesses it tracks is FoodNet (Figure 2.3). There have been sustained and important decreases in the reported incidence of *Campylobacter*, *Yersinia*, *Listeria,* and *Salmonella* infections since 1996 (CDC, 2002a). These declines are not accounted for by changes in diagnostic procedures or in the surveillance system itself; the declines were significant even when the considerable regional variation in these infections was

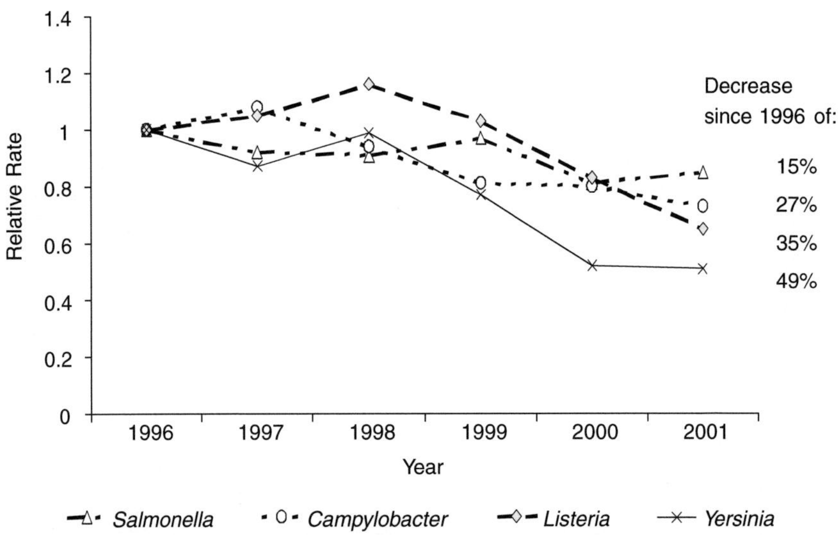

FIGURE 2.3 Trends in relative incidence of selected foodborne infections, FoodNet 1996–2001. SOURCE: CDC (2002a).

taken into account. Such declines coincided with the implementation of food safety assurance measures by USDA, including the PR/HACCP rule, in meat and poultry slaughter and processing plants. Additional interventions that have been introduced in the past several years include consumer safety warnings on raw meat and poultry, education efforts for the public, egg-quality assurance programs for *S.* Enteritidis (see below), increased attention to fresh produce safety, implementation of HACCP in the seafood industry, application of HACCP to juice processing, and heightened awareness about the importance of food safety controls for imported foods.

Changes in slaughter and processing procedures and sanitation are likely to have played an important role in reducing the incidence of four important foodborne diseases between 1996 and 2001. *Y. enterocolitica* infections, often associated with pork (Lee et al., 1990; Tauxe et al., 1987), have declined the most: 49 percent (CDC, 2002a; FDDB, 2002a). This decline may have resulted in part from changes in pork carcass-dressing practices such as tying the bung (large intestine) early in the process. Because there have been no targeted public health control efforts for this infection in recent years, this decrease may also have been achieved partly as a result of basic food safety education and implementation of the PR/HACCP rule in pork processing. *L. monocytogenes* infections showed the second greatest decline: 35 percent. Outbreaks and sporadic cases of illness caused by this pathogen are most frequently associated with ready-to-eat and processed meats and raw-milk cheeses (Mead et al., 2002). The recent decline in *Listeria* infections occurred as the ready-to-eat meat industry focused on improving factory sanitation and implementation of HACCP programs in the wake of a large listeriosis outbreak in 1998 that was traced to hot dogs (CDC, 1998). The 27 percent decline in *Campylobacter* infections, which are often associated with poultry, occurred alongside changes in poultry processing-plant operations that were introduced with the objective of reducing *Salmonella* contamination. These changes included the PR/HACCP rule implementation, as well as general food safety information dissemination efforts to increase public awareness (Shane, 2000). The overall decline in *Salmonella* infections of 15 percent echoes the trends seen in national *Salmonella* surveillance. It includes declines in both *S.* Typhimurium (down 24 percent) and *S.* Enteritidis (down 22 percent), so it reflects more than the control of egg-associated *S.* Enteritidis infections. The overall decline in salmonellosis would be even greater except for the concurrent increase in infections due to *S.* Newport (up 32 percent; Figure 2.2).

The decline in the incidence of *Salmonella* infections in humans from 1996 to 2001 coincided with a decline in the prevalence of *Salmonella* isolated from FSIS-regulated products, according to comparisons of the baseline studies performed by USDA before (1994 to 1996) and after (2000) the PR/HACCP rule was implemented (Rose et al., 2002). Similarly, the declines observed in the frequency of the four most common serotypes of *Salmonella* found in broiler chicken samples are matched by significant declines in the frequency of infections in humans with three of the four serotypes (*S.* Heidelberg, *S.* Typhimurium, and *S.* Hadar); the fourth serotype (*S.* Kentucky) was already rare among humans (RTI, 2002b). It is difficult to ascribe these trends to any one specific control measure because they are occurring in the setting of many simultaneous changes and improvements; nevertheless, the committee believes that these trends indicate that, collectively, the food safety efforts are making progress toward the national public health goals for 2010 (Table 2.2).

Infections with *E. coli* O157:H7 do not show a sustained decline. Although their number decreased 21 percent in 2001 as compared with 1996, this decline is the result of a decrease only between 2000 and 2001 that does not imply a consistent trend; it may simply represent year-to-year variation and perhaps the effect of case-finding activities associated with specific outbreaks (Bender et al., in press). Trends in meat contamination from 2000 to 2002 indicate that the prevalence of this microorganism in ground beef has not changed. The trend, in percentage of positive samples, is flat at approximately 0.8 percent of tested samples (FSIS, 2003).

Among other pathogens tracked by FoodNet, *Shigella*, which has a human reservoir and is predominantly transmitted from person-to-person and only sometimes via food, did not decrease significantly. *Vibrio* infections—typically transmitted via undercooked shellfish—increased by 83 percent. This increase coincided with the recognition of a new epidemic strain of *V. parahaemolyticus* in 1997 (Daniels et al., 2000). The incidence of parasitic infections with *Cyclospora* and *Cryptosporidium*, for which surveillance began in 1997, also decreased by 2001, although statistical trends were not calculated for *Cyclospora* because of the small number of cases and the shorter time of observation (CDC, 2002a).

The committee recognizes that, ironically, because of some improvements in surveillance programs, the food safety problem in some cases may appear to have worsened. For example, the number of foodborne outbreaks reported to CDC increased sharply in 1998 from 400 to 500 per year (1990–1993) to 1,300 to

TABLE 2.2 Incidence of Selected Foodborne Diseases in FoodNet, 2001, and the *Healthy People 2010* Goals

Pathogen	Incidence, 2001[a] (per 100,000)	National Goals 2010[b] (per 100,000)
Campylobacter	13.8	12.3
Salmonella	15.1	6.8
E. coli O157:H7	1.6	1.0
Listeria	0.3	0.25
Total	30.8	20.4

[a] Preliminary FoodNet data (CDC, 2002a).
[b] *Healthy People 2010* goals (HHS, 2000).

1,400 per year (Figure 2.4). As described earlier, this increase followed a revision of the reporting system and therefore largely reflects the impact of the new reporting procedures. In addition, better surveillance using PulseNet means that some outbreaks that were missed in the past are now being detected.

For example, in the year following the introduction of PulseNet subtyping for *E. coli* O157:H7 in Minnesota, four of ten common-source outbreaks caused by that pathogen were detected that would likely have been missed otherwise (Bender et al., 1997). Similarly, more *Listeria* outbreaks are being detected since the implementation of routine molecular subtyping; where these outbreaks used to be detected once every 5 years, they are being detected approximately twice a year (Mead et al., 2002).

Long-term trends can also be observed in reported foodborne outbreak investigations. Since 1967, the number of outbreaks of staphylococcal and *Clostridium perfringens* food poisoning has decreased substantially (Bean and Griffin, 1990). Outbreaks of *S.* Enteritidis infections increased in the 1980s to a peak in the mid-1990s, but have since declined, as have the number of sporadic infections (FDDB, 2002c).

Linking Pathogens to Specific Foods: Allocating the Burden of Disease

Many foodborne pathogens are associated with a specific reservoir, either a food, an animal, or a human, and consequently the illnesses they cause are also

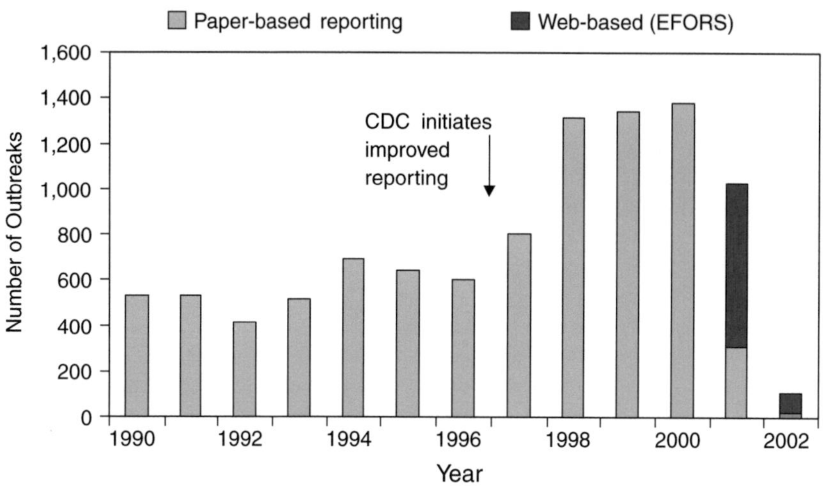

FIGURE 2.4 Foodborne disease outbreaks reported to the Centers for Disease Control and Prevention, January 1, 1990, through March 15, 2002.
SOURCE: FDDB (2002a).

often associated with a characteristic food group or reservoir. The current state of knowledge about the association of common food groups and common foodborne agents is summarized in Table 2.3.

The data that link a pathogen to a specific reservoir often come from outbreak investigations. For many pathogens, a series of investigated outbreaks provides the best information to define the association of the illness with specific foods. For example, the first investigation of *E. coli* O157:H7 infections identified the pathogen and linked the distinctive illness to eating undercooked hamburgers (Riley et al., 1983). Trace-back from an outbreak caused by ground beef and from sporadic cases caused by drinking raw milk led to identification of the bovine reservoir for *E. coli* O157:H7; this finding is particularly noteworthy because infected cows are usually asymptomatic (Martin et al., 1986; Wells et al., 1991). More recently, outbreaks of this infection have been associated with an expanding array of foods (Griffin et al., 2002). Early investigations of *Campylobacter* outbreaks identified raw milk, undercooked poultry, and contaminated water as common sources (Blaser et al., 1979; Deming et al., 1987; Vogt et al., 1982).

Pathogens that have human reservoirs can also be linked to specific foods, depending on the most characteristic mechanisms of contamination. In 1924, a large epidemic of typhoid fever was linked to raw oysters that were harvested and held near sewage sources (Lumsden et al., 1925). More recently, outbreaks of Norwalk-like virus infection, which also has a human reservoir, have been linked to shellfish (and to direct contamination from ill fishermen) and to foods such as cold salads and sandwiches that are handled extensively in the kitchen (and to direct contamination from ill food handlers) (Kohn et al., 1995; Parashar and

TABLE 2.3 Specific Association of Commodity Food Groups and Pathogens

Food Group	Pathogens
Beef	*Salmonella, Escherichia coli* O157:H7
Poultry	*Campylobacter, Salmonella*
Pork	*Staphylococcus aureus, Yersinia enterocolitica, Salmonella, Toxoplasma, Trichinella*
Ready-to-eat meats	*Listeria monocytogenes*
Dairy	*L. monocytogenes, E. coli* O157:H7, *Salmonella, Campylobacter*
Eggs	*Salmonella*
Fresh produce	Norwalk-like virus, *Salmonella, Shigella, E. coli* O157:H7, Hepatitis A, *Cyclospora*
Finfish	Histamine fish poisoning (scombroid), ciguatera poisoning, helminth parasites
Shellfish	*Vibrio* spp, Norwalk-like virus, Hepatitis A

SOURCE: Doyle et al. (2001).

Monroe, 2001). For pathogens that rarely cause outbreaks, studies of sporadic cases and comparison with healthy controls can define associations with particular foods. For example, *V. vulnificus* infection was definitively associated with consumption of raw oysters soon after it was first described (Blake et al., 1979). Studies of *E. coli* O157:H7 infections linked sporadic cases of infection with this pathogen to eating undercooked ground beef, thus supplementing the data from outbreaks (Kassenborg et al., 1998; Mead et al., 1997; Slutsker et al., 1998). Studies of sporadic *Campylobacter* infection have linked it to eating poultry and other meats, as well as to drinking untreated water and to other sources. Around the world, poultry remains the dominant reservoir for this pathogen (Friedman et al., 2000a, 2000b; WHO, 2000).

Allocating the burden of infections quantitatively across specific food groups is a complex challenge that has been approached using several strategies. A main strategy draws from epidemiological and public health investigations. Data on outbreaks associated with foods, supplemented with data from sporadic cases, provide the most readily available public health information for allocating the burden of specific infections across food groups. For example, between 1993 and 1997, 1,152 foodborne disease outbreaks with a determined food vehicle, which involved 46,453 illnesses, were reported in the United States (updated from Olsen et al., 2000). Among the 713 outbreaks for which the implicated food could be assigned to a single food group, 21 percent of the illnesses were associated with meat, 11 percent with poultry, 28 percent with produce, 15 percent with seafood, and 26 percent with other foods. These findings indicate that food safety concerns exist for all major food groups. For those illnesses that rarely appear in outbreak form, data from individual case series or from case-control studies can be used to allocate the burden.

Epidemiological investigations of outbreaks and cases can also provide important insight into the precise mechanisms of exposure and the variations in human behavior that contribute to it. For example, illness in an outbreak was particularly associated with tasting raw ground beef in the process of seasoning and cooking it (Fontaine et al., 1978). In an investigation of *Campylobacter* infections in Colorado, illness was associated particularly with handling and preparing chicken, rather than with eating it (Hopkins and Scott, 1983). In an assessment of sporadic ground beef-associated *E. coli* O157:H7 infections in New Jersey, ill persons were no less likely to have noticed the new meat handling recommendations on the meat wrapper than those who were well, but they were less likely to have washed their hands after handling raw beef (Mead et al., 1997).

Another strategy to help allocate the burden of foodborne disease relies on systematic sampling data from many foods. For example, the patterns of molecular subtypes in strains of *Salmonella* isolated from people can be compared and matched to those of strains isolated from a variety of foods. This can help relate specific pathogenic subtypes and diseases to specific foods. To be successful, this strategy depends on extensive and systematic sampling of many foods and on the use of standardized subtyping methods on a large number of strains. This strategy has been routinely applied in Denmark to track the burden of salmonellosis associated with various foods (Hald and Bronsted, 2002).

Finally, if data on pathogen prevalence are available for a large number of foods, a risk allocation can be constructed using the methods of risk analysis that have been used for *L. monocytogenes* (FSIS/CFSAN, 2001). This approach depends on the assumptions that all strains of a pathogen are equally likely to cause disease, and that the distribution of the pathogen in foods can be reliably estimated from studies using a broad range of methods and conducted over a substantial time span.

Once a food is implicated as a common source of a pathogen, a detailed review of its production process may reveal the likely points in the process where the food became contaminated. This is an important phase of intensive outbreak investigations that often involves tracing back along the production process from the implicated food the ill persons ate. Such a review may identify where the contamination was likely to have originated and where it may have been further amplified or controlled. This information, of particular interest to risk assessors, is only gathered in a minority of foodborne outbreak investigations and requires a multidisciplinary approach.

Index of Consumer Behavior

Surveys of consumer behavior can provide a useful index of behavior, subject to the limitations associated with reporting by consumers. The 12-state BRFSS survey of 1995 to 1996 showed that in the preceding 12 months, 50 percent of those interviewed ate undercooked eggs, 20 percent ate pink ground beef, 19 percent did not wash their hands after handling raw meat or chicken, 8 percent ate raw oysters, and 1.4 percent consumed raw milk (Yang et al., 1998). The frequency of consumption of pink hamburgers was higher in men, increased with education and salary, but decreased with age. As the correlation between hamburger color and degree of doneness is imperfect, these data do not mean that the persons interviewed necessarily ate undercooked hamburger (Berry et al., 1998; Hunt et al., 1999; Killinger et al., 2000). In the most recent cycle of FoodNet population surveys, 27 percent of respondents reported that they ate a raw or runny egg dish in the preceding month, 26 percent ate pink ground beef, and 2.5 percent ate raw oysters. This survey also included questions about thermometer use in cooking (recommended by USDA to measure an internal temperature of 160°F as an indication of doneness); only 3 percent reported using a thermometer when cooking hamburgers (Yang et al., 1998).

Other food safety surveys were conducted by FDA in 1988, 1993, 1998, and 2001 to gather data on consumer food-safety practices related to cross-contamination and consumption of potentially risky foods (Consumer Studies Branch, 2002). The data showed large improvements consisting of the reduction of cross-contamination and the decreased consumption of potentially risky foods between 1993 and 1998 that were maintained at the time of the 2001 survey. However, notable exceptions to this trend were an increase in the consumption of raw clams, raw oysters, and raw fish from 1998 levels. The proportion of the population who reported not washing their hands after touching raw meat or after cracking eggs decreased from 29 percent and 66 percent, respectively, in 1993, to 15 percent and 55 percent in 2001. Although the proportion of the population who reported eating pink hamburger declined from 24 percent in 1993 to 16 percent in 2001, research (Berry et al., 1998; FSIS, 1998a, 2000; Hunt et al., 1999) has demonstrated that cooked ground-meat color is not an indication of safety. Based on this research, in the late 1990s USDA began recommending the use of a thermometer to check the internal temperature of cooked hamburgers.

Analysis of existing surveys, focus groups, and observational data, conducted by the Research Triangle Institute for USDA, also indicated improved food safety knowledge and practices, as reported by consumers (RTI, 2002a). For example, this analysis indicated that the proportion of the population using thermometers when cooking hamburger doubled from 3 percent in 1998 to 6 percent in 2001. A certain degree of disparity between consumer-reported practices and observed behavior was also noted. RTI recommended additional educational efforts to encourage consumer changes in behavior concerning proper cleaning, heating, refrigeration, and use of thermometers.

Overall, consumer behavior surveys indicate that although some changes in consumer behavior have occurred, consumer habits are still frequently less than optimal. The committee recommends periodic repetition of such surveys to help document behavioral changes concerning food safety in the population at large as a result of consumer education efforts, and to target food safety messages to subgroups of the population that engage in risky food-preparation and consumption behavior.

MONITORING HAZARDS IN THE FOOD CHAIN

Systematic Monitoring

Routine systematic monitoring at various points of the food supply is the main form of surveillance for many toxic hazards for which the associated human illnesses are hard to diagnose and are persistent in nature. For example, FDA conducts a systematic pesticide residue monitoring program (CFSAN, 2002), shellfish beds are routinely monitored for evidence of fecal contamination, and imported shellfish are sampled for pathogens. As new foodborne hazards emerge, a system for rapid assessment of their prevalence at various points in the food supply is critical to developing prevention measures. For example, brains of cattle with evidence of neurological disease are tested for the presence of bovine spongiform encephalopathy just after slaughter, providing an indication of the likely absence of the infectious prion in the food supply (APHIS, 2002).

For infectious pathogens, few systematic sampling programs exist in the public sector, although internal monitoring by industry is common. Although the PR/HACCP rule requires the monitoring of generic *E. coli* on carcasses in slaughter plants, these data are not publicly available and thus cannot be used to measure the overall effectiveness of the PR/HACCP rule or to compare contamination levels among individual producers or groups of producers. Because systematic monitoring is a powerful tool for tracking specific microbial hazards, particularly if coupled with molecular subtyping, the committee recommends expansion of this type of monitoring to all high-risk food groups.

For meat and poultry, although not designed to be an optimal surveillance system, product sampling as part of PR/HACCP verification provides some information about the frequency of *Salmonella* in specific meat and poultry products, about the impact of plant size on contamination levels, and about trends in specific serotypes (Rose et al., 2002; RTI, 2002b). The committee believes that the value of this information would increase if such data were collected systematically throughout the year, analyzed in ways that accounted for various processing plant characteristics, and used by the various plants to benchmark their performance compared with that of their peers. Further, anonymous linking of the library of subtype patterns thus generated for detected pathogens to public health subtyping systems could also provide valuable information regarding sources of contamination (e.g., to risk assessors). To this end, the committee suggests that a third-party repository be established for environmental and product testing data from industry, using subtyping methods comparable to those used in public health, and maintained in an anonymous fashion and with voluntary subscription.

Disease-causing microorganisms and other hazards in the food chain can be tracked in targeted surveys of the environment, food animal reservoirs, and foods themselves. These surveys can be used to estimate risks associated with certain foods and to identify or design strategies to control or mitigate these risks. When systematically gathered, such information can also be used to monitor trends in contamination and to measure the impact of control strategies. In addition to the final public health surveillance outcome, this information can provide an indication of the effectiveness of specific control measures.

The committee concluded that systematic sampling of animals at the farm, and especially immediately before slaughter, may be particularly useful to measure the frequency of the presence of important human pathogens such as *S.* Newport and *E. coli* O157:H7 in animal populations.

Given that the potential importance of pre- and postharvest infection of live animals needs to be assessed to obtain a clear understanding of contamination routes, the committee recommends that systematic sampling of animals for pathogens at the point of slaughter be undertaken, analogous to the National Animal Health Monitoring System (NAHMS) surveys of producers conducted by

USDA's Animal and Plant Health Inspection System (APHIS). The results of this sampling should be linked to those of other systematic sampling programs in existence, such as the NAHMS surveys and PR/HACCP monitoring. In addition, the sampling should be concurrent with an enhancement of the capacity of food and agriculture laboratories to rapidly subtype *Salmonella* and *E. coli* O157:H7 isolates from the various systematic sampling programs. FSIS and FDA, in turn, should conduct periodic, systematic microbiological surveys of food-processing plants, with sampling at various points in the production chain. The results of these surveys should serve as the basis to revise baselines on the prevalence of pathogen and indicator microorganisms and to better characterize the structure of the industry and its pathogen reduction practices. The committee also recommends that, for all surveys, collection of samples for *Salmonella* be conducted within the same time frame each year, completed without interruptions or delays, and reported annually, in aggregate form, by size of establishment.

In addition, the committee believes that further studies of farm, production, transport, and lairage-related risk factors for microbiological contamination of food animals are urgently needed to better define control points and strategies at these levels. Conducting additional studies on pathogen prevalence in animals arriving at processing plants would be a critical component for progress in foodborne disease prevention. The contamination is not likely to be random. By comparing sources, transport routes and conditions, and other characteristics of the incoming live animals, the factors that predict higher contamination levels could be defined. This information could target further research into how contamination occurs and how it may be prevented on the farm, in the feedlot, or during transportation. It could also be used to channel into special processing the animals most likely to be contaminated.

For example, though unusual, it is standard practice for an individual animal on a slaughter line to be "passed for cooking" when a veterinary inspector identifies a lesion that indicates localized tuberculosis (9 C.F.R. §311.2). The carcass is removed from the main slaughter line and sent on a different path to receive a fully supervised cook. In recent years, egg farms that are known to have *S.* Enteritidis on the premises routinely send their eggs for pasteurization under voluntary Egg Quality Assurance Programs. In a new program, the Norwegian Agriculture Department is testing broiler flocks for *Campylobacter* and requiring positive flocks to be slaughtered after negative flocks to avoid cross-contamination at the plant; carcasses from positive flocks are then cooked or frozen under supervision (Norwegian Zoonosis Centre, 2002). Therefore, in the future, groups of animals most likely to be contaminated may be designated for uses other than sale in raw form or may be processed in particular ways to minimize the contamination of raw final products.

For produce, recent FDA surveys of imported and domestic items identified *Salmonella* or *Shigella* on 4.4 percent (44 out of 1,003 samples) of imported items (OPDFB, 2001) and on 1.6 percent (12 out of 767 samples) of domestic produce items (CFSAN, 2001). Among the latter, 0.8 percent (6 samples) were positive for *Salmonella* and an equal percentage were positive for *Shigella*.

Considering the increasing importance of raw produce as a vehicle of foodborne infections in the United States, the committee recommends that high-risk (i.e., known to be frequently associated with foodborne infections) raw produce, both domestic and imported, be systematically monitored for such indicators of fecal contamination as generic *E. coli*, and for prevalence of such pathogens as *Salmonella* and *Shigella*. The results of this monitoring should be linked to studies of the specific determinants of such contamination and of the relationship between indicator organisms and pathogen prevalence.

Periodic Monitoring

In addition to systematic surveys, periodic surveys can also provide useful information. Following the release of a National Academies report (NRC, 1985), NAHMS began conducting surveys on food-animal production that provide snapshots of the prevalence of animal and human pathogens and of management practices on farms (Wineland and Dargatz, 1998). For example, a NAHMS survey of layer-hen farms conducted in 1999 showed that 7.1 percent of farms had *S.* Enteritidis on their premises, that farms having high rodent populations were much more likely to be *S.* Enteritidis-positive, and that 56 percent of the farms participated in major egg quality assurance programs. Encouragingly, farms that practiced careful hen-house cleaning and disinfection between flocks did not have *S.* Enteritidis in their environments (APHIS, 2000). Similar periodic, targeted surveys at other points in the food chain could provide important information. For example, although it is known that animal feeds may be contaminated with *Salmonella*, the source and frequency of contamination of specific feed ingredients remains undefined (Crump et al., 2002). Pigs free of *Salmonella* at the farm were shown to acquire *Salmonella* infections in temporary holding pens just before slaughter, indicating that it was not the nonspecific stress of transport or holding, but specific exposure to *Salmonella* after the animals left the farm that was the most important determinant of carriage at slaughter (Hurd et al., 2001). Similarly, a recent study of dairy animals at slaughter in the United Kingdom suggested that 75 percent of the *E. coli* O157:H7 on their hides were the result of contamination that occurred after the animals had been transported to slaughter (Avery et al., 2002).

Standardization of Monitoring Methods

Food hazard surveillance is usually a shared responsibility of the food industry and local, state, or federal regulatory agencies. Data generated are not standardized and thus are difficult to compare. Lack of standardization of foodborne, microbial-hazard surveillance data hinders the development of nationwide hazard assessments and reduces the value of much of the surveillance.

A consortium of state and federal regulatory agencies known as the National Food Safety System (NFSS) has begun to address the interrelated issues of laboratory accreditation, methods validation, and national data-sharing standards. Currently, clinical, environmental, and food microbiology laboratories are accredited by a variety of bodies, each with different standards and evaluation criteria. An NFSS workgroup is encouraging the accrediting bodies to accept the International Organization for Standardization 17025 standard, so that they abide by a single standard. To address methods validation, AOAC International is developing an electronic compilation of analytical methods (e-CAM) to serve as a repository of validated methods and is providing peer review for validating new methods (AOAC, 2002). Finally, development of technical standards for the electronic exchange of data between food safety laboratories has begun with the electronic laboratory exchange network (eLEXNET), which was pilot tested in September 2000 and connected 38 laboratories in 26 states by 2002.

The committee recommends that compatible subtype and antimicrobial resistance surveillance data from humans, animals, farms, and food products should be linked among such agencies and services as CDC, APHIS, FSIS, FDA (including its Center for Veterinary Medicine), and other state and federal laboratories. To facilitate these linkages, NFSS plans should be implemented to (1) provide for uniform accreditation of food safety laboratories, (2) promote the use of validated methods and the rapid validation of new methods, and (3) expand the scope of participation by food safety laboratories in eLEXNET.

Association of Human Diseases with Specific Reservoirs

Comparing information from monitoring and surveillance in animals, foods, and humans can document and even quantify the flow of specific pathogens from particular reservoirs to humans. For example, Denmark has established a comprehensive surveillance system that includes extensive, systematic sampling of many foods and animal groups for *Salmonella*, and subtyping of *Salmonella* strains, which allows it to define the annual contribution of each of the animal reservoirs to human illness in that country (Hald, 2001; Hald and Bronsted, 2002). These data provide a clear illustration of the link between the contamination of food and the resulting infections in humans and the effectiveness of targeted *Salmonella* control programs. In Denmark, these data drive the prevention strategies from farm to table. Hence, screening pork for antibodies to *Salmonella* on the farm has been used to identify pork herds that have a high prevalence of *Salmonella*. These animals are slaughtered separately from animals that come from herds with a low prevalence of *Salmonella* in order to avoid cross-contamination during slaughter and dressing; they are also used only in cooked products (Hald, 2001).

In the United States, strains of *Salmonella* from NAHMS surveys, from HACCP monitoring, and from veterinary diagnostic laboratories are referred to USDA's Agricultural Research Service for determination of antimicrobial resistance as part of the NARMS system (ARS, 2000).

Routine characterization of *Salmonella* from the NARMS system using molecular fingerprinting and comparison of these data to similar data on the human isolates from foodborne outbreaks would make it possible to connect human infections with specific subtypes of *Salmonella* to specific animal reservoirs, similar to the Danish model. The committee recommends that *Salmonella* continue to be tracked in foods as an important foodborne pathogen. It is the only pathogen for which human surveillance systems are widely distributed.

While food safety policy may be guided by monitoring hazard levels in animals or foods, and contaminated food certainly is associated with human illness, the relationships that link contamination levels in foods at processing with incidences of human illness is likely to be more complex than a simple one-to-one linear correspondence. Factors such as multiplication of microorganisms during distribution and preparation undoubtedly affect this relationship. Although careful cooking may eliminate many pathogens from the final food, cross-contamination in the kitchen may easily transfer microbes from raw products to other foods (Redmond et al., 2002). Moreover, the state of the host may make exposure to a low dose of a pathogen highly problematic or inconsequential (see later section, "Pathogenesis"). Risk assessment can attempt to model this complex series of relationships, but major uncertainties will still remain. Documenting the level of a hazard in foods and comparing changes in that level with the final incidence of disease can empirically define the nature of the relationship.

Thus, allocating the burden of illness to different foods and defining the points at which contamination occurs is a complex and imperfect process. It would be helpful to have a mathematical model that allocates hazards of foodborne illness across all food groups and allocates risks across all consumers, but the available data do not permit the development of such a complete and rigorous model. In the absence of such a model, the committee believes that monitoring microbiological contamination at various points in the food production and distribution chain can provide benchmarks to develop standards based on performance and current understanding of risk. These benchmarks and standards must be updated as new information emerges.

The level of processing needed to make a food safe may depend on the likelihood that the product is contaminated. As mentioned before, microbiological methods are used to determine which flocks should send their eggs to pasteurization and whether to open or close shellfish beds to raw oyster harvest. In the future, scientific studies of sources and frequencies of contamination at several points in the process may differentiate various levels of contamination. This information could help identify sources with a higher risk of contamination, to target additional production and processing control steps, and to produce and evaluate a continually safer food supply (Guerrant and Theno, 1995).

PATHOGENESIS

Whether a person is infected by a microorganism depends on a wide range of microbial and host factors. Numerous microbial virulence factors determine infectious doses and pathogenicity, while host susceptibility is determined by genetics, special conditions (e.g., pregnancy), immunity (e.g., vaccination, acquired immune deficiency syndrome), and behavior (e.g., hygiene, education, culture, food preparation methods). These factors and their estimates would contribute to the information required to make risk assessment modeling (as described later in Chapter 3) more complete and accurate.

There is a dose–response relationship for many foodborne infections. The dose level at which 50 percent of exposed individuals will be infected will be much higher than the dose level at which only 5 percent of exposed individuals will be infected. In the context of an outbreak, dose–responses may correlate with attack rates. Thus, in many *Salmonella* outbreaks in which the food was contaminated with only a few organisms, the attack rates were similarly small (Blaser and Newman, 1982). However, even with a low attack rate, large-volume production can mean that the number of infected people, and therefore the outbreak itself, is very large. For example, in a large nationwide outbreak associated with ice cream, only 6 percent of persons who ate the ice cream became ill, perhaps because the ice cream was contaminated with only six or fewer *Salmonella* cells per serving (Hennessy et al., 1996). Because of the large volume of production and its nationwide distribution, however, an estimated 224,000 cases occurred during this outbreak.

Microbial-Related Factors

Microbial threats to our food and water supplies range from toxins and viruses to bacteria, molds, and parasites. While many of these are easily inactivated or killed by sanitizers, heat, or radiation, or removed by filtration, others are resistant to these and other control measures. Unlike viruses and parasites that do not multiply outside their animal hosts, small numbers of bacteria typically multiply to large numbers when conditions permit.

Infectious doses that cause disease in the majority of healthy hosts may range from over 1 million organisms for certain bacteria such as *V. cholerae* to as few as one to ten organisms for pathogens such as *Cryptosporidium* or *Shigella* (Guerrant and Steiner, 1999). Many bacteria have the capacity to increase their resistance to acid, heat, drying, and peroxides through a range of inducible mechanisms. Bacteria stressed by one environmental challenge may become more resistant to a range of other environmental stresses and may become even more invasive (Humphrey et al., 1996). Furthermore, mobile genetic elements, sometimes transmissible as plasmids, phages, or even as naked deoxyribonucleic acid, enable microorganisms to rapidly acquire new virulence and resistance properties.

Host-Related Factors

Host-related factors also influence microbial infectious doses. For example, neutralization of gastric acidity (e.g., higher stomach pH) reduces the infectious doses of *Vibrio*, *Salmonella,* and *E. coli* (Gitelson, 1971; Hornick et al., 1971). This fact places the gastrectomized patient taking antacids at greatest risk when exposed to a potential pathogen (Baine et al., 1974). Similarly, when critical defenses provided by normal bacterial flora are altered by antibiotics, a resistant pathogen may be favored and may complicate therapy for other infections (Barza and Travers, 2002). For example, people taking antibiotics were at a sixfold higher risk than others of acquiring a resistant *Salmonella* infection in the 1985 Chicago outbreak of salmonellosis (Ryan et al., 1987). An earlier report involving Norwegian tourists visiting Spain in the 1960s showed that those who took prophylactic antibiotics were more likely to acquire salmonellosis than those who did not (Mentzing and Ringertz, 1968). Furthermore, immunocompromised patients are not only at greater risk of acquiring enteric infections, but also of suffering from them more severely and experiencing difficulty in overcoming them; examples include salmonellosis and cryptosporidiosis in patients immunocompromised by age, chemotherapy, or immunodeficiency (Navin and Juranek, 1984; Sperber and Schleupner, 1987). Finally, host educational, cultural, and behavioral factors also profoundly influence the risk of acquiring foodborne infections (Mead and Mintz, 1996). Knowledge about food choices, cleanliness, storage, preparation, cooking, and serving practices can help reduce the risk posed to the host by microbial hazards in foods.

USE OF PUBLIC HEALTH DATA TO IMPROVE FOOD SAFETY: SPECIFIC EXAMPLES

Preventing foodborne disease is complex, requiring attention and intervention from farm or fishery to table (IOM/NRC, 1998). There are no vaccines for the pathogens that are most commonly transmitted through foods, and while education of the consumer provides an important final safety barrier, it is not by itself sufficient. Making food safer before it reaches the consumer is critical to maintain confidence in the food supply. The consumer eats many foods without cooking them; prepares raw foods of animal origin with the same hands that prepare uncooked salads; is instructed by tradition and by cookery texts to prepare many meat, poultry, egg, and seafood dishes with more concern about overcooking than undercooking; and is told routinely to season dishes "to taste" during the preparation process.

When new foodborne hazards are identified, the knowledge base for defining effective preventions may be quite limited (Holmberg and Feldman, 1984). Public health surveillance, with detailed investigations of outbreaks, can identify new and emerging hazards, can help define the likely points of control and the questions in need of further research, and can track the effectiveness of control measures. For some hazards, the control measures seem obvious and immediate. For example, requiring toilets with holding tanks on oyster boats made it less likely that oyster gatherers would contaminate the oyster beds with Norwalk-like virus (Kohn et al., 1995). Similarly, providing appropriate toilet and hand washing facilities for field workers, and ensuring that such facilities are properly used, would likely reduce the incidence of workers contaminating produce with enteric pathogens. Providing restaurant kitchens with dedicated hand washing stations, in turn, would be expected to reduce the risk of microbiological cross-contamination of foods. For other situations, the relative merits of potential strategies to minimize or fully prevent microbial contamination of foods are less obvious at the outset, and development of controls must proceed by an iterative process. As more is learned about the settings of outbreaks, prevention strategies are progressively refined. Five examples are presented below to illustrate how this process can lead to improved prevention.

Salmonella and Precooked Roast Beef

From 1975 to 1977, surveillance detected repeated outbreaks of *Salmonella* infection associated with precooked deli roast beef (Parham, 1984). Evaluation of cooking temperatures revealed that they were sometimes insufficient to kill *Salmonella* present in raw beef, and consequently, an improved approach that used specific temperature requirements was applied as an emergency regulation in 1977. In 1981, outbreaks of salmonellosis were again traced to precooked roast beef prepared under these new regulations, showing that these measures were still insufficient (CDC, 1981). In addition to time and temperature of cooking, further studies identified humidity inside the oven as a critical cofactor in determining *Salmonella* survival (Parham, 1984). Since further regulations have been promulgated, outbreaks traced to precooked roast beef have become extremely rare.

Escherichia coli O157:H7 and Apple Cider

In 1992, investigation of an outbreak of *E. coli* O157:H7 infections in Massachusetts linked this pathogen to apple cider for the first time (Besser et al., 1993). This traditional beverage was often pressed from fallen apples, with minimal cleaning, but was long believed to be sufficiently acidic to be safe. However, assessment of survival of the microorganism in apple cider revealed that *E. coli* O157:H7 was unusually acid tolerant and could easily survive in cider having a pH lower than the value that was considered safe until then (pH 4.5) (Zhao et al., 1993). Investigators of the Massachusetts outbreak thought that the apples were probably contaminated before they were pressed, possibly in the orchard, which was visited by deer. The first control measures adopted by the industry were simply to wash and brush the apples before pressing them. Yet recurrent outbreaks of *E. coli* O157:H7 and *Cryptosporidium* infections occurred that were traced to cider made from apples that had been brushed and washed, which showed that even with cleansing of the apples, cider could be hazardous (CDC, 1997; Cody et al., 1999; Millard et al., 1994). It was also shown that *E. coli* O157:H7 could, under some circumstances, be internalized into apples and thus be protected from washing, brushing, or external disinfection (Buchanan et al., 1999; Burnett et al., 2000). The occurrence of outbreaks of *Salmonella* infections also attributed to fruit juices, as well as recent related research, has led to the promulgation of juice regulations requiring a pathogen-reduction step such as pasteurization (FDA, 2001). To date, no further commercial juice- or cider-associated outbreaks have been reported.

Salmonella Enteritidis and Shell Eggs

In the 1980s, dramatic outbreaks of *S.* Enteritidis infections were traced to Grade A shell eggs (St. Louis et al., 1988). This was surprising, as the egg grading and disinfection process instituted in the 1960s (as a result of egg-associated salmonellosis related to contamination of the outside of the shell by *Salmonella* in chicken feces) had appeared to be effective. It was suggested that the new problem might reflect internal contamination of eggs, possibly as a result of infection of the hen's reproductive tissues. Sporadic cases of *S.* Enteritidis infections were also increasing, first in the Northeast, and later over most of the country (CDC, 1993). It was possible to relate these cases to eggs and even to show a gradient of risk according to the degree of cooking, from hard-boiled and hard-cooked through over-easy, to soft-boiled and sunny-side-up (Hedberg et al., 1993; Passaro et al., 1996). The *Salmonella* strains in the birds on farms that were the source of contaminated eggs were the same as the strains found in the affected humans, confirming that the source of contamination was the birds themselves (Altekruse et al., 1993; Mishu et al., 1991). Experimental feeding of *Salmonella* to birds demonstrated that the birds developed silent ovarian infection and then laid normal-looking eggs that had contaminated contents (Gast, 1999).

In the early 1990s, a pilot project to develop flock-based screening and control measures was begun: the Pennsylvania Egg Quality Assurance Program (Schlosser et al., 1999). This project became the model for other states' egg quality assurance programs. The incidence of *S.* Enteritidis infections in mid-Atlantic states, for which Pennsylvania was the main egg source, began decreasing, followed later by decreases in other states (FDDB, 2000). Microbiological screening of farms for *S.* Enteritidis is an integral part of an egg quality assurance program, with voluntary diversion of the eggs to liquid egg pasteurization if they are found positive. Thus, many potentially tainted eggs are sent for safe processing before they enter the shell egg market. As the epidemic among egg-laying flocks spread from the Northeast to virtually the entire country, outbreak investigations and the attendant trace-backs demonstrated the spread of this problem into new areas and stimulated local authorities to develop their own quality assurance programs for *S.* Enteritidis in eggs and egg products (Burr et al., 1999; CDC, 1993).

A risk assessment was completed in 1998 (Baker et al., 1998). The sustained epidemic prompted further measures, such as the refrigeration requirement for eggs in 1998 and 2000 (FDA, 2000; FSIS, 1998b) and the commercialization of a new in-shell pasteurization process. Current control policies of egg-associated *S.* Enteritidis appear to be having an impact. By 2000, the incidence of *S.* Enteritidis had decreased to 2 per 100,000, down from the peak of nearly 4 per 100,000, although it remains above the pre-epidemic incidence of 1 per 100,000 (Figure 2.2). However, egg-associated outbreaks continue to occur (CDC, 2003). The surveillance data clearly show that progress is being made in slowing the *S.* Enteritidis problem in eggs, but further efforts are needed to completely control it.

Salmonella, E. coli O157:H7, and Alfalfa Sprouts

Like *S.* Enteritidis in eggs, the new food safety problem with alfalfa sprouts is not an emerging pathogen, but rather the emergence of well-known pathogens in a different food. In 1995, shortly after the statistical outbreak detection algorithm was developed for the *Salmonella* surveillance system, a large, 22-state outbreak of infections caused by a rare serotype, *S.* Stanley, was detected in the United States (Mahon et al., 1997). Simultaneously, public health officials in Finland identified an outbreak caused by the same organism. Both outbreaks were linked to the consumption of alfalfa sprouts, sprouted from the same batch of seeds (Mahon et al., 1997). Research showed that the sprouting process could greatly amplify the number of salmonellae originally present in the seed and that the pathogen could be inside the sprout, where it might not be affected by washing or disinfecting (Itoh et al., 1998; Jaquette et al., 1996). The next three years witnessed at least seven outbreaks in the United States, caused by several serotypes of *Salmonella* and *E. coli* O157:H7 in sprouts, often from contaminated seeds (Taormina et al., 1999). Japan experienced a devastating outbreak traced to radish sprouts that affected 6,000 school children (Michino et al., 1999; Watanabe et al., 1999). Alfalfa and other seeds for sprouting are produced as raw agricultural commodities and may be easily contaminated in the field or warehouse, where they may be held for years before being sprouted (Breuer et al., 2001).

After researchers determined that disinfecting seeds with 20,000 ppm calcium hypochlorite could reduce contamination and preserve the ability of seeds to germinate, FDA promulgated guidelines on seed disinfection (FDA, 1999), and the major seed distributors put these instructions on the seed packages. Since then, outbreaks of salmonellosis have been linked to a sprout producer that reported disinfecting the seeds following those guidelines (Proctor et al., 2000), as well as to a sprout producer using less chlorine than recommended (Winthrop et al., 2003). Another recent outbreak involved a single lot of clover seed shipped to two sprout producers in Colorado (Brooks et al., 2001). The first did not disinfect the seed before sprouting and caused 1.13 documented infections per 50 lb-bag of seed sprouted, whereas the second did disinfect the seeds and caused only 0.29 infections per bag of seed. These outbreaks show that the disinfection strategy works partially, but is by itself insufficient to completely protect the public. In addition to disinfection, FDA also recommended lot-by-lot testing of the irrigation water for *Salmonella* (FDA, 1999). One outbreak occurred that was linked to sprouts that had passed such a test, suggesting that false negative tests may occur (Winthrop et al., 2003). Continued surveillance and investigation indicate that the challenge of preventing outbreaks of salmonellosis from sprouts has been partially met, but complete prevention has still not been achieved.

Multidrug-Resistant *Salmonella* Newport and Foods of Bovine Origin

One of the latest food hazards to emerge in the United States is a new and highly resistant strain of *S.* Newport (Zansky et al., 2002). This strain was first identified through NARMS surveillance in 1998, and its detection increased rapidly in 1999 and 2000. The strain is resistant to at least nine antibiotics because it possesses a large plasmid bearing several resistance genes, including an unusual gene, the AmpC *cmy2* gene, which confers resistance to most cephalosporins. In 2001, a retrospective study of these strains in Massachusetts identified the same strains in ill and dying dairy cattle, and showed that visiting or working on dairy farms was a risk factor for illness (Gupta et al., 2001). Later that year, an outbreak in Connecticut was traced to traditional cheese made from insufficiently pasteurized milk from Massachusetts dairy farms (McCarthy et al., 2002). In 2002, an investigation of a multistate cluster of cases in the Northeast linked the illness to eating ground beef traced to meat from a single slaughter plant (Zansky et al., 2002). Surveillance of human infections indicates a sharp increase in *S.* Newport infections, which in 2001 represented 10 percent of human salmonellosis (FDDB, 2002c). Many of the *S.* Newport strains are multidrug resistant (CDC, 2002b). The same organism has been detected since 1998 among isolates from animals, including bovines (Fedorka-Cray et al., 2002). Among *S.* Newport isolated from cattle in 2000, 74 percent had the AmpC multidrug resistance profile (ARS, 2002). The evidence to date indicates that this strain has spread in epidemic fashion among cattle herds and that it affects the animals themselves, persons in contact with the animals, and consumers of bovine products (including meat, cheese, and other foods). Once control measures begin, success can be measured by monitoring animals and meat for this strain, by trends in human illness, and by outbreak surveillance. Surveillance activities in animals, meat, and poultry can also provide early warning of the spread of this strain or its plasmid to other food-animal populations.

ANTICIPATING THE FUTURE

In the future, it can be expected that new pathogens and new foodborne modes for transmission of such pathogens will continue to be recognized. New diagnostic strategies will identify some pathogens that currently are often or completely missed. Globalization of the food supply and concentration of food production, in turn, will create new challenges for detection, investigation, control, and prevention of microbial foodborne hazards.

The committee concludes that enhanced public health surveillance for human foodborne illnesses will be vital to identify and investigate these new challenges. In addition, it believes that a flexible monitoring system is needed that permits comparison of information from multiple points in the food supply. Just as monitoring individual cattle at slaughter is an important strategy for documenting the continuing absence of bovine spongiform encephalopathy, a system for documenting the frequency of microbial or other foodborne hazards at the point of slaughter or processing could be critical to assessing and controlling these hazards in the future. Systematic surveys of potential hazards, such as the appearance of antibiotic resistant microbial strains in live animals in production, already provide information useful to industry, regulators, and the public health sector. In the future, similar systematic surveys of microbial contamination in various categories of processing plants and at various points along processing lines could be equally useful for risk assessors. Preventing or minimizing contamination early in the chain, as well as identifying foods at higher risk of being contaminated so that they can be diverted out of the raw product market and into safer processing, may become the norm. For some foods, irradiation and other terminal microbial decontamination steps hold great potential (Tauxe, 2001). High-pressure processing, for example, is already commercially available. Preventing foodborne disease means preventing contamination before food reaches the consumer. Risk-management policies applied throughout the food system—on farms, fisheries, and orchards; in slaughter facilities and processing plants; during transportation and storage; and in retail food stores, food service establishments, and homes—are all key parts of food safety.

For certain products, it may be possible to define varying levels of processing depending on microbiological and other markers of the risk that they are contaminated. Already, eggs that are cracked or that come from farms contaminated with *S.* Enteritidis are routinely approved for marketing after pasteurization; milk for manufacturing purposes meets standards that are different from Grade A milk; and an occasional carcass is passed for cooking rather than being allowed to go through standard slaughter. In the future, such treatments of higher-risk food may be a useful tool for achieving pathogen reduction in other foods.

REFERENCES

Altekruse S, Koehler J, Hickman-Brenner F, Tauxe RV, Ferris K. 1993. A comparison of *Salmonella* Enteritidis phage types from egg-associated outbreaks and implicated laying flocks. *Epidemiol Infect* 110:17–22.

Angulo FJ, Swerdlow DL. 1999. Epidemiology of human *Salmonella enterica* serovar Enteritidis infections in the United States. In: Saeed AM, Gast RK, Potter ME, Wall PG, eds. Salmonella enterica *Serovar Enteritidis in Humans and Animals: The Epidemiology, Pathogenesis and Control*. Ames, IA: Iowa State University Press. Pp. 33–41.

AOAC (Association of Analytical Communities). 2002. A vision: The National Food Safety System and the three-legged stool. *Inside Laboratory Management* May/June:e7–e12. Online. Available at http://www.aoac.org/AOAC_e-CAM.pdf. Accessed January 19, 2003.

APHIS (Animal and Plant Health Inspection Service). 2000. *Highlights of Layers '99 Study Results*: Salmonella enterica *serotype Enteritidis*. Online. U.S. Department of Agriculture (USDA). Available at http://www.aphis.usda.gov/vs/ceah/cahm/Poultry/lay99SEhi.htm. Accessed September 11, 2002.

APHIS. 2002. *Bovine Spongiform Encephalopathy*. Online. USDA. Available at http://www.aphis.usda.gov/lpa.pubs/fsheet_faq_notice/fs_ahbse.html. Accessed December 5, 2002.

ARS (Agriculture Research Service). 2000. *National Antimicrobial Resistance Monitoring System (NARMS)—Animal Veterinary Isolate Data*. Online. USDA. Available at http://www.arru.saa.ars.usda.gov/narms/narms.htm. Accessed September 5, 2002.

ARS. 2002. *NARMS— EB 2000; Veterinary isolates. Figure 18. Resistance among Salmonella serotypes for isolates from cattle*. Online. USDA. Available at http://www.ars-grin.gov/ars/SoAtlantic/Athens/arru/narms_2000/2000_figure_18.pdf. Accessed September 11, 2002.

Avery SM, Small A, Reid CA, Buncic S. 2002. Pulsed-field gel electrophoresis characterization of Shigatoxin-producing *Escherichia coli* O157 from hides of cattle at slaughter. *J Food Prot* 65:1172–1176.

Baine WB, Zampieri A, Mazzotti M, Angioni G, Greco D, Di Gioia M, Izzo E, Gangarosa E, Pocchiari F. 1974. Epidemiology of cholera in Italy in 1973. *Lancet* 2:1370-1381.

Baker AR, Ebel ED, Hogue AT, McDowell RM, Morales RA, Schlosser WD, Whiting R. 1998. Salmonella *Enteritidis Risk Assessment: Shell Eggs and Egg Products*. Washington DC: Food Safety and Inspection Service, U.S. Department of Agriculture.

Barza M, Travers K. 2002. Excess infections due to antimicrobial resistance: The "attributable fraction." *Clin Infect Dis* 34:S126–S130.

Bean N, Griffin P. 1990. Foodborne disease outbreaks in the United States, 1973–1987: Pathogens, vehicles, and trends. *J Food Prot* 53:804–817.

Bean N, Martin S, Bradford H. 1992. PHLIS: An electronic system for reporting public health data from remote sites. *Am J Public Health* 82:1273–1276.

Bell BP, Goldoft M, Griffin PM, Davis MA, Gordon DC, Tarr PI, Bartleson CA, Lewis JH, Barrett TJ, Wells JG, Baron R, Kobayashi J. 1994. A multistate outbreak of *Escherichia coli* O157:H7—Associated bloody diarrhea and hemolytic uremic syndrome from hamburgers. The Washington experience. *JAMA* 1349–1353.

Bell BP, Shapiro CN, Alter MJ, Moyer LA, Judson FN, Mottram K, Fleenor M, Ryder PL, Margolis HS. 1998. The diverse patterns of hepatitis A epidemiology in the United States—Implications for vaccination strategies. *J Infect Dis* 178:1579–1584.

Bender JB, Hedberg CW, Besser JM, Boxrud DJ, MacDonald KL, Osterholm MT. 1997. Surveillance for *Escherichia coli* O157:H7 infections in Minnesota by molecular subtyping. *N Engl J Med* 337:388–394.

Bender JB, Hedberg CW, Boxrud DJ, Besser JM, Wicklund JH, Smith KE, Osterholm MT. 2001. Use of molecular subtyping in surveillance for *Salmonella enterica* serotype Typhimurium. *N Engl J Med* 344:189–195.

Bender J, Smith K, McNees A, Rabafsky-Ehr T, Segler S, Hawkins M, Spina N, Keene W, VanGilder T, Kennedy M, Hedberg C. In press. Surveillance for *E. coli* O157:H7 infection in FoodNet sites, 1996–1999. *Clin Infect Dis*.

Berry BW, Lyon BG, Soderberg DL, Philipo T, Bakowski R, Henry C, Dreas J, Powell S, Agmata E, Yee C, Clinch N, Vanlonkhuyzen D. 1998. *Visual and Instrumental Evaluations of Color in Beef Patties Obtained Nationwide and Cooked to Four Internal Temperatures*. Presented at the Reciprocal Meats Conference, American Meat Science Association, Indianapolis, IN, July 24–28.

Besser RE, Lett SM, Weber JT, Doyle MP, Barrett TJ, Wells JG, Griffin PM. 1993. An outbreak of diarrhea and hemolytic uremic syndrome from *Escherichia coli* O157:H7 in fresh-pressed apple cider. *JAMA* 269:2217–2220.

Blake PA, Merson MH, Weaver RE, Hollis DG, Heublein PC. 1979. Disease caused by a marine vibrio. Clinical characteristics and epidemiology. *N Engl J Med* 300:1–5.

Blaser MJ, Newman LS. 1982. A review of human salmonellosis. I. Infective dose. *Rev Infect Dis* 4:1096–1106.

Blaser MJ, Cravens J, Powers BW, Laforce FM, Wang WL. 1979. *Campylobacter* enteritis associated with unpasteurized milk. *Am J Med* 67:715–718.

Bresee JB, Widdowson M-A, Monroe SS, Glass RI. 2002. Foodborne viral gastroenteritis: Challenges and opportunities. *Clin Infect Dis* 35:748–753.

Breuer T, Benkel DH, Shapiro RR, Hall WN, Winnett MM, Linn MJ, Neimann J, Barrett TJ, Dietrich S, Downes FP, Toney DM, Pearson JL, Rolkalt H, Slutsker L, Griffin PM. 2001. A multistate outbreak of *Escherichia coli* O157:H7 infections linked to alfalfa sprouts grown from contaminated seeds. *Emerg Infect Dis* 7:977–982.

Brooks JT, Rowe SV, Shillam P, Heltzel DM, Hunter SB, Slutsker L, Hoekstra RM, Luby SP. 2001. *Salmonella* Typhimurium infections transmitted by chlorine-pretreated clover sprout seeds. *Am J Epidemiol* 154:1020–1028.

Buchanan RL, Edelson SG, Miller RL, Sapers GM. 1999. Contamination of intact apples after immersion in an aqueous environment containing *Escherichia coli* O157:H7. *J Food Prot* 62:444–450.

Burnett SL, Chen J, Beuchat LR. 2000. Attachment of *Escherichia coli* O157:H7 to the surfaces and internal structures of apples as detected by confocal scanning laser microscopy. *Appl Environ Microbiol* 66:4679–4687.

Burr R, Effler P, Kahana J, Kanenaka R, Balmer M, Angulo F, Barrett T, Hayes P, Nekomoto T, Nakata M, Sasaki D, Higa H, Sawa T, Choy B. 1999. *Emergence of* Salmonella *Serotype Enteritidis Phage Type 4 in Hawaii Caused by Locally Produced Contaminated Eggs*. Abstract presented at the 48th Annual Epidemic Intelligence Service Conference, Centers for Disease Control and Prevention (CDC), Atlanta, GA, April 19–23.

Buzby JC, Roberts T. 1996. ERS updates U.S. foodborne disease costs for seven pathogens. *Food Review* 19:20–25

CDC (Centers for Disease Control and Prevention). 1981. Multiple outbreaks of salmonellosis associated with precooked roast beef—Pennsylvania, New York, Vermont. *Morb Mortal Wkly Rep* 30:569–570.

CDC. 1993. Outbreaks of *Salmonella Enteritidis* gastroenteritis—California, 1993. *Morb Mortal Wkly Rep* 42:793–797.

CDC. 1997. Outbreaks of *Escherichia coli* O157:H7 and cryptosporidiosis associated with drinking unpasteurized apple cider—Connecticut and New York, October 1996. *Morb Mortal Wkly Rep* 46:4–8.

CDC. 1998. Update: Multistate outbreak of listeriosis—United States, 1998. *Morb Mortal Wkly Rep* 47:1085–1086.

CDC. 2001. Updated guidelines for evaluating public health surveillance systems: Recommendations from the Guidelines Working Group. *Morb Mortal Wkly Rep* 50:2–35.

CDC. 2002a. Preliminary FoodNet data on the incidence of foodborne illnesses—Selected sites, United States, 2001. *Morb Mortal Wkly Rep* 51:325–329.

CDC. 2002b. *2000 Annual Report. NARMS. National Antimicrobial Resistance Monitoring System: Enteric Bacteria*. Online. Available at http://www.cdc.gov/narms/annual/2000/NARMS_final_report_2000.pdf. Accessed April 15, 2003.

CDC. 2003. Outbreaks of *Salmonella* serotype Enteritidis infection associated with eating shell eggs—United States, 1999–2000. *Morb Mortal Wkly Rep* 51:1149–1152.

CFSAN (Center for Food Safety and Applied Nutrition). 2001. *Survey of Domestic Fresh Produce: Interim Results (July 31, 2001)*. Online. Food and Drug Administration (FDA). Available at http://www.cfsan.fda.gov/~dms/prodsur9.html. Accessed September 3, 2002.

CFSAN. 2002. *FDA Pesticide Program: Residue Monitoring, 1993–2001*. Online. FDA. Available at http://www.cfsan.fda.gov/~dms/pesrpts.html. Accessed January 22, 2003.

Cody SH, Glynn KM, Farrar JA, Cairns KL, Griffin PM, Kobayashi J, Fyfe M, Hoffman R, King AS, Lewis JH, Swaminathan B, Bryant RG, Vugia DJ. 1999. An outbreak of *Escherichia coli* O157:H7 infection from unpasteurized commercial apple juice. *Ann Intern Med* 130:202–209.

Consumer Studies Branch. 2002. *Food Safety Survey: Summary of Major Trends in Food Handling Practices and Consumption of Potentially Risky Foods*. Online. CFSAN, FDA. Available at http://www.cfsan.fda.gov/~dms/fssurvey.html. Accessed September 23, 2002.

Crump JA, Griffin PM, Angulo FJ. 2002. Bacterial contamination of animal feed and its relationship to human foodborne illness. *Clin Infect Dis* 35:859–65.

Dalton C, Mintz E, Wells J, Bopp C, Tauxe R. 1999. Outbreaks of enterotoxigenic *Escherichia coli* infection in American adults: A clinical and epidemiologic profile. *Epidemiol Infect* 123:9–16.

Daniels NA, MacKinnon L, Bishop R, Altekruse S, Ray B, Hammond RM, Thompson S, Wilson S, Bean NH, Griffin PM, Slutsker L. 2000. *Vibrio parahaemolyticus* infections in the United States, 1973–1998. *J Infect Dis* 181:1661–1666.

Deming MS, Tauxe RV, Blake PA, Patton C, Dixon SE, Fowler BS, Jones TS, Lockamy EA, Patton CM, Sikes RO. 1987. *Campylobacter* enteritis at a university: Transmission from eating chicken and from cats. *Am J Epidemiol* 126:526–534.

Doyle MP, Beuchat LR, Montville TJ. 2001. *Food Microbiology: Fundamentals and Frontiers*, 2nd ed. Washington, DC: American Society for Microbiology Press.

FDA (Food and Drug Administration). 1999. Guidance for industry: Reducing microbial food safety hazards for sprouted seeds and Guidance for industry: Sampling and microbial testing of spent irrigation water during sprout production. *Fed Reg* 64:57893–57902.

FDA. 2000. Food labeling, safe handling statements, labeling of shell eggs; Refrigeration of shell eggs held for retail distribution; Final rule. *Fed Reg* 65:76091–76114.

FDA. 2001. *FDA Publishes Final Rule to Increase Safety of Fruit and Vegetable Juices*. Online. Available at http://www.fda.gov/bbs/topics/NEWS/2001/NEW00749.html. Accessed September 9, 2002.

FDDB (Foodborne and Diarrheal Diseases Branch). 2000. *FoodNet Surveillance Report for 1999 (Final Report)*. Online. Division of Bacterial and Mycotic Diseases (DBMD), CDC. Available at http://www.cdc.gov/foodnet/annual/1999/pdf/FoodNet__1999_Annual_Report.pdf. Accessed September 11, 2002.

FDDB. 2002a. *Foodborne-Disease Outbreaks Reported to CDC January 1, 1990 through March 15, 2002*. Online. DBMD, CDC. Available at http://www.cdc.gov/foodborneoutbreaks/outbreak_satistics/cdc_reported.htm. Accessed October 20, 2002.

FDDB. 2002b. *FoodNet Data Sources. Population Survey*. Online. DBMD, CDC. Available at http://www.cdc.gov/foodnet/surveys/pop_cov.htm. Accessed September 11, 2002.

FDDB. 2002c. Salmonella: *Annual Summary, 2001*. Online. DBMD, CDC. Available at http://www.cdc.gov/ncidod/dbmd/phlisdata/salmtab/2001/SalmonellaAnnualSummary2001.pdf. Accessed September 11, 2002.

Fedorka-Cray PWF, Gray T, Hermosilla J, Ball T, Anandaraman M, Salamone B, Rose B, Dargatz D, Headrick M. 2002. Prevalence and resistance of *Salmonella enterica* serotype Newport 1997–2000: A NARMS Report. In: *Proceedings of the National Conference on Antimicrobial Resistance*. Bethesda, MD: National Foundation for Infectious Disease.

Fontaine RE, Arnon S, Martin WT, Vernon TM Jr, Gangarosa EJ, Farmer JJ 3rd, Moran JB, Silliker JH, Decker DL. 1978. Raw hamburger: An interstate common source of human salmonellosis. *Am J Epidemiol* 107:36–45.

Friedman CR, Neimann J, Wegener HC, Tauxe RV. 2000a. Epidemiology of *Campylobacter jejuni* infections in the United States and other industrialized nations. In: Nachamkin IJ, Blaser MJ, eds. *Campylobacter,* 2nd ed. Washington, DC: American Society for Microbiology. Pp. 121–138.

Friedman C, Reddy S, Samual M, Marcaus R, Bender J, Desai S, Shiferaw B, Helfrick D, Carter M, Anderson B, Hoekstra M, The EIP FoodNet Working Group. 2000b. *Risk Factors for Sporadic Campylobacter Infections in the United States: A Case-Control Study on FoodNet Sites*. Presented at the International Conference on Emerging Infectious Diseases, CDC, Atlanta, GA, July 16–19.

FSIS (Food Safety and Inspection Service). 1998a. *An FSIS/ARS Study: Premature Browning of Cooked Ground Beef.* Online. USDA. Available at http://www.fsis.usda.gov/OPHS/prebrown.htm. Accessed September 11, 2002.

FSIS. 1998b. Refrigeration and labeling requirements for shell eggs. Final rule. *Fed Reg* 63:45663–45675.

FSIS. 1998c. *Report to Congress. FoodNet: An Active Surveillance System for Bacterial Foodborne Diseases in the United States*. Online. USDA. Available at http://www.fsis.usda.gov/OPHS/rpcong98/rpcong98.htm. Accessed April 10, 2003.

FSIS. 2000. *Color of Cooked Ground Beef as it Relates to Doneness.* Online. USDA. Available at http://www.fsis.usda.gov/OA/pubs/colortech.htm. Accessed September 10, 2002.

FSIS. 2003. *Microbiological Results of Raw Ground Beef Products Analyzed for Escherichia coli O157:H7, Calendar Year 2003.* Online. USDA. Available at http://www.fsis.usda.gov/OPHS/ecoltest/ecpositives.htm. Accessed March 7, 2003.

FSIS/CFSAN. 2001. *Draft Assessment of the Relative Risk to Public Health from Foodborne Listeria monocytogenes Among Selected Categories of Ready-to-Eat Foods.* Online. USDA, FDA. Available at http://www.foodsafety.gov/~dms/lmrisk.html. Accessed September 9, 2002.

Garman R, Jones T, Bulens S, Tong S, Myers R, Gettner S, Mead P, Parashar U, EIP FoodNet Working Group. 2002. *A Pilot Study in FoodNet of the use of Stool Collection Kits Delivered to the Home to Improve Confirmation of Etiology in Gastroenteritis Outbreak Investigations.* Presented at the International Conference on Emerging Infectious Diseases, CDC, Atlanta, GA, March 24–27.

Gast R. 1999. Applying experimental infection models to understand the pathogenesis, detection and control of *Salmonella enterica* serovar Enteritidis in poultry. In: Saeed AM, Gast RK, Potter ME, Wall PG, eds. Salmonella enterica *Serovar Enteritidis in Humans and Animals: The Epidemiology, Pathogenesis and Control.* Ames, IA: Iowa State University Press. Pp. 233–243.

Gitelson S. 1971. Gastrectomy, achlorhydria, and cholera. *Isr J Med Sci* 7:663–667.

Griffin P, Mead P, Sivapalasingam S. 2002. *Escherichia coli* O157:H7 and other enterohemorrhagic *E. coli*. In: Blaser MJ, Smith PD, Ravdin JI, Greenberg H, Guerrant RL, eds. *Infections of the Gastrointestinal Tract*, 2nd ed. Philadelphia: Lippincott Williams and Wilkins. Pp. 627–642.

Guerrant RL, Steiner TS. 1999. Principles and syndromes of enteric infection. In: Mardell G, Bennet J, Dolin R, eds. *Principles and Practice of Infection Diseases*, 4th ed. Kent, UK: Churchill, Livingstone. Pp. 1076–1093.

Guerrant RL, Theno DM. 1995. *Escherichia coli* O157:H7. *N Engl J Med* 333:1711–1712.

Guerrant RL, Hughes JM, Lima NL, Crane J. 1990. Diarrhea in developed and developing countries: Magnitude, special settings, and etiologies. *Rev Infect Dis* 12: S41–S50.

Guerrant RL, Kosek M, Lima AA, Lorntz B, Guyatt HL. 2002. Updating the DALYs for diarrhoeal disease. *Trends Parasitol* 18:191–193.

Gupta A, Crowe C, Bolstorff B, Fontana J, Stout A, Montgomery S, McGuill M, Matayas B, Schoenfeld S, Angulo F. 2001. Multistate investigation of multi-drug resistant *Salmonella* serotype Newport infections in the Northeastern U.S., 2000: Human infections associated with dairy farms. In: *Proceedings of the Annual Meeting of the Infectious Disease Society of America.* Alexandria, VA: Infectious Disease Society of America. P. 36.

Hald T. 2001. Salmonella *in Pork—Epidemiology, Control and the Public Health Impact. Manuscript 3: Quantifying the Contribution of Animal-Food Sources to Human Salmonellosis in Denmark in 1999*. PhD Thesis. Copenhagen, Denmark: Royal Veterinary and Agricultural University.

Hald T, Bronsted T. 2002. *Annual Report on Zoonoses in Denmark, 2001*. Copenhagen: Ministry of Food, Agriculture and Fisheries.

Hall JA, Goulding JS, Bean NH, Tauxe RV, Hedberg CW. 2001. Epidemiologic profiling: Evaluating foodborne outbreaks for which no pathogen was isolated by routine laboratory testing: United States, 1982–9. *Epidemiol Infect* 127:381–387.

Hedberg CW, David MJ, White KE, MacDonald KL, Osterholm MT. 1993. Role of egg consumption in sporadic *Salmonella* Enteritidis and *Salmonella* Typhimurium infections in Minnesota. *J Infect Dis* 167:107–111.

Helms M, Vastrup P, Gerner-Smidt P, Molbak K. 2002. Excess mortality associated with antimicrobial drug-resistant *Salmonella* Typhimurium. *Emerg Infect Dis* 8:490–495.

Hennessy TW, Hedberg CW, Slutsker L, White KE, Besser-Wiek JM, Moen ME, Feldman J, Coleman WW, Edmonson LM, MacDonald KL, Osterholm MT. 1996. A national outbreak of *Salmonella* Enteritidis infections from ice cream. *N Engl J Med* 334:1281–1286.

Herikstad H, Motarjemi J, Tauxe RV. 2002a. *Salmonella* surveillance: A global survey of public health serotyping. *Epidemiol Infect* 129:1–8.

Herikstad H, Yang S, Van Gilder TJ, Vugia D, Hadler J, Blake P, Deneen V, Shiferaw B, Angulo FJ. 2002b. A population-based estimate of the burden of diarrhoeal illness in the United States: FoodNet, 1996–1997. *Epidemiol Infect* 129:9–17.

HHS (U.S. Department of Health and Human Services). 2000. *Healthy People 2010*. Vol.1. 2nd Ed. Washington, DC: U.S. Government Printing Office.

Holmberg SD, Feldman RA. 1984. New and newer enteric pathogens: Stages in our knowledge. *Am J Public Health* 74:205–207.

Hopkins RS, Scott AB. 1983. Handling raw chickens as a source for sporadic *Campylobacter jejuni* infections. *J Infect Dis* 148:770.

Hornick RB, Music SI, Wenzel R, Cash R, Libonati JP, Snyder MJ, Woodward TE. 1971. The Broad Street pump revisited: Response of volunteers to ingested cholera vibrios. *Bull NY Acad Med* 47:1181–1191.

Humphrey TJ, Williams A, McAlpine K, Lever MS, Guard-Petter J, Cox JM. 1996. Isolates of *Salmonella enterica* Enteritidis PT4 with enhanced heat and acid tolerance are more virulent in mice and more invasive in chickens. *Epidemiol Infect* 117:78–88.

Hunt MC, Soerheim O, Slinde E. 1999. Color and heat denaturation of myoglobin forms in ground beef. *J Food Sci* 64:847–851.

Hurd HS, McKean JD, Wesley IV, Karriker LA. 2001. The effect of lairage on *Salmonella* isolation from market swine. *J Food Prot* 64:939–944.

Hutwagner LC, Maloney EK, Bean NH, Slutsker L, Martin SM. 1997. Using laboratory-based surveillance data for prevention: An algorithm for detecting *Salmonella* outbreaks. *Emerg Infect Dis* 3:395–400.

IOM/NRC (Institute of Medicine/National Research Council). 1998. *Ensuring Safe Food from Production to Consumption*. Washington, DC: National Academy Press.

Itoh Y, Sugita-Konishi Y, Kusuga F, Iwaki M, Hara-Kudo Y, Saito N, Noguchi Y, Konuma H, Kumagai S. 1998. Enterohemorrhagic *Escherichia coli* O157:H7 present in radish sprouts. *Appl Environ Microbiol* 4:1532–1535.

Jaquette C, Beuchat L, Mahon BE. 1996. Efficacy of chlorine and heat treatment in killing *Salmonella* Stanley inoculated onto alfalfa seeds and growth and survival of the pathogen during sprouting and storage. *Appl Environ Microbiol* 62:2212–2215.

Jones T, Imhoff B, Deneen V, Samuel M, Mshar R, Gibbs-McCombs K, Kamer T, Cambridge M, Slutsker L, EIP FoodNet Working Group. 2000. *Limitations of Field Investigations: Etiology and Food Vehicle not Determined for a Substantial Proportion of Foodborne Outbreaks in FoodNet, 1998–1999*. Presented at the 2nd International Conference on Emerging Infectious Diseases, CDC, Atlanta, GA, July 16–19.

Kassenborg H, Hedberg C, Evans M, Chin G, Fiorentino T, Vugia D, Bardsley M, Slutsker L, Griffin P. 1998. Case-control study of sporadic *Escherichia coli* O157:H7 infections in 5 FoodNet sites. In: *Proceedings of the International Conference on Emerging Infectious Diseases*. Atlanta, GA: CDC. P.50.

Killinger KM, Hunt MC, Campbell RE, Kropf DH. 2000. Factors affecting premature browning during cooking of store-purchased ground beef. *J Food Sci* 65:585–587.

Kohn MA, Farley TA, Ando T, Curtis M, Wilson SA, Jin Q, Monroe SS, Baron RC, McFarland LM, Glass RI. 1995. An outbreak of Norwalk virus gastroenteritis associated with eating raw oysters: Implications for maintaining safe oyster beds. *JAMA* 273:466–471

Lee LA, Gerber AR, Longsway DR, Smith JD, Carter GP, Puhr ND, Parrish CM, Sikes RK, Finton RJ, Tauxe RV. 1990. *Yersinia enterocolitica* O:3 infections in infants and children, associated with the household preparation of chitterlings. *N Engl J Med* 322:984–987.

Lumsden L, Hasseltine H, JP L, Veldee M. 1925. A typhoid fever epidemic caused by oyster-borne infections (1924–1925). *Public Health Rep* 50:1–102.

Mahon BE, Ponka A, Hall WN, Komatsu K, Dietrich SE, Siitonen A, Cage G, Hayes PS, Lambert-Fair MA, Bean NH, Griffin PM, Slutsker L. 1997. An international outbreak of *Salmonella* infections caused by alfalfa sprouts grown from contaminated seeds. *J Infect Dis* 175:876–882.

Marano NN, Rossiter S, Stamey K, Joyce K, Barrett TJ, Tollefson LK, Angulo FJ. 2000. The National Antimicrobial Resistance Monitoring System (NARMS) for enteric bacteria, 1996–1999: Surveillance for action. *J Am Vet Med Assoc* 217:1829–1830.

Martin ML, Shipman LD, Wells JG, Potter ME, Hedberg K, Wachsmuth IK, Tauxe RV, Davis JP, Arnoldi J, Tilleli J. 1986. Isolation of *Escherichia coli* O157:H7 from dairy cattle associated with two cases of haemolytic uraemic syndrome. *Lancet* 2:1043.

McCarthy T, Phan Q, Mshar P, Mshar R, Howard R, Hadler J. 2002. *Outbreak of Multi-Drug-Resistant* Salmonella *Newport Associated with Consumption of Italian-Style Soft Cheese, Connecticut*. Presented at the International Conference on Emerging Infectious Diseases, CDC, Atlanta, GA, May 24–27.

Mead PS, Mintz ED. 1996. Ethnic eating: Foodborne disease in the global village. *Infect Dis Clin Pract* 5:319–323.

Mead PS, Finelli L, Lambert-Fair MA, Champ D, Townes J, Hutwagner L, Barrett T, Spitalny K, Mintz E. 1997. Risk factors for sporadic infection with *Escherichia coli* O157:H7. *Arch Intern Med* 157:204–208.

Mead PS, Slutsker L, Dietz V, McCaig LF, Bresee JS, Shapiro C, Griffin PM, Tauxe RV. 1999. Food-related illness and death in the United States. *Emerg Infect Dis* 5:607–625.

Mead P, Slutsker L, Gellin B. 2002. Listeriosis. In: Blaser M, Smith P, Ravdin J, Greenberg H, Guerrant R, eds. *Infections of the Gastrointestinal Tract*, 2nd ed. Philadelphia: Lippincott Williams & Wilkins. Pp. 802–811.

Mentzing LO, Ringertz O. 1968. *Salmonella* infection in tourists. 2. Prophylaxis against salmonellosis. *Acta Pathol Microbiol Scand* 74:405–413.

Michino H, Araki K, Minami S, Takaya S, Sakai N, Miyazaki M, Ono A, Yanagawa H. 1999. Massive outbreak of *Escherichia coli* O157:H7 infection in schoolchildren in Sakai City, Japan, associated with consumption of white radish sprouts. *Am J Epidemiol* 150:787–796.

Millard PS, Gensheimer KF, Addiss DG, Sosin DM, Beckett GA, Houck-Jankoski A, Hudson A. 1994. An outbreak of cryptosporidiosis from fresh-pressed apple cider. *JAMA* 272:1592–1596.

Mishu B, Griffin PM, Tauxe RV, Cameron DN, Hutcheson RH, Schaffner W. 1991. *Salmonella Enteritidis* gastroenteritis transmitted by intact chicken eggs. *Ann Intern Med* 115:190–194.

Murray C, Lopez A. 1997. *The Global Burden of Disease: A Comprehensive Assessment of Mortality and Disability from Diseases, Injuries, and Risk Factors in 1900 and Projected to 2020.* Cambridge, MA: Harvard University Press.

Nachamkin I, Allos B, Ho T. 2000. *Campylobacter jejuni* infection and the association with Guillain-Barré syndrome. In: Nachamkin I, Blaser M, eds. *Campylobacter*, 2nd ed. Washington, DC: ASM Press. Pp. 155–175.

NRC (National Research Council). 1985. *Meat and Poultry Inspection: The Scientific Basis of the Nation's Program.* Washington, DC: National Academy Press.

Navin T, Juranek D. 1984. Cryptosporidiosis: Clinical, epidemiologic, and parasitologic review. *Rev Infect Dis* 6:313–327.

Norwegian Zoonosis Centre. 2002. *Action plan—*Campylobacter *spp. in Norwegian broilers. Summary of results from the surveillance of broiler flocks 2001; Survey of broiler meat products 2001.* Available at http://www.vetinst.no/Zoonosesenteret/Camp_handlingsplan2002.pdf. Accessed September 11, 2002.

Olsen SJ, MacKinnon LC, Goulding JJ, Bean NH, Slutsker L. 2000. Surveillance for foodborne disease outbreaks—United States, 1993–1997. *Morb Mortal Wkly Rep* 49:1–62.

Olsen SJ, Bishop R, Brenner FW, Roels TH, Bean N, Tauxe RV, Slutsker L. 2001. The changing epidemiology of *Salmonella*: Trends in serotypes isolated from humans in the United States, 1987–1997. *J Infect Dis* 183:753–761.

OPDFB (Office of Plant and Dairy Foods and Beverages). 2001. *FDA Survey of Imported Fresh Produce: FY 1999 Field Assignment.* Online. CFSAN, FDA. Available at http://www.cfsan.fda.gov/~dms/prodsur6.html. Accessed September 3, 2002.

Parashar UD, Monroe SS. 2001. "Norwalk-like viruses" as a cause of foodborne disease outbreaks. *Rev Med Virol* 11:243–252.

Parham G. 1984. *Salmonellae* in cooked meat products. In: Snoeyenbos G, ed. *Proceedings of an International Symposium on* Salmonella. Kennett Square, PA: University of Pennsylvania. Pp. 275–280.

Passaro DJ, Reporter R, Mascola L, Kilmon L, Malcolm GB, Rolka H, Werner SB, Vugia DJ. 1996. Epidemic *Salmonella* Enteritidis infections in Los Angeles County, California. The predominance of phage type 4. *West J Med* 165:126–130.

Potter M, Archer D, Benson A, Busta F, Dickson J, Doyle M, Farber J, Finlay BB, Goldblatt M, Hedberg C, Hoober D, Jahncke M, Jaykus L-A, Kaspar C, Liang AP, Lindsay J, Pestka J, Pierson M, Slade P, Tompkin RB, Tortorello ML. 2000. *Emerging Microbiological Food Safety Issues: Implications for Control in the 21st Century.* Chicago: Institute of Food Technology.

Proctor M, Hamacher M, Tortorello M, Archer J, Barnett M, Ying M, Slutsker L, Davis J. 2000. Multistate outbreak of *Salmonella* Muenchen infections associated with alfalfa sprouts grown from seeds pretreated with calcium hypochlorite. In: *Proceedings of the 2nd International Conference on Emerging Infectious Diseases.* Atlanta, GA: CDC. P. 98.

Redmond E, Griffith C, Slader J, Humphrey T. 2002. Assessment of risks associated with consumer food handling practices using real-time microbiological analysis. In: *Proceedings of the Annual Conference of the International Association for Food Protection.* Des Moines, IA: International Association for Food Protection. P. 67.

Riley LW, Remis RS, Helgerson SD, McGee HB, Wells JG, Davis BR, Hebert RJ, Olcott ES, Johnson LM, Hargrett NT, Blake PA, Cohen ML. 1983. Hemorrhagic colitis associated with a rare *Escherichia coli* serotype. *N Engl J Med* 308:681–685.

Rose BE, Hill WE, Umholtz R, Ransom GM, James WO. 2002. Testing for *Salmonella* in raw meat and poultry products collected at federally inspected establishments in the United States, 1998 through 2000. *J Food Prot* 65:937–947.

Rosenberg C. 1987. *The Cholera Years: The United States in 1832, 1849, and 1866.* Chicago: University of Chicago Press.

RTI (Research Triangle Institute). 2002a. *PR/HACCP Rule Evaluation Report. Changes in Consumer Knowledge, Behavior and Confidence since the 1996 PR/HACCP Final Rule. Final Report.* Online. FSIS, USDA. Available at http://www.fsis.usda.gov/oa/research/HACCPimpacts.htm. Accessed September 23, 2002.

RTI. 2002b. *Revised Final Draft: PR/HACCP Rule Evaluation Report. Effect of the 1996 PR/HACCP Rule on Foodborne Illness: Young Chicken Salmonella Study.* Research Triangle Park, NC: RTI.

Ryan CA, Nickels MK, Hargrett-Bean NT, Potter ME, Endo T, Mayer L, Langkop CW, Gibson C, McDonald RC, Kenney RT, Purh ND, McDonnell PJ, Martin RJ, Cohen ML, Blake PA. 1987. Massive outbreak of antimicrobial-resistant salmonellosis traced to pasteurized milk. *JAMA* 258:3269–3274.

Samuel MC, Portnoy D, Tauxe RV, Angulo FJ, Vugia DJ. 2001. Complaints of foodborne illness in San Francisco, California, 1998. *J Food Prot* 64:1261–1264.

Schlosser W, Henzler D, Mason J, Kradel D, Shipman L, Trock S, Hurd S, Hogue A, Sischo W, Ebel E. 1999. The *Salmonella enterica* serovar Enteritidis pilot project. In: Saeed AM, Gast RK, Potter ME, Wall PG, eds. Salmonella enterica *Serovar Enteritidis in Humans and Animals: The Epidemiology, Pathogenesis and Control.* Ames, IA: Iowa State University Press. Pp. 353–365.

Shane SM. 2000. *Campylobacter* infection of commercial poultry. *Rev Sci Tech Off Int Epizoot* 19:376–295.

Sivapalasingam S, Kimura A, Ying M, Frisch A, Barrett E, Phan Q, Shillam P, Reddy S, Breslowsky T, Gould E, Van Duyne MS, Slutsker L. 2000. *A Multistate Outbreak of* Salmonella *Newport Infections Linked to Mango Consumption, November–December 1999.* Abstract presented at the 38th Annual Meeting of the Infectious Diseases Society of America, New Orleans, LA, September 7–10.

Slutsker L, Ries AA, Maloney K, Wells JG, Greene KD, Griffin PM. 1998. A nationwide case-control study of *Escherichia coli* O157:H7 infection in the United States. *J Infect Dis* 177:962–966.

Sperber SJ, Schleupner CJ. 1987. Salmonellosis during infection with human immunodeficiency virus. *Rev Infect Dis* 9:925–934.

St. Louis ME, Morse DL, Potter ME, DeMelfi TM, Guzewich JJ, Tauxe RV, Blake PA. 1988. The emergence of grade A eggs as a major source of *Salmonella* Enteritidis infections: Implications for the control of salmonellosis. *JAMA* 259:2103–2107.

Swaminathan B, Barrett TJ, Hunter SB, Tauxe RV. 2001. PulseNet: The molecular subtyping network for foodborne bacterial disease surveillance, United States. *Emerg Infect Dis* 7:382–389.

Taormina PJ, Beuchat LR, Slutsker L. 1999. Infections associated with eating seed sprouts: An international concern. *Emerg Infect Dis* 5:626–634.

Tauxe RV. 1997. Emerging foodborne diseases: An evolving public health challenge. *Emerg Infect Dis* 3:425–434.

Tauxe RV. 2001. Food safety and irradiation: Protecting the public health from foodborne infections. *Emerg Infect Dis* 7:516–521.

Tauxe RV, Vandepitte J, Wauters G, Martin SM, Goossens V, De Mol P, Van Noyen R, Thiers G. 1987. *Yersinia enterocolitica* infections and pork: The missing link. *Lancet* 1:1129–1132.

Thacker SB. 1994. Historical development. In: Teutsch S, Churchill R, eds. *Principles and Practice of Public Health Surveillance*. New York: Oxford University Press. Pp. 3–17.

Thacker SB, Berkelman RL. 1988. Public health surveillance in the United States. *Epidemiol Rev* 10:164–190.

Voetsch D, Angulo F, Shallow S, Marcus R, Farley M, Hedberg C, Cieslak P, Tauxe R, FoodNet Working Group. 1998. *Estimate of the Burden of Illness Caused by Nontyphoidal Salmonella Infections in the United States from FoodNet*. Presented at the American Public Health Association 126th Annual Meeting Exposition, Washington DC, November 15–19.

Vogt RL, Sours HE, Barrett T, Feldman RA, Dickinson RJ, Witherell L. 1982. *Campylobacter* enteritis associated with contaminated water. *Ann Intern Med* 96:292–296.

Watanabe Y, Ozasa K, Mermin JH, Griffin PM, Masuda K, Imashuku S, Sawada T. 1999. Factory outbreak of *Escherichia coli* O157:H7 infection in Japan. *Emerg Infect Dis* 5:424–428.

Wells JG, Shipman LD, Greene KD, Sowers EG, Green JH, Cameron DN, Downes FP, Martin ML, Griffin PM, Ostroff SM, Potter ME, Tauxe RV, Wachsmuth IK. 1991. Isolation of *Escherichia coli* serotype O157:H7 and other Shiga-like-toxin-producing *E. coli* from dairy cattle. *J Clin Microbiol* 29:985–989.

WHO (World Health Organization). 2000. *The Increasing Incidence of Human Campylobacteriosis. Report and Proceedings of a WHO Consultation of Experts*. Online. Available at: http://www.who.int/emc-documents/zoonoses/docs/whocdscsraph20017.pdf. Accessed April 11, 2003.

WHO. 2002. *Global Salm-Surv*. Online. Available at http://www.who.int/emc/diseases/zoo/SALM-SURV/index.html. Accessed September 9, 2002.

Wineland NE, Dargatz DA. 1998. The national animal health monitoring system: A source of on-farm information. *Vet Clin North Am Food Anim Pract* 14:127–139.

Winthrop KL, Palumbo MS, Farrar JA, Mohle-Boetani JC, Abbott S, Beatty ME, Inami G, Werner SB. 2003. P101 Alfalfa sprouts and *Salmonella* Kottbus infection: A multistate outbreak following inadequate seed disinfection with heat and chlorine. *J Food Prot* 66:13–17.

Yang S, Leff MG, McTague D, Horvath KA, Jackson-Thompson J, Murayi T, Boeselager GK, Melnik TA, Gildemaster MC, Ridings DL, Altekruse SF, Angulo FJ. 1998. Multistate surveillance for food-handling, preparation, and consumption behaviors associated with foodborne diseases: 1995 and 1996 BRFSS food-safety questions. *Morb Mortal Wkly Rep* 47:33–57.

Zansky S, Wallace B, Schoonmaker-Bopp D, Smith P, Ramsey F, Painter J, Gupta A, Kalluri P, Noviello S. 2002. Outbreak of multidrug-resistant *Salmonella* Newport—United States, January–April 2002. *Morb Mortal Wkly Rep* 51:545–548.

Zhao T, Doyle MP, Besser RE. 1993. Fate of enterohemorrhagic *Escherichia coli* O157:H7 in apple cider with and without preservatives. *Appl Environ Microbiol* 59:2526–2530.

3

Food Safety Tools

This chapter describes some of the major modern tools available to regulatory agencies for use in developing food safety criteria and standards. Some of these techniques or concepts are widely known and extensively used, whereas others are still in the developmental stage. The description of these tools and the discussion of their current or potential uses and applications to enhance food safety have been organized as a progression from the better known to the novel. In addition, the committee strived to circumscribe the material on each tool to that which is relevant to food safety, recognizing that some of the sections, such as "Statistical Process Control" and "The Economics of Food Safety Criteria," are not only foreign to many food processors and food safety regulators, but are technical and scientific fields that only recently have been brought into play in the food safety arena. Thus, in view of the limitations in space and time facing the committee, the reader is referred to specialized treatises that expand on these areas when additional information is desired.

HAZARD ANALYSIS AND CRITICAL CONTROL POINTS

Introduction

The Hazard Analysis and Critical Control Point (HACCP) system is a methodology that constitutes the foundation of the food safety assurance system in the modern world. Although a detailed history and description of HACCP principles and applications are beyond the scope of this report, the invaluable contribution that this food safety tool is making to improve public health, its central role in present-day food processing, and its inseparable relationship to the issues discussed in this report demand a short introduction and description of it.

HACCP history goes back to 1959, when the National Aeronautics and Space Administration (NASA) commissioned the Pillsbury Company to manufacture food products for use by astronauts during space missions. The stringent safety requirements imposed on these foods were a reflection of deep concerns in NASA about the potential consequences of foodborne sickness among astronauts in space, as well as of food particles interfering with flight systems (Stevenson and Bernard, 1995). Although HACCP made its debut at the 1971 National Conference of Food Protection (Stevenson and Bernard, 1995), analogous systems (not yet designated as HACCP) had been in existence and had been applied in practice in some food-processing operations, notably in the canning of low-acid foods and in milk pasteurization. These operations included: (1) identification and assessment of the hazards: *Clostridium botulinum* spores in canned low-acid foods and milk-borne pathogens such as *Mycobacterium tuberculosis*, *Brucella* spp., and *Coxiella burnetii*; (2) identification of the critical control point for these hazards: heating at specified temperatures and for similarly specified times in either of these operations; and (3) a system to monitor the critical control point: time and temperature recorders. Despite the fact that these food-processing operations had built-in notions of HACCP, the efforts of the Pillsbury team in articulating the fundamentals of present-day HACCP and testing its effectiveness, followed by additional contributions from the U.S. Army's Natick Laboratories, are nothing short of landmarks in food safety history.

HACCP is well established in the food-processing regulations of the United States. However, its introduction proceeded slowly, beginning in the 1970s and accelerating only until the mid-1990s. The migration of HACCP from textbooks into the U.S. Code of Federal Regulations came about, in part, as a result of a National Academies report (NRC, 1985a) that recommended the adoption of HACCP ". . . universally in food protection programs . . ." and of subsequent, instrumental efforts by the International Commission on Microbiological Specifications for Foods (ICMSF, 1988) and the National Advisory Committee on Microbiological Criteria for Foods (NACMCF, 1998). Other reports of the National Academies (IOM, 1990, 1991; IOM/NRC, 1998; NRC, 1985a, 1985b) have further endorsed the introduction or expansion of HACCP into the processing and inspection of meat, poultry, seafood, and, in general, throughout the food industry.

Implementation of HACCP by the food industry has been a slow—and at times painful—process that still is in progress. To facilitate implementation of HACCP by the food industry and help standardize HACCP training, a coalition of industries and trade organizations in the United States formed the International Meat and Poultry HACCP Alliance in 1994. This group has since endeavored to "train the trainers" by conducting training courses and certifying HACCP trainers who can further train personnel at the processing-plant level. In addition, the

International HACCP Alliance has contributed to the development of generic HACCP plans for use by regulatory agencies in facilitating the preparation of specific HACCP plans by food processors. There is also a Seafood HACCP Alliance and a Juice HACCP Alliance. The committee recognizes the multiple technical, financial, and educational efforts made by the food industry to implement HACCP, including the development and adoption of various interventions to enhance the microbiological safety of the food supply—often in anticipation of regulations—and commends such efforts.

National food safety regulatory agencies and international institutions have published procedures for the development and implementation of HACCP plans. Some of these are established national food regulations, such as those mandated by the Food and Drug Administration (FDA) (21 C.F.R. part 114) and the U.S. Department of Agriculture (USDA) (FSIS, 1996), while others, such as the Codex Alimentarius guidelines on HACCP (CAC, 1997), play a central role in international food trade despite the fact that their adoption by Codex Alimentarius member countries is voluntary.

There are numerous HACCP training manuals, including a few that are international in nature (WHO, 1999), as well as a wealth of information on HACCP from various sources. An example of these sources is a joint USDA/FDA website that offers a variety of training materials (USDA/FDA, 2002).

Continued training in HACCP principles to attain proper implementation by industry personnel and consistent interpretation and monitoring of compliance by inspectors from the regulatory agencies is necessary.

The Principles of HACCP

Unlike the traditional model for food safety assurance that has been used for decades, HACCP does not rely on end-product testing to ensure the safety of food batches, but on continuous control and monitoring of Critical Control Points (CCPs) along the production and processing continuum. It is, therefore, a preventive food safety assurance system in that it focuses on ensuring control of known potential hazards before the product reaches the end of the line, as opposed to the traditional corrective system that focuses on examining the final product and determining whether any hazard of concern is present.

CCPs, in general, are defined in HACCP language as "those points where loss of control would result in an unsafe food product," and more specifically as "those points where the identified hazard(s) may be prevented from entering the food, eliminated from it, or reduced to acceptable levels" (Stevenson and Bernard, 1995). It is noteworthy, however, that an intrinsic weakness of HACCP is that it does not provide information on what these acceptable levels are or a guide on how to set them. Linkage between public health goals and HACCP, through a developing concept of Food Safety Objectives (described later in this chapter), may enable regulators in the future to define numerical levels of tolerance for foodborne hazards in foods at the point of consumption that could be translated into "acceptable levels" at CCPs in food-processing plants.

The methodology for developing a HACCP plan calls for the systematic application of seven principles:

1. Hazard analysis
2. Identification of CCPs
3. Establishment of critical control limits for each CCP
4. Establishment of monitoring procedures for each CCP
5. Establishment of corrective actions
6. Establishment of record-keeping procedures
7. Establishment of verification procedures

The process begins with the formation of a team that includes plant management and personnel, as well as individuals who have expertise in foodborne hazards and the particular product and process being used. The team prepares a flow diagram of the production process and physically examines each of its steps in the actual premises where production takes place. Points along the flow diagram where the hazard may be prevented, eliminated, or reduced to acceptable levels, and for which a control exists that can be established and monitored, are designated as CCPs. Critical limits are then set for the parameters that can be measured to determine that the control at each CCP is being effectively applied. Monitoring procedures are then established, and corrective actions are predetermined to be taken if a loss of control is indicated by a deviation from the critical limits. The HACCP plan, along with records demonstrating that the controls at each CCP have performed successfully and have been continuously monitored during processing, are organized for ease of access by the processor and by inspectors from the regulatory agency charged with ascertaining compliance with the regulations. Finally, internal and external verification procedures are defined to periodically assess the performance of the system and to revise the HACCP plan whenever changes are introduced in the production process that could compromise the effectiveness of the system. Internal verification procedures may involve such activities as instrument calibration, periodic product testing, and records review, while external verification may involve expert audits and external product testing.

Full compliance with Good Manufacturing Practices (GMPs) and the preexistence of Standard Operating Procedures for plant sanitation are assumed to be in place when introducing HACCP into a food-processing plant. Therefore, HACCP is not a stand-alone methodology, but part of a larger set of manufacturing practices that include these preconditions. In addition, the HACCP plan is specific for each processing plant, processing line, and product manufactured in each line. As a result of discussions held during information-gathering meetings, the committee has been made aware that inappropriate identification of CCPs and inappropriate HACCP plans have caused problems in complying with HACCP regulations. Similarly, the committee recognizes that inconsistency in the interpretation and enforcement of HACCP rules between and within regulatory agencies has hampered a smooth transition to the new food-processing inspection model and monitoring of compliance with HACCP rules.

HACCP has revolutionized food safety assurance by bringing about a radical change in the roles of regulators and regulated industries regarding food safety responsibilities, as described in Chapter 1. The committee believes that despite some continued disagreements between these sectors—and some widely publicized failures of the system notwithstanding—the balance of progress in food safety after implementation of HACCP in various sectors of the food industry is decidedly favorable and commendable. The committee, therefore, endorses the recommendations made by previous reports of the National Academies (IOM, 1990, 1991; IOM/NRC, 1998; NRC 1985a, 1985b) and strongly recommends that the regulatory agencies continue to introduce and audit the implementation of HACCP in all sectors of the food industry as appropriate.

RISK ASSESSMENT

Various techniques have been examined for their potential to provide a scientific basis for improving public health and to address emerging foodborne diseases. Risk assessment has surfaced as one key method to embark upon these challenges. The use of quantitative and qualitative risk assessments for biological issues has emerged from the use of quantitative risk assessments for chemical and environmental toxicology (Dourson et al., 2001; IFT, 2002; Neubert, 1999; Paustenbach, 2000). In simple terms, quantitative risk assessment uses mathematical equations, numerical data, and expert opinion to create a computer simulation of reality. These computer models allow interested individuals to explore various risk-management options. Quantitative risk assessment is useful because it allows risk managers to see the entire situation related to a hazard without being an expert on each one of the component factors. Risk managers can rapidly examine various technical solutions to a problem using computer-based models, while using their expert judgment on the social, political, and economic factors that also influence how policies are perceived.

Risk assessment is usually presented as part of the overall risk analysis paradigm, where risk analysis consists of risk assessment, risk communication, and risk management (Figure 3.1) (Vose, 2000). Quantitative risk assessment is a scientific process that addresses the magnitude of the risk and identifies factors that control it. Risk communication is a social and psychological process that promotes dialogue among different affected individuals regarding the risk. Finally, risk management is a process that combines science, politics, economics, and proper timing to arrive at a decision regarding what to do about the risk.

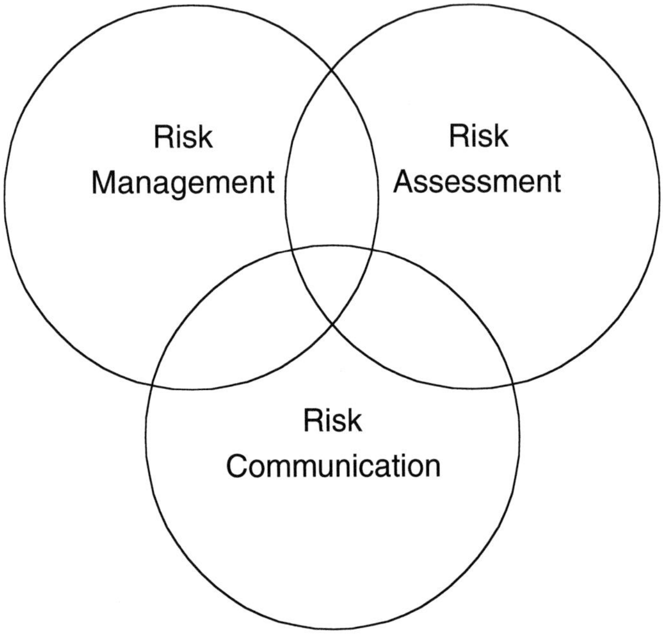

FIGURE 3.1 Components of a risk analysis.

Differences and Similarities Between Chemical and Microbial Risk Assessment

Chemical risk assessment is a relatively mature field compared with that of microbial risk assessment. This is due in part to the requirement for drugs and chemicals to be approved or registered by either FDA or the U.S. Environmental Protection Agency (EPA) prior to human exposure. Rigid guidelines have been established and quantitative approaches to assessing adverse effects in humans have been developed. Despite the differences in maturity, the overall paradigm of chemical risk assessment has remarkable similarities to the emerging practice of microbial risk assessment. A comparison of key differences and similarities may benefit both fields.

In both fields, risk assessment is a component of the larger field of risk analysis that also encompasses risk management and risk communication. A variety of diagrams have been used to explain the interaction of these components, including that shown in Figure 3.1. Chemical (and microbial) risk assessments are typically divided into four parts: hazard identification, dose–response assessment (or hazard characterization), exposure assessment, and risk characterization (Lammerding and Paoli, 1997; Neubert, 1999; Paustenbach, 2000).

Hazard Identification

Hazard identification involves assessing whether the agent (chemical or microbial) produces adverse effects in biological systems. Historically, this was assessed for chemicals through the use of animal bioassay screens, but now it is largely accomplished using in vitro systems and, recently, by techniques targeted to advances in genomic sciences. Microbial risk assessments are typically initiated in response to a public health concern, and hazard characterization in microbial risk assessment typically uses epidemiological or outbreak data (*Escherichia coli* O157:H7 Risk Assessment Team, 2001; *Salmonella* Enteritidis Risk Assessment Team, 1998).

The hazard characterization step in microbial risk assessment includes identifying the organism that caused the public health concern and summarizing the details regarding the exposure pathway and the microbial ecology of the particular hazard (see Chapter 2).

Dose–Response Assessment

Once an agent is identified as potentially injurious, the next phase is to define the dose–response relationship. The techniques for chemical dose–response assessments are well defined, while the same cannot be said for their microbial counterparts.

Studies conducted in laboratory animals form the basis of the field of toxicology and are readily used in chemical risk assessment. There is an extensive experimental database of well-designed laboratory animal studies, all conducted under agreed upon Good Laboratory Practice (GLP) guidelines (40 C.F.R. §160.1). GLP guidelines ensure that all tests conducted for regulatory action on a drug or for chemical registration are conducted according to acceptable practices and generate an auditable paper trail. The validity of this approach to chemical risk assessment has a proven track record: FDA uses essentially these same techniques in preclinical studies of human drugs. The determination of dose for a human drug is based on knowledge of the dose–response relationship for both beneficial and adverse effects. The extensive pre- and postmarketing drug approval process validates the accuracy of these approaches.

Tolerances for man-made chemicals introduced into the food supply are based on extrapolation of no-effect data from laboratory animal studies. Experiences with FDA drug approval would indirectly support the validity of this approach, as stated above. Microbial risk assessment is qualitatively quite different, for microbial hazards are not man-made and usually are introduced into the food supply only naturally or accidentally. Because of the host–pathogen specificity differences, animal studies are of only limited use in microbial risk assessment. Additionally, no microbial equivalent of the FDA human-drug approval process exists to validate any proposed dose–response relationships, although if properly collected, outbreak data may help in this regard.

Experimental designs in chemical risk assessment are specific for different toxicological endpoints (e.g., acute, subacute, chronic, reproductive, carcinogenic). The mathematical form of the dose–response relationship is assessed based on the biological mechanism of action of the chemical being studied. The end result is a definition of a dose that does not produce adverse effects in laboratory animals: the no-observed-adverse-effect level (NOAEL). There are many variations on how this is determined and on how data from multiple studies are combined (Neubert, 1999). However, for the purpose of this discussion, the key point is that in chemical risk assessment, the end product (derived from standard toxicological testing protocols) is a defined dose considered safe by the scientific community.

Microbial dose–response relationships have been derived from human feeding trials (many done on volunteer prisoners in the early part of the twentieth century), animal studies, and, increasingly, data from foodborne disease outbreaks, as noted. As with chemical risk assessment, various endpoints can be used, ranging from mild diarrhea to death; also, data from multiple studies can be combined (Holcomb et al., 1999). A variety of mathematical forms for microbial dose–response has been proposed. Microbial dose–response equations do not have as clear a link to a biological mechanism as in chemical risk assessment, due in part to the complexity of the underlying biology.

The committee believes that defining microbial dose–response relationships for foodborne pathogens is important if more accurate risk assessment results are desired. Allocation of resources to fund basic research studies defining these relationships would help to remedy this deficiency.

The host side of the dose–response relationship may also be different for microbial and chemical risk assessments. Some researchers have suggested that in the case of microbial risk assessment, a population's response to an infectious pathogen is more variable than it is to acutely toxic chemicals and rivals the complexity seen with carcinogens. This variability is due to altering immune status as a function of genetics, environment, age, concurrent diseases, and a host of other factors (ICMSF, 1998). However, the response of an individual to a chemical exposure is also variable based on many of the same factors and individual differences in the inherent receptor sensitivity, pharmacokinetics (including metabolism), and simultaneous exposure to a myriad of drugs and chemicals. In both scenarios, the large degree of interindividual variability makes the risk assessment process prone to large degrees of uncertainty.

In the drug arena, the development of population pharmacokinetic techniques has partially reduced this uncertainty by identifying subpopulations that vary significantly from the norm. Perhaps the most important difference is that microbial dose–response assessment for infectious pathogens does not produce any concept analogous to the NOAEL, since a single microbial cell may (under the right circumstances) produce illness. It may, however, be possible to use a risk assessment term analogous to the NOAEL for organisms like *Staphylococcus aureus* or *Bacillus cereus* that cause illness through formation of a toxin in the food, or for *Listeria monocytogenes* in healthy adults. Because microbial dose–response assessment does not typically produce a NOAEL, the key point in microbial risk assessment is that for many pathogens there is no safe dose. Even if a microbial NOAEL could be determined, it might not be adopted. USDA's Food Safety and Inspection Service (FSIS) has taken the position with respect to *Escherichia coli* O157:H7 that it is an adulterant, and hence, it is not allowed in raw ground beef in any number (see Chapter 4). While the agency could change its position in this regard, it might be difficult to explain such a change to the public, and so it might hesitate to do so. If a firm scientific basis for determining no-effect levels for some pathogens existed, along with appropriate detection and enumeration methods to ensure that microbial NOAELs are not exceeded, it would still be necessary to convince the public that their safety would be sufficiently assured by the implementation of the microbial NOAELs.

Exposure Assessment

The next step in either microbial or chemical risk assessment is to estimate human exposure to the agent. For chemicals such as pesticides, environmental compounds, and food additives, potential modes of exposure must be assessed. These include assessing whether the primary routes are inhalation, dermal, or, in the case of food chemicals or microorganisms, oral. Aggregate exposure must be determined where multiple routes may contribute to human exposure. This often occurs in the case of pesticides, where exposure may occur by inhalation after spraying in a home or place of work, orally in food, or dermally by physical contact with a sprayed surface. For chemicals, a major task of exposure assessment is to determine the fraction of the dose that is actually absorbed into the body, that is, the bioavailability. Additionally, it is important to determine if this absorbed dose is metabolized, either to an inactive moiety or to an active and potentially toxic metabolite.

An arena where risk assessment is routinely applied to chemicals is in the drug approval process. Pharmaceutical drugs are somewhat different in this respect than other chemicals because hazard characterizations and dose–response assessments are conducted in the preclinical phases of drug development in order to estimate a tolerable dose for humans. Hazard identifications for pharmaceuticals are essentially validated in the first phase of human testing. The appropriate dose is finally determined after the second and third phases of human testing, which seek to determine effectiveness and obtain additional safety information. When the drug's sponsor applies to FDA for approval of its application to market the drug, a determination is made on whether it is safe and effective and may be released to the marketplace. The approval process necessitates balancing the potential benefits of the drug to the patient population against the risks that it might pose. Through the initial testing or postmarket surveillance, information may arise that suggests that certain specific patient populations are more at risk than others for adverse effects or treatment failures; such information may be reflected in labeling information that guides proper drug use. If information is developed later that changes the risk/benefit ratio significantly, FDA may require that the drug be withdrawn from the market.

Exposure assessment in quantitative microbial risk assessment (QMRA) involves modeling movement of the pathogen through the production system. Both temporal (in time) and spatial (in space) exposure data are relevant to this step. Exposure assessment results in an estimate of the likelihood of pathogen ingestion by the consumer.

Exposure assessment for microorganisms is quite different from that for drugs or other chemicals, primarily because (at least with bacterial pathogens) some microorganisms can increase or decrease in number in the food under suitable conditions. Aggregate exposure to multiple chemicals is often considered, especially with carcinogens. Although each chemical exposure to an individual in a given time period might not produce illness, such exposures may produce subclinical organ damage, induce metabolic changes, or result in accumulation that could modify subsequent responses. In contrast, if repetitive exposure to low levels of infectious microbes occurs, host immunity may decrease risk (ICMSF, 1998), but counterexamples also exist (Maijala et al., 2001). Unlike a chemical that has a constant potency (unless degraded), a microbe is dynamic and adaptable. Virulence factors acquired from other organisms could change the inherent infectivity and pathogenicity of a foodborne microorganism (ICMSF, 1998).

In food-processing operations that combine raw materials from multiple sources, microbial or chemical contamination in some of these raw materials would have differing effects on contamination in the resulting product. While a chemical contaminant would be diluted during mixing, similar dilution of bacterial contaminants would mean that the bacteria are spread throughout the mix (e.g., by breakup of microbial colonies that initially may be highly localized into what is referred to as "point source" or "hot spots" in the incoming raw material). For example, consider the mixing of meat trimmings in a grinding operation where a point source of either a chemical or a bacterial pathogen occurs. Dilution of the chemical from a point source to a larger mass of product would be expected to reduce the hazard by decreasing the concentration of the chemical a consumer would ingest. In the case of bacteria, mixing meat trimmings from multiple sources (animals, producers, packing plants, states, countries) would increase the volume of contaminated ground product and, because of bacterial growth, the potential number of consumers that might be affected.

The spread of bacterial contaminants would also seriously confound attempts to trace back the source of contamination to a specific supplier of raw material.

This effect is well known in the dairy industry, where milk that contains antibiotic residues from an individual cow will be diluted in the tank truck after mixing with milk containing no antibiotic residues. Thus, because of similar dilution effects, ground-meat products would be expected to raise no major concerns regarding chemical residues; but, unlike the situation in whole-muscle meat, chemical hot spots would likely be spread in ground meat. Therefore, the microbiological risk in ground meat may be expected to be greater than any chemical risk. The same logic could be extended to processing food from multiple sources or to consumption of a contaminated item in a multi-ingredient meal (e.g., vegetables, meat, and sauces).

There are also some differences in the analytical detection of microbes versus chemicals that may impact data used in exposure assessment calculations. Concerns about sampling strategies are fairly similar for both chemicals and microbes, although the latter may be more prone to localization from hotspots of point-source microbial contamination.

In the chemical residue arena, the development of multiple drug-class residue screening assays that would detect and quantify multiple contaminants in a single assay has been the focus of recent research efforts. Once considered cost prohibitive, these techniques are based on gas chromatography/mass spectrometry and are now feasible. Similar developments have begun to occur in the microbiological arena (see Chapter 1).

A similarity between chemicals and microbial pathogens is that all chemicals and pathogens do not have, qualitatively or quantitatively, the same propensity for causing human illness. Chemicals may exert a number of different types of toxicological reactions, including allergenicity, immunotoxicity, mutagenicity, carcinogenicity, and "classic" chemical toxicity (renal, hepatic, etc.) seen with many pesticides and drugs. A single chemical may exhibit the full spectrum of effects depending on the dose and length of exposure. Quantitative structure–activity relationships have also been developed that help in the prediction of these chemical effects. For microbes, a similar diverse spectrum of potential adverse effects can be observed depending on the species, serotype, strain, or host differences. For example, ingestion of foods contaminated with some strains of *E. coli* may produce a transient gastrointestinal disturbance, while exposure to strains such as O157:H7 may be fatal for some individuals. Finally, detection of a chemical allows one to estimate whether the sample exceeds tolerance. Techniques such as polymerase chain reaction (PCR), which amplifies deoxyribonucleic acid (DNA), can detect—and in some cases can also quantify—pathogens (Hein et al., 2001a, 2001b; Li and Drake, 2001). However, rapid tests that determine microbial viability and infectivity are just becoming available (see Chapter 1).

The issue of multiple points of contamination within a food-processing establishment is also different for some chemical classes versus microorganisms because of the ability of some of the latter (e.g., bacteria, molds) to multiply and cross-contaminate. Antibiotics or pesticides that occur either in animal or plant products will not likely result in cross-contamination in a processing plant. Control of the raw product at the producer or harvest level is essential. Approved chemical or drug tolerances in meat or produce serve as effective performance standards to control these hazards.

However, the same cannot be said for microbial contamination because bacteria can be transferred from one to other parts of a production line. Data on microbial cross-contamination rates suitable for quantitative risk assessment are only now becoming available. Precise localization of where such cross-contamination occurs would require multiple sampling points in the production system.

The committee calls on USDA and FDA to undertake or fund studies on food–pathogen combinations for which insufficient knowledge has prevented intervention to characterize the points in the production system where control would be most effective and could have the greatest impact on reducing foodborne disease. Such information is essential in the application of appropriate controls at critical points and for the development of future microbiological criteria for foods.

Risk Characterization

The risk characterization phase of a chemical risk assessment differs depending on the type of chemical involved and on the regulatory agency that has jurisdiction (e.g., EPA vs. FDA for an animal drug). However, all chemical risk characterization approaches are conceptually similar, and can be quite different from microbial risk characterizations. Chemical risk characterization involves determining the dose of a chemical that is essentially not harmful to humans, based on the dose–response data from laboratory animal studies and exposure assessments. In contrast, most microbial risk assessments have been undertaken with full knowledge that a particular pathogen is harmful. Microbial risk characterization involves estimating the risk to the consumer population (or in some cases a subset of the consumer population) and prioritizing effective control strategies.

Chemical risk characterization is used to determine some "risk value," which is a point on a dose–response curve with some probability of occurrence. Data such as the NOAEL or a benchmark dose from laboratory animal studies are reduced to adjust for uncertainty (e.g., species to species extrapolation, experimental shortfalls, increased sensitivity of the young) through the use of safety or uncertainty factors ranging from 100 to 1,000. For many pesticides and environmental compounds, the result is a reference dose or reference concentration. For a drug used in food-producing animals, an allowable daily intake is computed. Alternate endpoints, such as those related to allergenicity or inducement of microbial resistance, may be employed. The potential amount of food consumption is then estimated and the allowable daily intake or reference dose is partitioned across all food items to arrive at a tolerance or a maximum contaminant level goal below which food consumption or exposure is assumed to be safe. In the European Union and in the Codex Alimentarius, a similar process is used to calculate a maximum residue level. These are all variants of a theme of acceptable exposure or tolerable intake. Recent work has attempted to directly determine these endpoints using human data that would eliminate the uncertainty of interspecies extrapolations. A threshold of toxicological concern approach that uses a threshold based on chemical structure–activity relationships in an attempt to integrate all adverse effects has recently been proposed (Kroes and Kozianowski, 2002). If the compound is a potential carcinogen, the allowable concentration in food may be restricted to that which can be detected analytically using the most sensitive method. Finally, when the exposure is widespread, the question is often related to estimating the risk to the human population from this ubiquitous exposure (e.g., dioxin, mercury). In this case, exposure and the dose–response data are used to estimate risk to the human population of exposure to specific concentrations, which are then employed in remediation and risk-management strategies to reduce exposures to an acceptable level (Dourson et al., 2001).

Microbial risk characterization is not as well defined as its chemical counterpart. The goal of finding a risk value endpoint is similar and, in some cases, the methods by which this is obtained are also similar. In the absence of human- or animal-feeding models, a number of dose–response models based on epidemiological data, animal studies, expert opinions, or combinations thereof are evaluated to determine an endpoint or risk value. The highly variable nature of the microbial dose and the human response, as well as the fact that each model is based on different biological endpoints, make it extremely difficult to find one model that fits every situation. For example, the Joint FAO/WHO Expert Consultation on Risk Assessment of Microbiological Hazards in Foods suggests that it is not possible to endorse a single dose-response model for *L. monocytogenes* in ready-to-eat foods (FAO/WHO, 2000).

A variety of data gaps have been identified that must be addressed before microbial risk characterization will be as effective as chemical risk characterization. As more accurate dose–response models become available, it should be possible to identify the risk-value endpoint needed to achieve a desired public health outcome.

Compliance with chemical residue tolerances in meat, poultry, and eggs in the United States is monitored through the FSIS National Residue Program (FSIS, 1999). This dynamic residue surveillance program monitors domestic, as well as imported, food-animal carcass and egg products for a number of drug, pesticide, and environmental residues. This surveillance, based on a random statistical sampling protocol for a list of target drugs determined by a multidisciplinary, interagency working group, is designed to assess prevalence and define areas that need further attention. In addition, the National Residue Program undertakes a number of special projects to target specific residue concerns. Samples for these programs are usually collected from healthy animals to provide surveillance data. Because the surveillance sampling is conducted to develop databases for future reference and the product is not traceable, if a violating residue is found, recall does not occur.

The final component of the National Residue Program is enforcement testing, where samples are collected from individual animals or lots that appear suspicious to FSIS inspectors. This program is also used to follow-up on producers who have a history of violations or to verify HACCP performance. Violative products detected using this system are removed from the food supply because they are considered adulterated. If the product has been distributed into commerce, it may be subject to market recall. It should be noted that the analytical techniques used for these programs are not the same. Enforcement testing may use rapid screening methods that, if positive, force the carcass to be held until confirmatory tests are conducted at an approved laboratory. FSIS maintains a record of such violations in its Residue Violation Information System that is shared with FDA for follow-up investigations. The results of these investigations are then stored in the Tissue Residue Information Management System (Paige and Pell, 1997).

No data from a system analogous to the National Residue Program exist for use in microbial risk assessments. Typically, the results of each microbial risk assessment are validated based on a comparison with current Centers for Disease Control and Prevention estimates for the pathogen of interest. The National Residue Program may represent a useful working model on which a national pathogen system could be based. Just as the National Residue Program can be used to validate chemical risk assessments, such a national pathogen program would be invaluable in validating microbial risk assessments.

The strength of the chemical risk assessment approach is that there is a defined process whereby an acceptable exposure or tolerable intake of a chemical, based on a public health endpoint, can be defined and calculated from either experimental animal or human data. A specific dose–response relationship is defined for the chemical and adverse effect being modeled. In food safety applications, this allows definition of a tolerance below which lifetime human exposure is not deemed to be of concern to public health. In a HACCP environment, this tolerance can be directly employed as a performance standard (Taylor, 2002).

Microbial risk assessment currently suffers from a lack of a standardized process and from a perception that such a process would be expensive and very time consuming. The form of the dose–response relationship is not known and thus is difficult to quantify. Microbial risk assessment is also hampered by the infectious nature of microorganisms, such that some exposure almost always poses some risk. The current level of exposure of the population to a pathogen may be tolerated by most of the population because most people do not experience adverse consequences from the foods they consume every day. In light of current morbidity and mortality statistics, however, the level of exposure should be less than it is today.

Microbial risk assessment may provide the tools needed to help identify the most effective solutions for lowering consumer exposure to foodborne microbiological hazards. In fact, this is the philosophy behind setting microbiological performance standards as a percentage reduction of baseline data that should reduce overall levels of microbial contamination.

From the above discussion, it is clear that QMRA can benefit from accomplishments in chemical quantitative risk assessments in that the lessons learned from the latter can be applied to the new challenges of developing the former. Risk assessment offers a systematic approach to estimating the impact of pathogenic microorganisms in the food chain. In this way, risk assessment may assist public health decision-making and thus help improve overall public health by reducing the burden of foodborne illness.

Dealing with Microbial Risk Assessment Data Gaps

Several areas where data gaps exist in current microbial risk assessments have been identified by various groups studying this technique (Cassin et al., 1998; FAO/WHO, 2001; IOM, 2002; Whiting and Buchanan, 1997b). During hazard identification, gaps in data can significantly impact the resulting risk assessment. These gaps include, but are not limited to, microorganism variability regarding pathogenicity and infectivity in human hosts; variability of human hosts' susceptibility to illness; complete epidemiological data from outbreak studies, including organism dose and environmental factors of both organism and host; and data on the prevalence of pathogenic microorganisms throughout the food chain.

Exposure-assessment data gaps, in turn, include information on routes of animal infection; prevalence in animal groups (e.g., flocks); dynamics of within-animal group transmission of organisms; microbial stress adaptation; and cross-contamination within the production, processing, and consumption segments of the food chain.

There are also data gaps in dose–response assessment. These include data on the number of cells of particular microorganisms required to constitute an infective dose, as well as detailed information concerning the dose and the corresponding response of human hosts who are infected.

Finally, risk characterization data gaps include association of risk with human health effects, identification of potential risk mitigation strategies, and costs and benefits of mitigation strategies once the strategies are identified.

Some of the information listed above is available for a few microorganisms, whereas for others the data gaps are more significant. Nevertheless, despite these data gaps, there have been and will continue to be advances in the development of microbial risk assessments in foods (Cassin et al., 1998; FAO/WHO, 2001; Whiting and Buchanan, 1997a). Each new risk assessment adds to the information already in place and increases our understanding of the issues, while further defining what information is still lacking.

The list of identified data gaps available at the completion of a microbial risk assessment can assist government and industry in targeting funds to generate missing information. If data are not available for part of a food production chain, it may be possible to simplify the QMRA model such that this part of the chain is excluded. For example, if data on prevalence of a particular pathogen in a live food-animal population were not available, a QMRA could be constructed such that the start of the process was postslaughter. This assumes, of course, that pathogen prevalence and concentration data are available for the carcasses. If a QMRA were constructed in this way, important factors that affect pathogen prevalence and concentration in the live animal population obviously would be accounted for in the final assessment results.

Predictive models for the growth and inactivation of pathogens as influenced by environmental conditions have gained increased visibility in the last decade (Whiting and Buchanan, 1997b). If information on the behavior of a pathogen in a particular part of the food chain is not available, and a predictive model exists that could represent that part of the chain, then model predictions, rather than actual data, could be used. For example, data are seldom available on the levels of pathogens in a food just prior to consumption, but if data are available from an earlier part of the chain, and temperature and food composition data are available, predictive models could be used to estimate pathogen levels just prior to consumption. Limitations of predictive models include the use of models that have not been fully validated and a lack of information on prediction uncertainty.

It may be possible to use surrogate data if neither actual data nor predictive models are available. Surrogate data are data from a related organism that experts believe to be "close enough" to the unknown behavior of the actual pathogen to stand in its place. Examples might be the use of cross-contamination data for generic *E. coli* as a surrogate for *E. coli* O157:H7 cross-contamination and the use of dose–response data on *Shigella dysenteriae* as a surrogate for *E. coli* O157:H7 (*Escherichia coli* O157:H7 Risk Assessment Team, 2001; IOM, 2002).

Data gaps may not mean just the lack of a point estimate (e.g., mean, mode, or median), but also a lack of knowledge regarding the uncertainty and/or variability associated with the point estimate. The amount of effort needed to adequately fill a data gap either by combining data from a multitude of sources or conducting original research can make the elimination of data gaps a long process.

Another method to reduce and eliminate some of the existing data gaps in QMRAs could be stochastic simulation using probabilistic distributions to replace the data-gap information. In published risk assessments, probability distributions have been used to estimate the parameters associated with various parts of a QMRA, for example, the dose–response curve (Cassin et al., 1998; FAO/WHO,

2001; Whiting and Buchanan, 1997a). It follows that in places where data gaps exist, probabilistic models could be useful in providing information that helps to fill the data gap. In order to accomplish this, one of two conditions would need to be met. One requires the modeler to make an assumption about the shape of the probability distribution from estimates based on somewhat qualitative previous experience or other more quantitative data (FAO/WHO, 2001). The other condition relies on the use of probability distributions where variance—which arises from both uncertainty and variability—is large (e.g., exponential or beta distributions) to accommodate for the unknown information in the data gap. If either of these conditions were met, then the use of a probability distribution would be a valid method to fill a data gap.

Some data gaps can be filled through the use of expert opinions and consults (sometimes referred to as qualitative risk assessment) (IFT, 2002). Some opponents of using qualitative risk assessment as a component of a QMRA state that the former dilutes the latter's effectiveness, scientific basis, and end use of the resulting risk estimate. However, without the use of these qualitative expert consults, it is likely that some of these data gaps would continue to exist for some time. Waiting for "hard" scientific data would postpone the development of QMRAs that could be instrumental and effective in public health decision-making despite their qualitative or "soft" expert opinion content. Those involved in qualitative consults often have a qualitative feel for the data needed that is based on previous experience that has a foundation in quantitative research (Busta, 2002; IFT, 2002). Therefore, to include qualitative information from expert consults in a QMRA where data gaps exist and are difficult to fill seems both reasonable and scientifically sound. It should be noted that it is best to use standardized methods for eliciting expert opinion to enhance transparency and avoid introducing any potential bias into the process, and that techniques are available for pooling different opinions from a range of experts (Vose, 2000).

As noted above, most QMRAs will have data gaps. These data gaps should not prevent a risk assessment from being initiated and completed and from serving a useful purpose. However, these data gaps must be communicated to those requesting the QMRA, so that they will be aware of its limitations. The inherently iterative nature of risk assessments allows continual updating as more and better-quality data become available, thereby increasing their effectiveness as a qualitative tool for policy-making.

Using Microbial Risk Assessment as a Policy Tool

Each of the large QMRAs commissioned by the United States has been initiated with the objective of guiding policy. Table 3.1 provides the relevant quotation from each of these risk assessments.

Since the field of microbial risk assessment as applied to food is relatively new, there are few case histories that detail how QMRA can successfully impact

TABLE 3.1 Quantitative Microbial Risk Assessments Commissioned by the United States Government and Their Policy-Guiding Objectives

Risk Assessment	Objective	Reference
Salmonella Enteritidis Risk Assessment. Shell Eggs and Egg Products	"The risk assessment results detailed in this Final Report will be used by the agency, working in conjunction with economists from within and from outside the agency, to conduct cost-effectiveness studies and cost-benefit analysis in order to set forth recommendations for policy."	*Salmonella* Enteritidis Risk Assessment Team, 1998
Preliminary Pathways and Data for a Risk Assessment of *Escherichia coli* O157:H7 in Beef	"The baseline risk assessment is intended to inform a distinct FSIS policy analysis that will identify feasible risk mitigation options for further comparative analysis."	*E. coli* Risk Assessment Team, 2001
Draft Assessment of the Relative Risk to Public Health from Foodborne *Listeria monocytogenes* Among Selected Categories of Ready-to-Eat Foods	"The scientific evaluations and the mathematical models developed during the risk assessment, provide a systematic assessment of the scientific knowledge needed to assist both in reviewing the effectiveness of current policies, programs, and practices, and new strategies to minimize the public health impact of foodborne *L. monocytogenes*."	CFSAN/FSIS/CDC, 2001
Draft Risk Assessment on the Public Health Impact of *Vibrio parahaemolyticus* in Raw Molluscan Shellfish	"FDA anticipates that periodic updates to the risk model will continue to reduce the degree of uncertainty associated with risk estimates, and that these updates will assist FDA in making the best possible decisions and policies for reducing the risk posed by *V. parahaemolyticus* in raw molluscan shellfish."	Posnick et al., 2001
The Human Health Impact of Fluoroquinolone Resistant *Campylobacter* Attributed to the Consumption of Chicken	"The modeling approach we have used has been designed to address the effect of specific risk management actions [i.e. policies], while also providing the facility to take into account the effect of the most important future changes in the physical system . . ."	CVM, 2001

continued

TABLE 3.1 Continued

Risk Assessment	Objective	Reference
Draft FSIS Risk Assessment for *Listeria* in Ready-to-Eat Meat and Poultry Products	"By changing in-plant practices such as the frequency of testing and sanitation of food contact surfaces, the effectiveness of pre- and post-packaging interventions, the effectiveness of growth inhibitors, effectiveness of enhanced sanitation, etc., including combinations, this risk assessment can provide numerous outputs to address specific risk management questions. This risk assessment model was also developed with user-friendly interfaces to allow users to change scenario conditions and assumptions. As a result, this risk assessment model can be used as a tool to explore a variety of risk management scenarios beyond those developed for this report."	Gallagher et al., 2003

policy-making. In a few short years, QMRA has become the new way of organizing and interpreting data to enhance food safety. The definitive example of a "full-blown" QMRA for the U.S. food supply was the USDA *Salmonella* Enteritidis risk assessment for shell eggs and egg products (*Salmonella* Enteritidis Risk Assessment Team, 1998), although an example from Canada was published earlier the same year (Cassin et al., 1998), and an example from water microbiology predates these by several years (Rose et al., 1991).

The Salmonella *Enteritidis Risk Assessment (SERA): Shell Eggs and Egg Products* was the first of the major government-commissioned QMRAs, so it has the longest history that can be used to track any possible policy impact. Following the publication of the SERA in 1998, the President's Council on Food Safety (1999) published the document *Egg Safety from Production to Consumption: An Action Plan to Eliminate* Salmonella *Enteritidis Illnesses Due to Eggs*. The action plan attributes the FSIS final rule on shell eggs storage, transportation, and consumer labeling (*Salmonella* Enteritidis Risk Assessment Team, 1998) and the FDA proposed rule for shell egg safe handling statements and retail refrigeration requirements (FDA, 1999a) to the SERA. The action plan also states that the SERA predicts that multiple interventions could achieve a more substantial reduction in *S.* Enteritidis illnesses than could any one intervention alone, and then goes on to lay out such a broad-based policy approach. Finally, the action plan also indicates that the research needs identified in the SERA have been incorporated into the plan.

The policy implications of the *Draft Assessment of the Relative Risk to Public Health from Foodborne* Listeria monocytogenes *Among Selected Categories of Ready-to-Eat Foods* (CFSAN/FSIS/CDC, 2001) were laid out in a U.S. Department of Health and Human Services-USDA Joint Action Plan (FDA/FSIS, 2001) based on, and released concurrently with, the risk assessment (FDA/FSIS, 2001). This plan includes a number of areas for policy change, including redirection of enforcement and microbial product sampling strategies; proposal of new regulations and revisions to existing regulations; and support of additional research on exposure assessment, treatment strategies, safety-related date marking, and improved detection and quantification (FDA/FSIS, 2001).

Internationally, the World Health Organization/Food and Agriculture Organization of the United Nations has led the microbial risk assessment effort and has many projects underway, including risk assessment for *Salmonella* spp. in eggs and broilers, *L. monocytogenes* in ready-to-eat foods, *Vibrio* spp. in seafood, and *Campylobacter* spp. in broiler chickens. Various European countries have also developed risk assessments suited to various products, pathogens, and processing systems. Plans are underway to catalog and index European risk assessments through a European concerted research effort known as COST Action 920 (COST Action 920, 2002).

Clearly, each of these major risk assessments was undertaken to help make sound policy. In some cases, policy decisions have been made or proposed in the United States that are based on QMRA results. If one considers the pace with which QMRAs are being conducted around the world, the next decade should provide some interesting examples of their impact on the promulgation of sound science-based food safety policies.

FOOD SAFETY OBJECTIVES

Food Safety Advances with No Quantitative Measure of Impact on Public Health

Historically the major advances in consumer protection have resulted from the development and implementation of selected, targeted control measures at one or more steps along the food continuum. However, more often than not, the goal of such control measures has not been expressed in a numerical value (e.g., a specified reduction in the prevalence of a particular foodborne infection), or the relationship between hazard and risk has not been determined. This does not mean that control measures cannot be taken. Some examples of measures that might result in safer food without quantitative performance criteria include binomial slaughtering, where pathogen-free herds are slaughtered before those that are infected to prevent cross-contamination; vaccination programs to prevent infection in animals; and consumer information programs that target high-risk populations.

Efficient communication to all stakeholders of the reason for, and expected outcomes of, food safety control measures has been an important aspect of the acceptance of the measures. Any food safety criterion, the effectiveness of which is not readily observable, should be coupled with some sort of verification measure to ensure that the criterion actually has an effect.

The Need for Regulatory Flexibility

Because the pace of the regulatory process seldom matches that of innovation and scientific advancement, regulatory policies should ideally be designed with this understanding in mind. Good science-based policies should allow flexibility and encourage innovation, with minimal regulatory revisions. This implies a regulatory framework that specifies results, but not the methods used to achieve these results. It also implies a flexible, moving "results target" that can be easily changed in response to changing public health goals.

Food Safety Objectives and Traditional Microbiological Criteria

One approach that could provide this changeable regulatory structure is that of Food Safety Objectives (FSOs). FSOs are also important because they allow translation of public health goals (e.g., reduce the incidence of foodborne disease *x* by 50 percent in a specified period of time) into measurements that food processors are directly able to effect (e.g., ensure that no more than *y* cells per gram of the microorganism causing foodborne disease *x* are present in product *z* at the time of consumption). This is a novel approach that may allow regulators to address the inherent weakness of HACCP, that defines a CCP as any point, stage, or step along the food production and processing chain where a hazard can be prevented, eliminated, or reduced to an acceptable level, but it leaves the acceptable level undefined. An FSO provides the basis for defining this level.

An FSO is a statement of the maximum frequency or concentration of a microbiological hazard in a food at the time of consumption that provides the appropriate level of protection (ICMSF, 2002). FSOs are specified at the point of consumption, and they provide flexibility to food processors because various means of meeting an FSO may be practical and available for the same product. FSOs are quantitative and verifiable, are limited to food safety, and do not address concerns for quality. Regulatory agencies could use FSOs to define the level of control of a hazard expected in a food product at the time of consumption. They could also be used to subsequently evaluate the adequacy of a facility's control system to achieve the FSO given all the relevant assumptions about transportation and retail and consumer handling of the product.

FSOs differ from the microbiological criteria that have been traditionally used to determine the acceptance of food products. Traditional microbiological criteria specify details such as a sampling plan and the method of sample preparation and analysis, whereas FSOs do not prescribe a particular analytical method. Microbiological criteria are typically used to determine the safety or quality of a batch of food products, and as such provide a snapshot limited to the time the food was produced, but are not typically used in such a way as to provide information on process stability and capability. A review of any individual plant's food safety management system using an FSO approach could provide an assessment of long-term control.

How Are Food Safety Objectives Established?

Regulatory agencies may find that FSOs represent a useful concept for establishing a theoretical framework to relate performance standards to public health objectives. Conceptually, an FSO would be established on the basis of a quantitative risk assessment of the hazard of interest and would be consistent with the level of consumer protection that the regulatory agency deems appropriate to fulfill the public health objective. The reasoning followed in setting the FSO would be: no more than x mg/kg (chemical hazard) or no more than y cfu/g (microbial hazard) can be present in a given food product at the time of consumption to keep the number of illnesses attributable to the hazard below the preset public health objective. From there, the regulatory agency could establish a performance standard that would ensure control of the hazard at the processing plant so that the product would be consistent with the FSO when it reached the consumer. It would then be the processor's decision what process or combination of processes to apply and what additional parameters (e.g., antimicrobial food additives, packaging, and refrigeration and cooking protocols) to introduce or modify to ensure that the performance standard is met at the processing plant, and through it, that the product meets the FSO at the time of consumption.

FSOs offer one practical, if yet unproven, means to convert public health goals into values or targets that can be used by regulatory agencies and industry. For example, a public health goal may be to reduce the incidence of foodborne illness attributed to pathogen *a* by 50 percent (e.g., from 30 to 15 cases per 100,000 people per year). A regulatory agency or manufacturer could not design a control system that would be certain to meet such a goal. However, if this goal were translated into a numerical measure of the microbial hazard's frequency or concentration at the time of consumption (e.g., less than 100 cfu/g of pathogen *a* or less than 15 mg/kg of aflatoxin), industry could design control processes at the plant necessary to achieve this FSO and the regulatory agency could then establish inspection procedures at the plant to ensure processes are under control.

For newly emerging food safety concerns, however, there may be so little information available that it is difficult or impossible to relate the public health objective to an eventual FSO. In such a situation, qualitative risk assessments and, in some cases, simple dose–response estimates, could be used to set an FSO.

In this manner, depending on the urgency or the complexity of the situation, an FSO may be derived from a quantitative risk assessment or from expert opinion. The FSO may be based on a realistic estimate of the risk. However, if time is short, it could also be based on a detailed examination of the frequency or levels of a hazard that can be expected to protect consumers. FSOs should be considered interim standards that could be adjusted to be more or less stringent as more information becomes available.

Examples of criteria that are continually updated include the International Organization for Standardization (ISO) standards, which are reviewed every five years. Following review, these standards are accepted, revised, or eliminated (Cianfrani et al., 2002). Another example is FDA's model Food Code, which is revised every two years by the Conference for Food Protection (FDA, 2002).

FSOs can play an important role in modern food safety management by linking information from the risk assessment processes with measures to control the identified risk. As more information becomes available, risk assessments should be updated and FSOs adjusted accordingly. Thus, the FSO concept may be a useful tool for developing policies that are consistent with current science and could offer an alternative approach to food safety management focusing on the protection of human health, while offering flexibility in achieving that goal.

The Food Safety Objective Equation

The level of a microbial contaminant in a food at the point of consumption is related to (1) the initial level of that contaminant in the food, (2) the sum total of contaminant reductions occurring up to the point of consumption, and (3) the sum total of contaminant increases up to the point of consumption.

A simple equation summarizes the relationship between these three concepts and FSOs:

$$H_o - \sum R + \sum I \leq \text{FSO}$$

Here, FSO = Food Safety Objective, H_o = initial level of the hazard, $\sum R$ = cumulative (total) decrease (reduction expressed as positive) in the level of the hazard up to the point of consumption, and $\sum I$ = cumulative (total) increase in the level of the hazard up to the point of consumption.

It is very important to note that FSO, H_o, R, and I are expressed in $\log_{10}$ units, so if the initial level of a hazard is 100 cfu of a microorganism per gram of product, this is represented as $H_o = \log_{10} 100 = 2$. It also should be noted that controlling initial levels, preventing an increase in levels, and reducing levels of the hazard are all important in meeting the FSO, and that increases can occur from growth as well as from recontamination.

Hypothetical examples of FSOs are the following:

- The level of a potential bacterial pathogen in a certain food must not exceed *x* cfu/g at the time of consumption.
- The concentration of a certain enterotoxin in a certain food must not exceed *y* μg/100 g at the time of consumption.
- The concentration of a certain mycotoxin in a certain food must not exceed *z* μg/kg at the time of consumption.

Integrating Food Safety Objectives into the Food Safety Management System

The FSO is a new concept that builds on, rather than replaces, existing food safety terminology and concepts. FSOs have been discussed by a number of countries around the world, and internationally within Codex Alimentarius, specifically by the Codex Committee on Food Hygiene (Woteki, 2000).

ICMSF recently proposed an approach to food safety management that involves a series of seven steps that incorporate Codex Alimentarius principles (ICMSF, 2002). This approach, outlined below, integrates risk assessment and current hazard-management practices into a framework that could be used to achieve public health goals in a science-based, flexible manner. This approach also shows how FSOs relate to many existing food safety concepts:

1. Assemble epidemiological information indicating a need for improved control.
2. Conduct a qualitative or quantitative risk assessment, as appropriate.
3. Assess possible risk-management options, including an appropriate level of protection (ALOP).
4. Establish an FSO.
5. Confirm that the FSO is achievable through Good Hygienic Practices (GHP, GMP in the United States) and HACCP.
6. Establish process/product requirements.
7. Establish acceptance procedures.

Food Safety Objectives and Appropriate Level of Protection

The FSO concept was first introduced because of the difficulty in using public health goals (e.g., an ALOP) to establish control measures. An FSO is an intermediate step in the conversion of the ALOP into other parameters (i.e., performance standards) that can be controlled by food producers and monitored by government agencies. The ALOP is an expression of a public health risk—that is, the achieved or achievable level proposed following consideration of public health impact, technological feasibility, economic implications, and comparison with other risks in everyday life—while an FSO expresses the level of a hazard in relation to this risk.

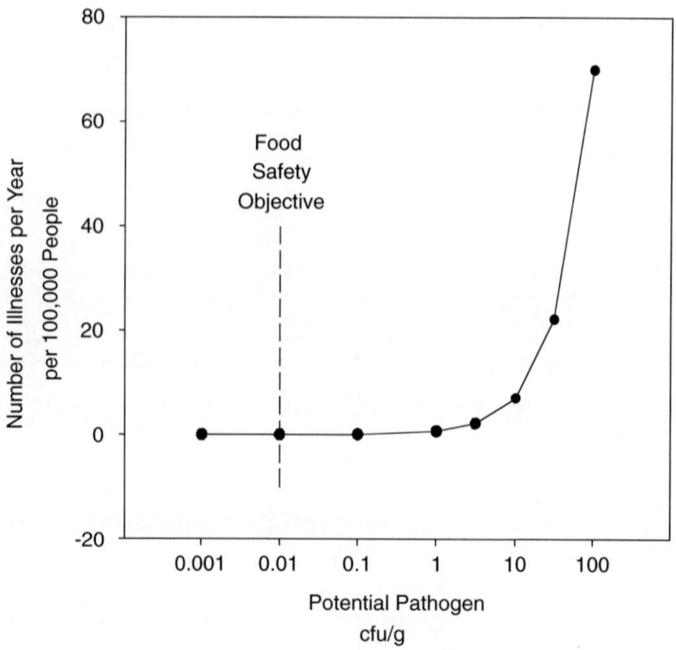

FIGURE 3.2 Relating a food safety objective and a hypothetical dose–response curve for a pathogen.

A hypothetical dose–response curve for a certain infectious pathogen is shown in Figure 3.2. In this figure, the estimated number of foodborne illness cases per 100,000 individuals increases as the concentration of the causative pathogen in the food exceeds 1 cfu/g. The FSO has been established at 100-fold less than this dose (i.e., 0.01 cfu/g at the time of consumption). This example could be representative for *E. coli* O157:H7 in products submitted to heat treatment or other processing steps.

Food Safety Objectives, Good Manufacturing Practices, Good Agricultural Practices, and HACCP

Once an FSO has translated a public health goal into a quantifiable standard, hazard control and monitoring practices must be developed. The ICMSF scheme recognizes that it is most effective to emphasize the design and control of food operations through the application of GHPs (or GMPs in the United States) and HACCP. However, it is important to note that other food safety concepts can be combined with this scheme to achieve the desired results in the farm-to-table approach to food safety; for example, implementing good agricultural practices may provide microbiologically safer foods.

GMPs, in turn, are important to minimize the hazard and prevent recontamination after processing. HACCP manages the application of control methods, ensuring that the process is effective.

As mentioned earlier, one of the long-standing limitations of HACCP is that the actual level of hazard control may not be clearly stated in the HACCP plan. Additionally, there is little or no guidance on the level of hazard control expected in an adequately designed and implemented HACCP plan. As is currently done with performance standards, use of the FSO concept could help remedy this problem by clearly indicating the level of control needed for adequate GMP and HACCP systems. Table 3.2 provides examples of how the FSO approach might be used to address a specific microbiological food safety issue.

Because the FSO must be met at the time of consumption, but regulatory action must take place at other locations in the food production and distribution chain, it may be necessary to introduce additional terms that represent various microbiological objectives throughout the food-processing chain. These examples might include slaughter safety objectives, processing safety objectives (analogous to the current *Salmonella* performance standard), transportation safety objectives, or retail safety objectives. For example, if the FSO is less than 100 cfu/g of a certain potential pathogen at the point of consumption and 1 $\log_{10}$ cycle of growth is projected during transportation, retail, and home storage, a hypothetical processing safety objective is calculated as no more than 10 cfu/g of the pathogen. Alternatively, if no growth of the pathogen is projected, the processing safety objective would be the same as the FSO. The processing safety objective can then be used to develop the performance and process/product criteria and to establish verification and acceptance procedures in the HACCP plan.

Food Safety Objectives and Performance Criteria or Standards

At certain points in the processing of a food, control measures can be applied to prevent an unacceptable increase in a hazard, eliminate it, or reduce it to an acceptable level. Each CCP must include parameters with defined critical limits. For example, pasteurization of milk at 72°C for 15 seconds inactivates recognized pathogens. Similar critical limits would define the degree of hazard control necessary to meet a processing safety objective (i.e., a performance standard) derived from an FSO. Process or product criteria, respectively, would define the process variables or product characteristics that will achieve the performance criteria or standard. Default criteria also play a very important role in the food safety system by providing one or more "safe harbor" sets of criteria (processes) for food operators lacking either the resources or the desire to develop a HACCP plan suited to their specific operation or product. Finally, microbiological criteria

TABLE 3.2 Framework for Food Safety Management

Action	Process
Formulate Public Health Goal to establish targets for improvement in the food safety system.	*Example:* Healthy People 2010 Objectives Reduce infections caused by key foodborne pathogens. Cases per 100,000 — 1997 Baseline — 2010 Target *Escherichia coli* O157:H7 — 2.1 — 1.0 *Salmonella* spp. — 13.7 — 6.8
Perform Risk Assessments (RAs) to apportion risk across food groups and estimate risk associated with various levels of contamination for specific foods.	Establish expert panels representing public health, regulatory agencies, industry, and academia to identify issues, available data sources, and knowledge gaps. Assemble scientific teams to conduct qualitative or quantitative RA and to develop surveillance and monitoring plans to address knowledge gaps.
Establish Food Safety Objectives (FSOs) for specific foods needed to reach public health goals given apportionment of risk across food groups.	Assemble scientific teams to establish FSOs for specific foods at the point of consumption, to develop monitoring plans for compliance with the FSOs, and to identify foods for which FSOs cannot be reasonably formulated due to the nature of the food.
Establish Transportation and Retail Safety Objectives (TRSOs) for specific foods needed toreach food safety objectives, orto reach public health goals in the absence of FSOs.	Assemble scientific teams to establish TRSOs for specific foods at the point of distribution or retail sale, to develop monitoring plans for compliance with the TRSOs, and to identify foods for which TRSOs cannot be reasonably formulated due to the nature of the food.
Establish Processing Safety Objectives (PSOs) for specific foods, needed alone or in combination with available TRSOs to reach food safety objectives, or to reach public health goals in the absence of FSOs.	Assemble scientific teams to establish PSOs for specific foods at the point of processing, to develop monitoring plans for compliance with the PSOs, and to identify foods for which PSOs cannot be reasonably formulated due to the nature of the food.
Establish Farm Safety Objectives (FarmSOs) for specific foods, needed alone or in combination with available PSOs and TRSOs to reach food safety objectives, or to reach public health goals in the absence of FSOs.	Assemble scientific teams to establish FarmSOs for specific foods at the point of production or harvest, to develop monitoring plans for compliance with the FarmSOs, and to identify foods for which FarmSOs cannot be reasonably formulated due to the nature of the food.

NOTE: This framework for food safety management establishes relationships between public health goals and measures or indicators of microbial contamination at each level of the food system from farm to table. The framework recognizes the wide variety of production, processing, and marketing practices that exist for different foods and can accommodate a range of different risk management options. The monitoring plans required for verifying compliance with the various Safety Objectives should be compatible with the development of Hazard Analysis and Critical Control Point systems, and will provide feedback for the periodic re-evaluation of the public health goals and the specific Safety Objectives needed to achieve these goals.
SOURCE: Adapted from IFT (2002).

and testing may be used to further verify that a processing safety objective has been met.

Examples Relating Performance Criteria to Food Safety Objectives

As many of these concepts are relatively new, there is clearly a need for further discussion relating to the terminology to be used in this area. The following examples show various ways in which FSOs can be related to performance criteria.

Example 1

Although FSOs should be quantitative and verifiable, this does not always imply that they must be verified by microbiological testing. For example, an FSO for low-acid canned foods could be established in terms of the probability of a viable spore of *C. botulinum* being present (< 0.000000001 per can). It is obviously impossible to verify this by end-product testing, and therefore it is done by measuring time/temperature protocols that are based on a performance criterion.

Example 2

A performance criterion could be used to limit recontamination and growth of a particular pathogen at any point after processing. Assume that the FSO for a certain potential pathogen in a food product is < 100 cfu/g (see Figure 3.3). Also assume that the greatest expected concentrations postslaughter and on arrival are both 1 cfu/g. If the heating step produces a 3-$\log_{10}$ reduction, the greatest expected concentration after heating will be 0.001 cfu/g or 1 cfu/1,000 g. The criterion (limit) for recontamination could be less than 0.1 cfu/g and the limit for growth could be less than a 3-$\log_{10}$ cfu/g increase, thereby meeting the FSO.

Example 3

In this example, the initial bacterial population (H_0) in the raw material is estimated to be as high as 10^3 cfu/g, but growth (I) can be prevented (e.g., $\Sigma I = 0$). The FSO is 1 cfu/100 g of product. The required performance criterion would be expressed as:

$$H_0 - \Sigma R + \Sigma I \leq \text{FSO}$$
$$3 - \Sigma R + 0 \leq -2$$
$$-\Sigma R \leq -5$$

Therefore, based on these calculations, the process must result in an overall reduction of greater than or equal to 5 $\log_{10}$ (i.e., 5-D reduction) to meet the FSO.

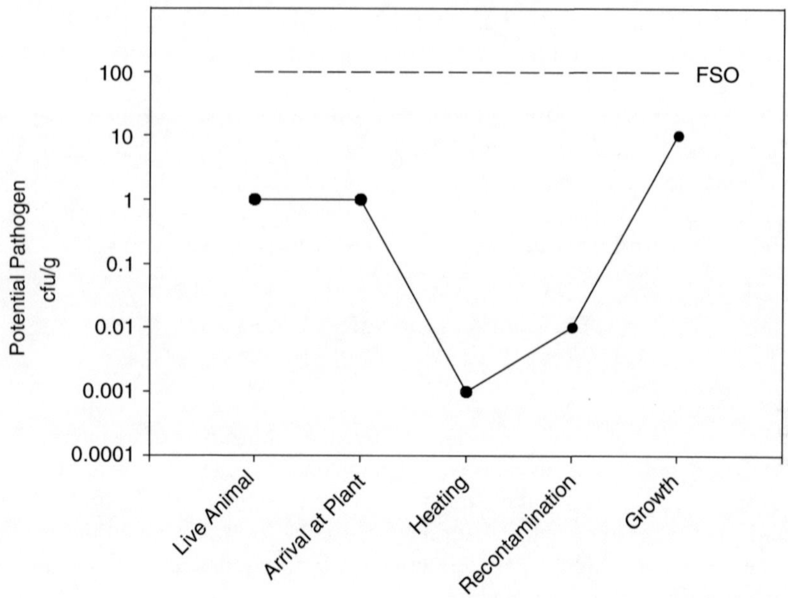

FIGURE 3.3 Relating a Food Safety Objective (FSO) and a performance criterion.

This corresponds to a performance criterion of a 5-D reduction of the pathogen and could be achieved by one control hurdle (measure) or a combination of hurdles.

Example 4

A 5-D reduction is currently required for the control of enteric pathogens such as salmonellae and *E. coli* O157:H7 for nonshelf-stable juice in the United States. It might be useful to consider what an appropriate FSO for such a product might be. If the initial level of salmonellae or *E. coli* O157:H7 could be as high as 100 cfu/mL of juice, then a 5-D reduction step theoretically would result in a level of 0.001 cfu/mL of juice or 0.1 cfu/100 mL of juice (100 mL is an assumed normal serving size). This would not be adequate to ensure the safety of the juice considering the total quantity of juice consumed on a daily basis by a diverse population of consumers, including some who may be at higher risk. The alternatives would be either to control the incoming juice to maintain a lower initial pathogen level or to apply a reduction step that would achieve greater than a 5-D reduction.

The question then is, "What level of microbial hazard would be considered tolerable for juice?" NACMCF (1997) has suggested that a level of ≤ 1 cfu of salmonellae or *E. coli* O157:H7 per 10 L of juice (≤ 1 cfu /10,000 mL or ≤ 0.00001 cfu/mL) would be considered adequate to provide an appropriate level of protection.

Returning to the FSO-based scheme for the management of food safety, an FSO for fresh juice could be expressed as: "The level of enteric pathogens, such as salmonellae and *E. coli* O157:H7, must not exceed 1 cfu/10 L of juice." This value should be considered when assessing the adequacy of a 5-D process and establishing control measures through the application of GMPs and HACCP.

When to Use Food Safety Objectives

On an Interim Basis

In the case of a new or emerging pathogen, establishment of an interim FSO could be an initial step to communicate to the food industry or to countries exporting food products to the United States the acceptable maximum level of a hazard. As further knowledge about the hazard, the food, and conditions leading to illness become available, and effective control measures can be determined, the interim FSO can be adjusted.

To Promote Industry Change

In the past, governments have used various mechanisms to bring about the changes necessary to reduce or eliminate the risk of disease. In some cases, modifications in commercial practices are necessary, including the adoption of new or more reliable technologies. These approaches are not inconsistent with the use of FSOs.

As is currently done with some performance standards, FSOs also could be used to promote change in an industry and enhance the safety of certain products. Many examples could be cited where epidemiological data have linked certain foods to foodborne illness. Government risk managers could use an FSO to communicate the level of control expected and thereby compel change on the part of the industry. A particular FSO may require some processors to modify their operation, implement more effective technologies, adopt tighter control systems, or even cease operation.

Limitations of Food Safety Objectives

FSOs are not a panacea, much in the way that HACCP, GMPs, novel processing technologies, or improved consumer education have not been able to solve all food safety problems. FSOs are simply the latest tool available in a growing food safety toolkit. There may be situations where FSOs are not appropriate. Such would be the case if the potential microbiological hazards associated with a food represent so little risk that an FSO is not needed (e.g., granulated sugar, most breads, carbonated drinks). In other cases, the sources of a pathogen are so variable that identifying the foods for which FSOs should be set is not possible. An example of the latter is shigellosis, which can be transmitted by many routes, many of which are more important than food (e.g., waterborne, person-to-person). Further, if a particular industry has been operating successfully for many years without FSOs, their introduction may offer no significant public health advantage. Examples of such industries include the pasteurized milk industry and the low-acid canned food industry.

The introduction of FSOs may lead to additional regulatory confusion, as FSOs for different products, developed at different points in time or by different expert groups, are compared. For example, if one set of FSOs were developed from the USDA *Salmonella* performance standard for raw meat and poultry—which allows some level of contamination—while another set of FSOs were developed from the FDA *Salmonella* performance standard for raw seafood—which does not allow any contamination—these two FSOs for the same pathogen in different products would be different.

There are also examples of foods recently regulated by performance standards, such as the 5-D process performance standard for fresh juice and the *Salmonella* performance standard for raw meat and poultry. It is reasonable to expect that both these performance standards have resulted (or will result) in improved public health, even though the interventions—at the processing plant—are separated in time and space from the effect—at the point of consumption. If these products were to be processed in ways that achieve an FSO, which is by definition at the point of consumption, this would introduce an additional layer of complexity.

Consider the following example with two fresh juice producers, both trying to meet a fresh juice FSO of ≤ 1 cfu of salmonellae or *E. coli* O157:H7 per 10 L of juice (≤ 1 cfu/10,000 mL, ≤ 0.00001 cfu/mL, or –4 $\log_{10}$ cfu/mL).

Juice producer 1: This producer squeezes the juice on site using tree-picked apples. Historical data collected by the processor over a number of years indicates that generic *E. coli* is occasionally present but always at levels of less than 10 cfu/mL (i.e., $H_o = \log_{10} = 1$). The pH of the juice is always 4.0 or below and he knows from published research that *E. coli* will not multiply in the juice at any storage temperature. The juicer applies a 5-D (i.e., $\Sigma R = 5$) thermal process.

$$H_o - \Sigma R + \Sigma I \leq -4$$
$$1 - (5) + 0 \leq -4$$

Juice producer 2: This juicer is producing a melon juice with a pH of 6.0. Although the juice is refrigerated, he has data demonstrating that, with temperature abuse (25°C), a maximum increase in *Salmonella* of 1 $\log_{10}$ (i.e., $\Sigma I = 1$) prior to spoilage of the product is possible. Historical data collected by the company over a number of years indicates that generic *E. coli* is occasionally present but always at levels of less than 100 cfu/mL (i.e., $H_o = \log_{10} 100 = 2$). He achieves a 7-$\log_{10}$ treatment using a 3-$\log_{10}$ thermal process combined with a 4-$\log_{10}$ ultraviolet treatment (i.e., $\Sigma R = 3 + 4 = 7$).

$$H_o - \Sigma R + \Sigma I \leq -4$$
$$2 - (3 + 4) + 1 \leq -4$$

While the net effect is identical, the additional complexity makes the regulatory verification of compliance significantly more difficult. The trade-offs between encouraging innovation and managing regulatory complexity will need to be evaluated carefully if FSOs are to be used successfully. Additional limitations to the rapid adoption of FSOs include the lack of definitive data on the initial level of the hazard (H_o) for many foods, and the lack of familiarity of many food-processing companies, particularly small- and medium-sized ones, with the FSO concept. Definitive instructions for food processors on what is needed to document achievement of an FSO are also lacking. The current situation regarding FSOs might be likened to that of HACCP 10 or 15 years ago.

Another limitation is that the measurements required to define whether an FSO is in fact working are rarely obtained directly. In order to validate or verify that a product meets an FSO or that overall progress has been achieved, the FSO needs to be linked to a contamination level in production, such as a processing safety objective, and that is where the level of contamination should be monitored. Government enforcement necessarily must focus on compliance at the level of production or retail sale because inspection is not possible literally at the point of consumption. One of the major benefits of the FSO concept is the flexibility it affords to producers to utilize different means of achieving the same ultimate level of food safety at the time of consumption. However, the practical need for government to measure compliance earlier in the product cycle than the point of consumption necessarily limits this flexibility.

FSOs may also be problematic because they introduce additional computational complexities and because the databases needed to calculate microbial concentrations at the point of consumption may not be adequate. For example, it is part of the definition of an FSO that it specifies pathogen concentrations at the point of consumption, yet very little data on pathogen concentrations at this point actually exist. Furthermore, the data on transportation, retail, and home storage and preparation practices needed to estimate pathogen concentration at the point of consumption are extremely limited and variable. Concentration at this point would typically be estimated using the techniques of QMRA described earlier, which introduces uncertainty and variability with every calculation. When all of the sources of variation are included in calculations of pathogen concentrations at the point of consumption, the overall range of possible concentrations can be quite large. Improvements in data quantity and quality may be needed to calculate useful estimates of expected FSOs.

In summary, the FSO concept may prove useful to both regulatory authorities and the food industry. FSOs could help to:

- Translate a public health goal into a measurable level of control upon which food processes can be designed.
- Validate food-processing operations to ensure that they will meet the expected level of control.
- Assess the acceptability of a food operation by regulatory authorities or other auditors.
- Highlight food safety concerns as separate from quality and other concerns.
- Compel change on the part of the food industry to improve the safety of a particular food commodity.
- Serve as the basis for establishing microbiological criteria for individual lots or consignments of food when the source or conditions of manufacture are uncertain.

To be used successfully, FSOs must:

- Be used only where appropriate.
- Be based on definitive data on the initial level of the hazard and be supported by sufficient data on transportation, retail, and home storage and preparation practices.
- Become familiar to food companies of all sizes.
- Include definitive instructions for food processors on what is needed to document achievement.
- Gain acceptance from the public, consumer organizations, and the public health community as a method to ensure safer food.

STRATEGIES FOR DEVELOPING CRITERIA AND PERFORMANCE STANDARDS

There are several strategies a regulatory agency can use to develop regulations, and care must be used in selecting the proper one to maximize the efficacy of food safety regulations. This procedure should be a transparent process in the gathering and analysis of data and in the development of the regulations. This section identifies some benefits and limitations of basic statistical approaches that may be used in developing food safety criteria and standards.

Food regulation should always be based on science. The President's Council on Food Safety, which was established in 1998 (E.O. 13040, 1998), directed regulatory agencies to use science-based approaches to develop new regulations. Therefore, a science-based approach must be used also in developing performance standards.

Depending on the quality of the data that are available or that can be generated in a pilot study, the committee defines a science-based approach as using one of the following strategies:

1. A statistically valid, controlled study in the laboratory or field, which might include risk assessment modeling (laboratory-based strategy).
2. The expertise and derived opinions from the best understanding of risk assessment, pathogenesis, and current food-processing techniques (expertise-based strategy).
3. A combination of a controlled study and expertise (combination strategy).

These strategies should not be seen as separate and individual, but as a continuum of a science-based approach. Each one has benefits and limitations, and lack of time is one limitation that recurs in the development of new regulations because many regulations are developed in response to a crisis. The actual approach will be dependent on the quality of data that are available or that can be generated through a pilot program or modeling approach. In most cases, strategy three (combination approach) presents the most effective and practical strategy to develop performance criteria. To improve the process of developing regulations, it is important to understand the limitations of each approach and select the best one.

Strategies to Develop Food Safety Criteria, Including Performance Standards

Laboratory-Based Strategy

A statistically valid, controlled-study strategy to develop regulations is one that applies the pure scientific method to develop regulations. An example of this strategy is the design and data analysis in standard laboratory experiments. This strategy can be summarized as follows:

1. Development of a hypothesis.
2. Design of a study (laboratory or field) to test the hypothesis.
3. Analysis of the results using appropriate statistical methods (such as analysis of variance) and use of these statistical results to determine if the hypothesis is accepted or rejected.

After these steps are followed, regulations may be developed on the basis of whether the hypothesis is accepted or rejected.

For efficiency in conducting a study, scientists study a sample of behavior or product and then generalize the results to the entire population or phenomenon. The following assumptions must be met to ensure validity of the statistical methods used to analyze the data from the study and apply the results to the entire population (Steel et al., 1997):

- The variation (either measured as standard deviation or variance) must be constant.
- There must be a defined population from which a sample can be selected.
- The sample size is a function of the standard deviation. The larger the standard deviation, the larger the sample size.
- The sampling method must assure a random sample.

When all of these criteria are met, it is possible to calculate the necessary statistics with a mathematically defined probability and known confidence, and then analyze the results. These statistics will define a probability that the hypothesis is correct at a known confidence level—a statistic that provides the experimenter with the probability that the answer is correct. In addition to the requirements stated above, if the data collected in the study are going to be extrapolated either beyond the population or into the future, the mean and the variation must remain stable and predictable over the period of time of the extrapolation.

If any of the requirements listed above is not met, numerical values can still be calculated; however, it is not possible either to accurately estimate the probability level or to determine the confidence level of the statistical data and resulting outcome. It can be safe to assume that most experiments conducted never meet all of the criteria and thus regulatory agencies must use some expertise in evaluating the results. Furthermore, the committee feels that there are probably no clear-cut examples of food safety regulations created under the strictest sense of the statistically valid, controlled study strategy as described. The greater the violation of the statistical criteria, the greater the likelihood that the statistics do not represent either the population or the sample. Such data, collected in a laboratory under a controlled environment, can still be used to develop regulations provided statistical gaps in the data are filled with scientific knowledge and derived scientific expert opinions. However, limitations exist if the pure science-based strategy is applied to the development of regulations to govern the food-processing industry. During the development of regulations, the actual laboratory is the field, and because of limited time and resources, there is often not enough data gathered to ensure statistical accuracy with a known certainty. In addition, it is not known whether the mean and standard deviation of the performance standard or criterion that is measured will remain stable over the period of time the regulation is enforced.

Thus, it is not possible for regulatory agencies to rely solely upon the statistically valid, controlled study strategy, as described above, to develop regulations. There will always be gaps in the knowledge, with subsequent gaps in the experimental design. In response to these gaps, the regulatory agencies must use expert knowledge to satisfy assumptions and develop knowledge bases.

Expert-Based Strategy

This approach can best be described as exclusively using expert opinions to develop the new regulation or performance standard, and this can be depicted in the following way: a group with broad-ranging expertise on a given food product, including regulators and outside experts, comes together, deliberates, and develops the performance standard or regulation. In this manner, the performance standard is developed using only the scientific-based expert knowledge present during the deliberations.

As with other strategies, this process has a number of limitations. First, the standard will be only as good as the knowledge of the experts who are gathered to develop the standard. Sccond, although experts may have an excellent knowledge of the situation, rarely do they have all of the needed knowledge to develop a robust performance standard. Therefore, the experts will have to fill in the knowledge gaps with assumptions, including how the regulation will perform in the future. Third, each expert works within a personal and professional paradigm. These are difficulties associated with the expertise-based method if the new standard requires a novel approach. Thus, if the standard requires thinking beyond the conventional framework and all of the participating experts have the same professional paradigm, it is likely that the expert group will not be able to develop an effective standard that is valid beyond that framework. In addition, if the assumptions change or if one assumption is slightly incorrect, a poor performance standard will result. (A poor performance standard can be defined as either not being effective in meeting the public health objective or generating a needless economic burden to one or more sectors of the food system.) A fourth limitation of this strategy is that the process is rarely transparent to the public, which may then question the validity of the performance standard.

The advantage of the expert-based strategy is that it requires the use of a minimal amount of resources such as time, money, and personnel. Therefore, regulations may be developed rapidly in response to a public health crisis.

In summary, although regulations derived exclusively using expert opinions require minimal resources, their success depends highly on the expert knowledge used to develop them.

Combination Strategy

The combination strategy uses both the laboratory-based and the expert-based strategies. It is a hybrid that includes the strengths of both strategies, while minimizing their weaknesses. Regulatory agencies must strive to develop regulations using the best available data. The general precept is that the more data (laboratory-based), the better; however, assumptions will always be made because rarely or never will there be enough appropriate data available to fully develop a regulation. Assumptions will need to be made using expert opinion. Consequently, this approach recognizes that expert knowledge will always be used to fill in the data and knowledge gaps. Currently, this approach is being used to some extent by regulatory agencies in developing new regulations and performance standards; for example, FSIS is using it in developing the performance standards for the HACCP-Based Inspection Models Project (HIMP) (FSIS, 2001). This approach is needed because it is impossible for a regulatory agency to utilize a pure laboratory-based approach in developing a regulation for the field.

The committee concludes that the combination strategy provides an appropriate means for managing food safety risks. Regulations must be developed in a timely manner by using the best available data—reflecting the pure laboratory-based approach—while taking into account that it is impossible to fill all data gaps without expert judgment—reflecting the use of expert-based knowledge. However, the committee recommends that when limitations in data occur, regulatory agencies should document these limitations and the assumptions used to fill in the data gaps, and make this information available to the public (reflecting a solid expert-based strategy). This process should include active involvement of the best scientists in the field. This can be accomplished through existing advisory committees or convening a temporary advisory committee to address the specific issue. Therefore, the following process should be used to develop regulations:

1. **Clearly document the public health objective and the appropriate level of protection.**
2. **Obtain or generate the best scientific knowledge through the use of laboratory or field studies, risk assessments, and similar food safety tools.**
3. **Minimize the amount of knowledge gaps by either conducting pilot programs of the proposed performance standard or by maintaining databases of critical information that can be used to develop performance standards, and including science-based expertise if necessary.**
4. **Explicitly state the nature, limits, and extent of the scientific uncertainties.**
5. **Explicitly identify the assumptions, criteria, and expertise used to address the uncertainties in formulating the performance standard.**

This process would have a high degree of transparency and would provide an appropriate strategy to establish a regulation in a timely manner.

Several dilemmas may be encountered during the development of regulations. For example, although the development of scientific knowledge is accelerating, corresponding advances in new technology development to either prevent or reduce the likelihood of a food safety hazard from occurring lag behind. In addition, the regulatory environment is such that it is exceedingly costly and time-consuming for the food safety regulatory agencies to implement new and innovative regulatory strategies to reduce the risk of foodborne illness. Once regulations are finalized, modifying them is time consuming and tedious. In addition, approval of new technologies for controlling pathogens (e.g., an additive or a new method for killing or reducing the numbers of a pathogen) is a very slow process.

To remedy this lack of flexibility and as previously recommended in the National Academies report, *Ensuring Safe Food from Production to Consumption* (IOM/NRC, 1998), Congress should grant the regulatory agencies the legal authority to develop, and the administrative process flexibility to update, food safety criteria, including performance standards. This flexibility includes incorporating new processing or assessment techniques and allowing the agencies the ability to improve a performance standard to align it with the best contemporary scientific knowledge.

Appropriate Data for Developing Performance Standards

Another dilemma that may be encountered during the development of regulations is that regulatory agencies, by mandate, must use a science-based approach (Presidents Council on Food Safety, E.O. 13100, 1998), and must usually do so within a very short time frame. Unfortunately, it normally takes time, in addition to other resources, to collect the appropriate data to make scientific decisions. One way to overcome this dilemma is to develop and maintain databases on critical information.

Regulatory agencies can develop and maintain databases on the prevalence of specific contaminants for critical commodities (e.g., ground meat). In addition, regulators can conduct or fund pilot studies to collect appropriate data if these data are not available. (Chapter 4 describes the particular need and justifications to maintain current databases on the major animal species that supply the majority of the meat consumed in the United States.) In addition to maintaining these databases, regulatory agencies must continually analyze these data using basic time series analysis (e.g., control charts, histograms, and capability analysis). Congress, in turn, should provide adequate resources to develop and maintain these databases.

Pilot studies are the preferred method for gathering the appropriate data to develop science-based regulations because they are designed to provide the specific data needed to develop a new regulation. A study of this type was conducted as part of the HIMP project (FSIS, 2001). In contrast, data analysis problems were identified when an old database was used to justify establishing a performance standard for stabilization of ready-to-eat meat (FSIS, 1998). Chapter 4 provides details of the analysis used to develop this performance standard.

Once the appropriate data are available through pilot studies or databases, there are two ways to proceed in developing a performance standard, depending on the desired outcome. The first assumes that all food-processing companies would be complying, that is, producing food of a predetermined acceptable level. If this strategy is used, the performance standard should be set at a level such that the lowest compliant processor will pass, while all of the noncompliant plants will fail. A second way is to set the performance standard at a level where only a portion of the plants will pass. This strategy is used to allow the regulatory agency to raise the bar of what is classified as acceptable performance. An example of the latter strategy was used in developing the HIMP performance standards, which were set at the 75th percentile of the plants that participated in the pilot study (FSIS, 2001). When this strategy is used, the regulatory agency must balance the benefits of raising the bar to meet the nation's public health goals with the economic consequences of strengthening the performance standard. Furthermore, flexibility must be incorporated into the development of performance standards so that the regulatory agencies may adjust a performance standard to meet future public health goals; that is, the regulatory structure should allow for review process flexibility.

In the absence of appropriate data or when only limited data are available, the only way to set a performance standard is to build in a safety factor of sufficient magnitude to ensure that any current or future process variation is of no public health significance. Such a safety factor may force the food processor to overprocess (e.g., cook excessively) a product to ensure that the performance standard is met, and thus may have a negative effect on the product. An example of this type of performance standard is the 12-D reduction of *C. botulinum* for low-acid canned foods (Karel et al., 1975).

STATISTICAL TOOLS TO VERIFY PROCESS STABILITY AND CAPABILITY

Manufacturing processes tend to vary over time. For example, in a canning operation, the temperature of the retort may vary by a degree or two from the target temperature. In a chicken processing operation, in turn, the weight of a dressed carcass can vary by as much as 20 percent. To assure that the outcome of the processing operation is predictable, it is critical for both processors and regulators to understand whether this variation is predictable or not. (Statistical Process Control [SPC] terminology uses the term "common causes of variation" when processes show only predictable variation, and the terms "special causes of variation" or "assignable causes of variation" when the process shows nonpredictable variation.)

Food-processing regulations should require that food processors and regulatory agencies analyze performance data to assure that the variation is stable. This can be done by using simple time-series analyses such as control charts, histograms, and process capability analysis, which are all tools to measure the stability of variation.

Capability indices are statistical calculations that relate the performance standard with both the amount of product variation and the relation of the process mean to the performance standard. There are three major types of performance indices: C_{pk}, C_{pl}, and C_{pu}. These indices provide the regulatory agency with information to determine if the food processor has the capability of meeting the performance standard. The C_{pk} is calculated when there is both a maximum and a minimum limit specification (i.e., performance standard); the C_{pu} is calculated when a performance standard has only an upper limit; and the C_{pl} is calculated when a performance standard has only a lower limit. SPC texts written by Kane (1989), Bothe (2001), and Montgomery (2001) provide details on the use and calculations of these indices. The indices provide a science-based approach for processors to demonstrate compliance with the performance standard and capability of their process, and for the regulatory agency to monitor such compliance.

SPC is a very robust scientific analysis that uses control charts and capability analysis to monitor process performance. When using SPC, all the tests that monitor the manufacturing process are linked into an appropriate process control plan that includes control charts, a simple but effective form of time series analysis. The charts are designed to measure process variation over time and to verify that the variation is stable and predictable. An example of the use of control charts in determining regulatory compliance is the current Pathogen Reduction (PR)/HACCP regulation in which the food processor has the choice of reporting generic *E. coli* carcass data either on a control chart or in tabular form (FSIS, 1996).

SPC processes are easy to audit by a trained investigator, which enables efficient regulatory oversight. In addition, it is difficult to falsify analytical data gathered through an appropriately designed system based on SPC, for the same analytical techniques that are used to control the process can be used by regulatory agencies to determine if the data accurately described the production process and, therefore, the safety of the product. SPC provides the signals that processors need to effectively improve their processes. Continuous improvement is a strategy that focuses on using a systematic process to identify and remove the root causes of variation in products and critical processes.

The international community recognizes the importance of continuous improvement as part of a quality management system. Section 8.5 of ISO 9001:2000 (Ketola and Roberts, 2001) requires that "organizations that are compliant to the standard must have a process that continually improves the quality management system." Continuous improvement is interpreted as both incremental improvements (small continuous improvement accomplishments) and breakthrough improvements (large, technology-driven improvement gains). Thus, it has been widely recognized that an effective SPC program must be linked to an effective continuous improvement program. Kume (1985) described a number of simple statistical tools that can be used to continuously improve manufacturing processes.

An example may help illustrate these concepts. Suppose a processor, to eliminate or reduce the population of a pathogen, is required to heat each unit of food product to *x* temperature and hold it at that temperature for *y* minutes. To assure the safety of each unit, the processor must plan to heat all units to a somewhat higher temperature to ensure that, with normal variation, no individual unit falls below that temperature. Using SPC techniques, the processor can map the variations in the process, thereby determining the optimal temperature at which to operate. It is in the processor's interest to minimize the amount of variation, because that will save energy costs and will also produce a more consistent product as no unit would be subjected to more heat than that necessary to ensure that each unit is adequately heated. If the process variation is $\pm 3°$ and an adjustment of the cooking equipment could reduce that variation to $\pm 1°$, the processor could save money and deliver better products by investing in such an adjustment. This is an example of continuous improvement.

The use of SPC linked to continuous improvement creates a situation where all involved parties—consumer, regulatory agencies, and industry—benefit: consumers will have safer food, industry will have lower production costs, and regulatory agencies will observe better regulatory compliance. It provides a logical, methodical way to establish process stability and capability analysis that is economically efficient for industry and is easy to review. In addition to its potential for facilitating regulatory compliance, the systematic, continuous process improvement focuses on eliminating the causes of foodborne disease and thus contributes to enhancement of food safety. Moreover, the actions taken to reduce a foodborne hazard will usually reduce waste and decrease product rework or loss in the plant, thus reducing production costs. It is generally believed that if a company does not have an active systematic continuous improvement process, the projected cost attributed to poor quality is at least 20 percent of the sales dollar amount (Breyfogle et al., 2001).

Therefore, food safety regulations should incorporate the concepts of SPC linked to continuous improvement, and require that food processors analyze and maintain records to ensure that their processes exhibit (1) stable and predictable variation (rather than unpredictable variation) and (2) are capable of meeting performance standards.

The regulatory agencies, in turn, must ensure that their professional staff assigned to either inspecting or auditing food-processing plants are appropriately trained so that they can determine if a processing plant is properly using SPC techniques to monitor performance standards and whether the plant is capable of meeting the performance standards.

Statistical Process Control: A Science-Based Approach to Ensure Regulatory Compliance

There are two methods by which food processors and regulators can determine conformance to a performance standard. The first method is to inspect either 100 percent of the product or a sample of the product. The second method is to rely on SPC. This section provides an overview of process control and process control as a tool for use in ensuring food safety, including a comparison between process control methods and the traditional inspection method used to verify compliance with food safety criteria and standards. This section does not cover in detail the statistical nuances of process control, an understanding of which, however, is required for proper development and implementation of SPC and continuous improvement procedures in the plant, and for the incorporation of SPC principles in regulations. Interested readers should refer to the numerous texts that have been published on the subject (Kane, 1989; Kume, 1985; Montgomery, 2001; Wheeler and Chambers, 1992).

Inspection

Inspection may be conducted on 100 percent of products or on a sample of the products. Neither strategy is practical or effective. One hundred percent inspection cannot guarantee that the product either meets specifications or is safe because no inspection technique is perfect (Konz et al., 1981). Many inspection techniques for food safety require the use of a destructive test. For example, if one wanted to use 100 percent inspection to ensure that all milk in a specific lot is free of pathogens, the only way this could be accomplished would be to open each container of milk, thus breaking the seal, remove a portion of the milk for microbiological analysis, conduct the analysis, and report the results. If this procedure were used, no package of milk tested would be acceptable for sale to the public.

An example of the ineffectiveness of 100 percent inspection was documented by the Research Triangle Institute (RTI) when conducting the baseline study for HIMP (RTI, 2000). RTI conducted a study that measured the effectiveness of the traditional inspection process used in poultry slaughter facilities. In this process, 100 percent of the chicken carcasses are inspected by an FSIS official to determine whether food safety defects or other consumer protection defects are present. RTI found that even after the FSIS inspector step, 1.9 percent of the carcasses contained a food safety defect or fecal contamination. In addition, a larger number of carcasses contained "Other Consumer Protection" (OCP) defects such as ingesta (13.8 percent), sores and scabs (16.0 percent), or pathological lesions (1.3 percent). The carcasses that contained OCP defects should have been removed from the line and reworked to remove the unacceptable tissue. In addition, RTI found that 12 percent of the carcasses that were condemned did not have either a food safety or OCP defect and thus should not have been condemned.

Because 100 percent inspection is often impossible, food processors and regulators instead use sampling techniques. In this method, a sample of the product is obtained and analyzed, and the test results are used to determine if the entire production lot is acceptable or unacceptable. This approach is called acceptance sampling.

Acceptance sampling assumes that the product characteristic that is being measured exhibits relatively stable variation or consistent variation within the lot. Thus, even using a true random sampling technique, acceptance sampling procedures are not designed to identify "hot spots" (i.e., when microorganisms or toxins are concentrated in a very small portion of the lot), sporadic food safety hazards, or food hazards that occur at very low levels in a production lot (like many microbial foodborne hazards).

The following example illustrates how acceptance sampling may be used to test for product safety when the hazard appears at a very low level. A person may need to know how many eggs must be sampled from a lot to be reasonably confident that the lot is not contaminated with *S.* Enteritidis. It can be assumed that the level of *S.* Enteritidis contamination in eggs is 1 egg in 20,000 (*Salmonella* Enteritidis Risk Assessment Team, 1998). An acceptable guideline to determine the sample size is to take a sample large enough that there is a chance that 8 contaminated eggs will be selected (LSRO, 1995); this guideline gives the investigator statistical confidence in the results of the test. Thus, the individual would have to sample 160,000 eggs and test them using an analytical method sensitive enough to detect one *S.* Enteritidis cell per egg. Obviously, a sample size of 160,000 eggs corresponds to a very large testing rate and is not practical in the food-processing industry. This sample size is independent of the size of the lot. Therefore, if the lot contained 120,000 eggs, each egg would have to be sampled and destroyed, making this sampling system very expensive; the cost to sample and analyze this number of eggs would be in excess of several million dollars and there would be no eggs left to sell at the end of testing.

When it is not possible to inspect 100 percent of a production lot, regulatory agencies may establish statistical criteria as an indication of the acceptable level of control of a potential food hazard. An example of this is the low-acid canned food performance standard, which requires an intervention capable of reducing the population of *C. botulinum* by 12 $\log_{10}$ in the final product (Karel et al., 1975).

Process Control

Process control is based on four premises: (1) product quality or product safety must be built into the manufacturing process, (2) the manufacturing process must be monitored and the data must be analyzed using appropriate measurement and statistical techniques, (3) the process must be managed to ensure its variation remains stable and predictable, and (4) the process is capable of delivering product that meets the performance standard. As described earlier, SPC relies on the appropriate generation and analysis of data by using control charts, histograms, and capability studies (Kane, 1989; Montgomery, 2001). When this is done, the data can be used to predict the performance of a process and the safety of a product.

SPC is the combination of these analytical procedures and it allows for the following assumption to be made: if the process exhibits stable variation or if the process is in statistical control, it will result in a product within a set of mathematically defined, predetermined limits. These limits are known as control chart limits and are calculated from process or product data. The control limits cannot be set by expert opinion.

Process Variation, Stability, and Capability

Control charts are used to determine if the variation of the process or product is predictable (stable variation) or nonpredictable (nonstable variation). When the variation is stable, the process is said to be in statistical control. If a process is in statistical control, it is possible to determine whether the process is capable of meeting performance standards by using process capability analysis. Then, if the process is found to be both capable and in statistical control, end-product inspection may become unnecessary.

On the other hand, if a process is not in statistical control, it is not possible to statistically determine the extent of the variation of the product or whether the product will meet a performance standard. To ensure product safety in this case, a very conservative performance standard must be developed, namely one that has a very large safety factor (which, as discussed earlier, may have a negative impact on the product).

If the process is not in statistical control, the food processor must take appropriate action to identify the causes of the problem (called in the literature "assignable causes") and eliminate them (Kane, 1989; Kume 1985). When properly designed, these actions can be taken in advance so that the risk of producing unsafe products is minimized. Regulatory agencies, in turn, need to monitor food processors to ensure that this task has been accomplished.

Therefore, SPC can be used to show process stability and, once the process is in statistical control, to show whether the process is capable of meeting a performance standard. A number of texts on SPC provide the details on creating control charts and evaluating the stability of a process (ASTM, 1976; Montgomery, 2001; Wheeler and Chambers, 1992).

The stability of a process is paramount in determining whether a process is in statistical control. Capability analysis, in turn, provides a statistical tool to determine if a process that is in statistical control can deliver product that meets the performance standard.

It must be noted that SPC requires conducting appropriate tests or measurements to predict the performance of a product. (These tests must show a correlation between process performance and specific product attributes.) If process variables measurable on the processing line do not exist for a particular process, then standard tests (microbiological or other) are necessary for process control evaluation and should be used as measures of performance. The results of these tests can then be used in control charts and capability analysis to evaluate process control. Control charts are used to demonstrate that a manufacturer has maintained control of the process. Histograms and capability indices are used to demonstrate that the product meets the performance standards.

The committee recommends that performance standards incorporate the analysis of appropriate data on process and product characteristics using SPC, and that the regulatory agencies define what constitutes the minimal acceptable process capability. In addition, it is recommended that performance standards link the SPC requirement to continuous improvement.

Examples of Other Process Control Approaches

Other methods may be appropriate to assure control of food-manufacturing processes. These control strategies include automation, education and training, procedures and check sheets, checks on incoming product quality (raw input acceptance sampling), or a combination of these. An automated process control has been used successfully in assuring that milk is properly pasteurized in accordance with the pasteurized milk ordinance (FDA, 1999b). Measuring and controlling a process parameter (i.e., temperature/time) using an electronic feedback control system accomplishes this objective (e.g., safe milk).

Another example is the combined set of process control strategies that has been successfully incorporated into the low-acid canned food regulations (21 C.F.R. part 114). The following is a summary of this process control strategy:

1. The processor determines the critical measures for the process.
2. The processor validates the thermal process.
3. The product is processed in accordance with the validated process.
4. The critical parameters are monitored.
5. The food processor verifies that the process was conducted in accordance with the validated process.

When all of the above steps are properly carried out, FDA declares that the low-acid canned food is safe and no final product testing is necessary to determine if *C. botulinum* is present (Gavin and Weddig, 1995).

The development of the Juice HACCP Final Rule is another example of a science-based approach that used both expert opinion and statistical studies to determine a sampling plan that provided the basis for the rule (the aforementioned combination strategy). One of the rule's supporting documents referencing the generic *E. coli* levels most likely to be found in juice states: "Data in this area are limited so certain assumptions were made" (Garthright et al., 2002). At the time the rule was being developed, there were no laboratory data that could substantiate the levels of *E. coli* O157:H7 that were found in juice. In the absence of such data, several assumptions had to be made using the best available expertise (expert-based strategy) of NACMCF. The resulting requirement of a 5-D reduction in pathogen numbers was a consensus value arrived at by NACMCF after reviewing comments received from the public (Personal communication, W. Garthright, Center for Food Safety and Applied Nutrition, FDA, October 2002).

In addition to the 5-D pathogen reduction performance standard subsequently established by FDA, producers of raw citrus juices that use surface decontamination to achieve the standard must conduct end-product testing to ensure that generic *E. coli* is absent. To this effect, a sampling protocol to be implemented by processors as part of their HACCP plan was developed. The two issues central to the sampling plan were sample size and testing window. The sample size for juice was determined to be 20 mL for each 1,000 gal of juice produced or, if the processor produces less than 1,000 gal in 5 days, a 20-mL sample must be taken every 5 days. This sampling procedure was developed using computer simulation techniques (Personal communication, W. Garthright, Center for Food Safety and Applied Nutrition, FDA, October 2002; Garthright et al., 2002), which is a science-based mathematical approach.

The next step in the development of this performance standard was the design of a sampling plan that would ensure absence of generic *E. coli*. An evaluation problem occurs in developing a performance standard when the variable to be tested, such as the presence of generic *E. coli* in juice, rarely occurs in the product, and yet the processor must determine whether there is a failure in its HACCP plan. A solution to this problem is to analyze the data using the moving window technique, which requires counting the number of positive samples within a specific time frame. FDA set the juice performance standard at no more than one generic *E. coli*-positive sample in any consecutive seven samples. If two or more samples test positive, FDA considers that there is a loss of process control and immediate corrective actions are necessary (FDA, 2001). FDA validated these statistics by means of a mathematical technique known as Monte Carlo Simulation that is used in many industrial analysis situations (Law and Kelton, 2000).

This example demonstrates the successful use of the combination strategy in developing a regulation. FDA used a combination of the best science-based expert opinion (expert-based strategy) and mathematical studies (laboratory-based strategy) to develop the sampling plan for the Juice HACCP Final Rule; however, the process could have benefited from more transparency regarding access to information on the assumptions that were made. The document stated that "as additional data become available, the agency [FDA] will consider those data and propose adjustments to the HACCP regulation and to the juice hazards guide as necessary" (FDA, 2001). The committee commends FDA's willingness to consider adjustments to performance standards as data become available, and recommends that the food safety regulatory agencies routinely conduct periodic, mandatory reviews of all performance standards.

Collecting the Appropriate Data

Any performance standard requires that monitoring and/or testing be conducted on the process or product. Ensuring that the monitoring and testing methods are validated and deliver the best data is essential when developing standards or verifying processes.

This need for adequate data is recognized at the international level and has brought about the development of international norms that describe standard and approved analytical techniques and GLPs (Singer, 2001). These principles require that a number of critical issues be addressed and controlled to ensure good analytical results, including sample collection, storage, and analysis; data management (collection, storage, analysis, and reporting); laboratory and testing facilities; calibration of equipment; and training of personnel. It is also critical that the proper test methods (i.e., having adequate specificity, sensitivity, precision, accuracy, and reproducibility) be used. This is ensured through validation of sampling and testing methods. Details on the application of GLPs are described in texts such as that by Singer (2001) and in federal regulations (40 C.F.R. §160.1).

When zero tolerance is used as a performance standard (see Chapter 1), unique methodology issues need to be considered. The concept of a zero tolerance performance standard is inextricably linked to the sensitivity of the method employed to detect the offending hazard, as well as the sampling strategy employed. Sampling protocols must take into account that a large sample is needed to ensure the absence of the hazard; also, the sample must be representative of the material being tested. The level that can be detected is a function of the sensitivity of the method as well as of the sample volume.

An assay's limit of quantitation and limit of detection are defined on the basis of measured performance of the specific assay being used and on agreed statistical criteria. When zero tolerance is applied in this context, zero is operationally defined as the limit of detection applied to the specific sample. It must be stressed that the hazard, be it chemical, microbial, or other, may still be present in the sample but not be detectable with the assay method being used. The limit of detection is a function of the precision of the analytical methodology.

In conclusion, regulatory agencies should use a science-based approach both to develop regulations and to measure compliance. Performance standards need to be based on appropriate data, to be possible to implement, and to be linked to public health objectives. This approach will require that the regulatory agencies use well-defined and current databases and/or conduct pilot studies. When data are limited, regulatory agencies need to make assumptions to fill any gaps. Subject-matter experts, using the best available knowledge, should make these assumptions. During the development of performance standards, regulatory agencies need to use a transparent process that publicly reports the data used, the statistical methods used to analyze the data, and the assumptions made to fill any data gaps.

The committee recommends that regulatory agencies adopt a transparent approach that uses a combination of controlled studies and expertise to develop science-based food safety criteria, including performance standards. Similarly, for flexibility, the periodic evaluation and updating of performance standards by the regulatory agencies is highly recommended by the committee.

The committee recognizes the value of SPC as a scientific method that can be used to (1) verify the control of a food-processing system, (2) provide a source of information to the food processor for properly controlling the manufacturing process, and (3) provide information that can be used to critically examine the food-processing system so that appropriate actions can be taken to reduce the likelihood of manufacturing unsafe food products. The committee also recognizes the potential benefit that could be derived from the use of SPC principles linked to continuous improvement by food processors, to continually reduce the risk of producing unsafe food products, and possibly also to reduce production costs. In addition, the committee concludes that the most effective procedure to determine whether a food processor is complying with a performance standard is to analyze process and product data using control charts, histograms, and process capability indices; therefore, the committee believes that SPC, linked to continuous improvement, provides a very robust methodology that is easy to monitor from a regulatory perspective.

Accordingly, the committee recommends the adoption by food processors of SPC principles linked to continuous improvement, as well as incorporation of such principles by the regulatory agencies into food safety regulations and into the agencies' compliance monitoring procedures.

THE ECONOMICS OF FOOD SAFETY CRITERIA

Any evaluation of food safety criteria needs to consider the costs and benefits incurred by government, companies, and consumers as a result of the regulation. Proposed new regulations are required to include a Regulatory Impact Assessment to evaluate their costs and benefits. Consequently, the charge to the committee included a request to examine the economics of food safety criteria. This section compares the effectiveness, efficiency, and equity of two broad sets of not-always mutually exclusive tools: process criteria and performance standards.

When regulation is deemed necessary, a target level (such as a performance standard) provides companies with flexibility in the manner of compliance. Surprisingly, however, the application of food safety policies based on this approach has become fashionable only over the last decade or so. Prior to this period, command-and-control or process criteria were more commonly adopted.

Effectiveness

Key questions that must be asked when evaluating the economics of food safety criteria include: Can a performance or process criterion be constructed to exactly fit with the stated aim? Because food safety regulations can be explicitly stated in terms of their quantitative public health goals (e.g., reduction in illnesses due to a particular foodborne pathogen by 10 percent over a number of years), is one form of criterion more naturally fitted to this goal than another? How can the effectiveness of a regulation be assessed once in place? Indirect and direct measures of effectiveness are being collected to assess risk reductions achieved by food safety policies, including performance standards. Examples include trends in foodborne illnesses and microbial sampling results, as described in Chapter 2. However, as stated earlier in the present chapter, without an understanding of attributable risk and clear links between hazard reductions at one particular stage (e.g., slaughter or processing for meat and poultry) and the reduction in illnesses, determination of the effectiveness of a regulation becomes complicated or even impossible.

Efficiency

How has a regulation been implemented? What are the monitoring/inspection costs surrounding it? Such questions focus on the technical efficiency of the manner of implementation.

With process criteria, compliance is assessed by determining whether companies are using the particular piece of equipment mandated by the standard and whether they are doing so correctly. With a performance standard, compliance may be more difficult to assess.

Government costs involved with implementation of a performance standard (e.g., from sampling for verification) may prove to be higher than with process criteria. For companies, performance standards may confer flexibility and reduced costs. However, if these savings are small and do not offset higher government costs, the overall societal costs may be lower for process criteria. Lower company costs may be seen over time given new technologies that achieve the process criteria. The determination of these cost reductions for use in cost–benefit analyses is a challenge. This may bias findings towards process standards.

Equity

When comparing performance and process criteria, the issue of equity centers on the incidence of costs and benefits placed upon, or derived by, a particular section of society as a direct result of the regulation under consideration. Theoretically, performance standards are more likely to be scale neutral compared with process criteria. However, a performance standard may cost large companies less to comply with because of economies of scale or scope. There may be a limited amount of research and development dedicated to providing interventions for smaller operations. The "safe harbor" strategy, whereby smaller operators are provided a set of validated interventions from which they may select, provides an example of how equity can be built into a regulation. However, there is an implicit inflexibility with the reliance on such safe harbor processes, and there may be a concern over the lack of plant-specific adaptation of the underlying HACCP plan. This echoes concerns stated earlier about the use of generic HACCP plans without a full appreciation of how appropriate these may be for the individual plant, line, and product.

The range of food safety criteria discussed in this report includes those that rely solely on performance standards (e.g., 5-D pathogen reduction in juice), mixed regulations that combine process and performance standards (e.g., the PR/HACCP rule), and process criteria (e.g., pasteurization of milk). Such broader aspects of the equity of food safety regulations as potential regional dimensions, distribution of costs along the supply chain, and equity dimensions on the benefits side in terms of greater risks incurred by particular subpopulations, are beyond the scope of this report. Given each of the economic concerns listed above, the individual regulation must be assessed for its impact on the balance of costs and benefits for each section of society (companies, consumers, government, and ideally subgroups of these such as small versus larger companies and immunocompromised populations versus the healthy), as well as the remaining incentives to innovate and therefore improve quality.

Costs and Benefits of Food Safety Regulations

The evolving field of food safety economics has focused significant attention on the tools necessary to first forecast and then track costs and benefits of regulations. This has led to many refinements in the methodology for forecasting benefits, including such impacts on specific populations as age-based morbidity and mortality calculations and early efforts to incorporate disability or quality adjusted life-year measures. Depending on the empirical method adopted for valuing such reductions in foodborne illness (e.g., cost-of-illness or willingness-to-pay [Kuchler and Golan, 1999]), large ranges in the estimates of a policy's hypothesized benefits generally result. Similarly, costs of compliance must be estimated ahead of time, often with limited knowledge of current industry practices or likely adoption of response strategies.

It should be noted that the bulk of food safety economics research does not focus on the impact of individual performance standards isolated from the overall food safety regulation or program under review (mostly HACCP-based regulations). As such, it is difficult to quantify the unique costs and benefits of performance standards implemented as part of broader regulatory change. In order to complete such evaluations it would be necessary to have representative, detailed cost data linked to actual microbiological improvements solely due to the particular performance standard under review. In this way, one could avoid (or at least minimize) incorrectly assigning costs and benefits to regulations (or parts of a regulation) that are more correctly due to a general trend in food safety enhancements that the plant, company, or industry may have performed in the absence of the regulation (MacDonald and Crutchfield, 1996). For example, if pathogen reduction resulted from an investment in a new piece of equipment purchased in response to customer demands and was not required by the regulation per se, then it would be incorrect to attribute this cost—and the resultant food safety benefit—to the regulation.

The scale of pathogen reductions used as inputs in benefit estimations also needs to be considered. Clearly, it is desirable for such food safety gains to be calculated from real-world changes in specified bacterial populations observed at the plant level. Based on this information, some form of aggregation would then provide a measure of the societal gain derived from the regulation. These pathogen reductions should not be laboratory-level performance evaluations of a strategy unless they have been validated in real-world applications. Challenge experiments often use inoculated samples with elevated populations of microorganisms and can bias results in favor of certain interventions, suggesting large pathogen reductions that may not be achieved in the processing plant.

Issues related to maintaining reductions in pathogens beyond the point or stage of application of a performance standard (e.g., the slaughterhouse or processing facility for meat and poultry), and to the optimal stages where these reductions were attained, remain understudied in the field of food safety economics. Thus, the benefits of large reductions in microbial loads on freshly slaughtered or processed meat and poultry may be diminished or even completely lost by downstream recontamination and thereby provide no risk reduction. When stage-specific risk-management strategies are assessed without the chain-wide determination of all economic implications, it is possible that, at best, an inefficient criterion may be selected and, at worst, that significant disincentives for companies to adopt proven food safety strategies will result.

Similarly, cost shifting among segments of the chain (transfers), as opposed to true cost reductions, may arise through the application of food safety criteria. An example could be a performance standard that leads to a requirement placed on input suppliers via a CCP at receiving that may drastically increase suppliers' costs and yet have limited public health benefits when compared with an end-point performance standard.

Innovation: Lessons from Environmental Regulations

The degree of innovation for food-processing companies can be thought of as a continuum between the two endpoints: (1) target standards (low degree of government intervention, such as sanitation guidelines), and (2) process criteria (a high degree of government intervention, such as pasteurization of milk). Performance standards lie somewhere in the middle of this continuum and are much less intrusive than process criteria. Most performance standards give requirements in terms of results (e.g., a 5-D reduction in bacterial numbers) and do not specify particular production or process methods. Therefore, they are more flexible than criteria. This flexibility should allow innovation and result in reduced costs. The thesis that flexibility allows innovation has been borne out in the area of environmental regulations. In fact, in the most general sense, successful companies innovate to fight pressures from competitors and customers, so this thesis may be amenable to extension into the food safety regulatory environment. If any lesson may be taken from environmental economics, it might be that properly designed regulations and standards can trigger innovations that lower the total cost of a product and improve its value (Porter and van der Linde, 1995). A highly competitive company may see compliance with a performance standard as a challenge and respond by creating innovative solutions to meet the standard.

The lessons learned from environmental regulations provide a basis for some general guidelines for setting performance standards (and subsequent regulations) in food safety systems, as described by Golan (2002):

> Regulate as close to the end user as possible, thus encouraging upstream innovation; choose strict, not simply feasible, standards to encourage efficiency and innovation; regulate along international trends; and select criteria for compliance verification that [are] informative, reliably measurable, and flexible.

These proposals are valid only if industry and regulators remove the contentious belief that regulations erode competitiveness (Porter and van der Linde, 1995). Therefore, if viewed as a challenge, a performance standard at the appropriate point could result in cost-reducing innovations that accrue for the entire food industry sector, while making food safer.

Innovation and Performance Standards

No regulation should be static. Every industry, regardless of its maturity, should be constantly challenged to innovate to reduce costs and improve quality. There is nothing implicit about either a process or a performance standard that either encourages or constrains innovation, so long as these standards are dynamic. This point was acknowledged by FSIS in the PR/HACCP rule (FSIS, 1996) and related collection of updated baseline data (see discussion in Chapter 4). Process criteria, however, by their nature as a preapproved form of production, may suffer from more "institutional friction" than performance standards. A great effort is thus required when implementing new, stricter, process criteria following an innovation such as the invention of a new piece of equipment designed to reduce pathogens in a food product.

Evidence of the impact on innovation of the introduction of food safety performance standards is unclear. There have been significant efforts placed on pathogen reduction strategies targeting carcasses (e.g., steam pasteurization, hot water and acid rinses, steam vacuum systems), meat products (e.g., irradiation), and other food products (e.g., high pressure and ultraviolet light treatment of juices). Further, many rapid pathogen tests have been developed to service the market created by performance standards and contractual specifications. Some of this research and development is subsidized by the public sector (e.g., universities, FDA, and USDA's Agricultural Research Service), whereas other efforts are solely in the private domain. In the United States, some of these innovations would likely have emerged without the implementation of performance standards, either because of international market demands or because these innovations lend themselves to becoming validated strategies for use in future processing of food—and perhaps even in process criteria. In relation to the PR/HACCP rule, the time period for evidence is still quite short (full implementation of HACCP in the meat and poultry industry is only three years old). Therefore, it is difficult to determine if innovation has been promoted by performance standards.

Based on these simple economic principles, the remaining challenge is how to design food safety regulations that help—within the framework of risk analysis—to link public health goals to scientifically valid and economically feasible performance standards. Risk management clearly serves the role of evaluating alternative food safety criteria to determine if they attain a prestated public health goal.

Risk-Management Economics

One economic approach that may highlight the connections among a public health goal, a specific food safety objective, and a performance standard consists of determining the relevant marginal social costs—changes in costs or benefits for the whole economy (companies, government, and consumers) as the level of food safety changes—and benefits uniquely due to the regulation (see Figure 3.4). This approach demonstrates that as the level of safety increases, so do social costs (borne by companies, the government, and consumers together). A 100 percent safe food supply is unachievable, and movement towards this goal leads to higher costs. Similarly, the benefits of additional increases in food safety decrease as the control of the food supply is progressively strengthened. However, most economists agree that without some form of government intervention, the market alone would not achieve the optimal level of food safety seen when marginal costs and

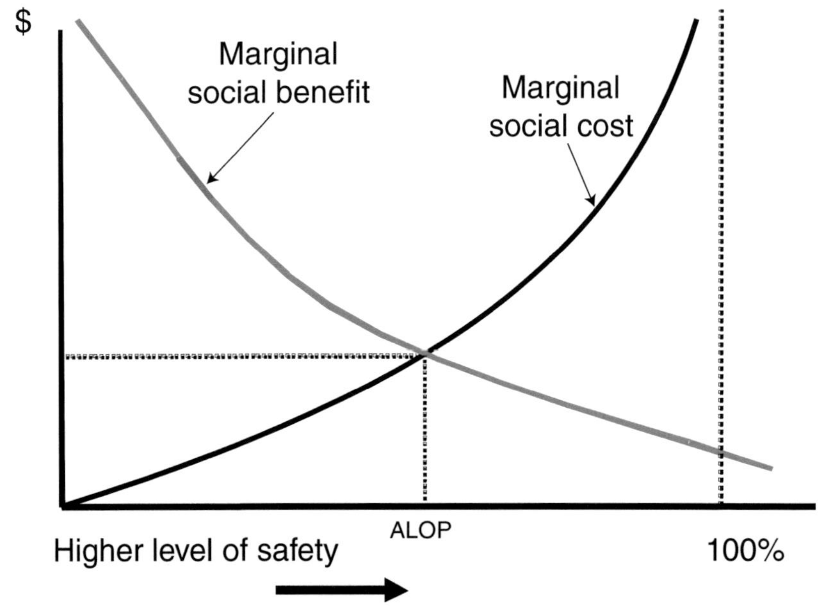

FIGURE 3.4 Toward a public health goal: relating an appropriate level of protection (ALOP) to marginal social benefit and cost.

benefits coincide (Figure 3.4). (As stated above, it is unlikely that definitive values can be provided of costs and benefits, and therefore such curves convey the most likely values around which confidence intervals must be built.) The inability of consumers to fully identify a product level of safety compared with the greater knowledge that processors have of the ability of a process to deliver safety (termed "imperfect and asymmetric" information problems in the literature) suggests that the market will fall short in providing the socially optimal level of protection for the particular product or pathogen under review.

Economic efficiency requires that the ALOP to aim for be at the point where marginal social costs equal marginal social benefits (Figure 3.4). Away from this equilibrium, either society desires a safer product and would benefit more than the additional costs of the stricter regime (points to the left of ALOP), or society is expending too many resources compared with the additional safety gains realized (to the right of ALOP). The ALOP can be related to the particular public health goal of the regulator because the model is stated in dollar terms but is partially based on population measures (benefit estimates). It is important to note that marginal social costs and marginal social benefits may change given the form of a regulation, the particular population and food product under assessment, and, over time, with a change in available technology or changing consumer demands or consumption patterns. Therefore, the ALOP and the most efficient food safety criteria are likely to be dynamic, given changing consumer tastes and preferences, risk tolerances, industry capabilities, and government oversight functions.

An example of how such marginal social costs can be calculated, highlighting costs to companies from the adoption of particular food safety strategies, is shown in Figure 3.5. Four possible strategies or combinations of efforts having various levels of effectiveness and cost are shown. Various interventions (single- or multiple-hurdle strategies) can be assessed based on their cost of implementation (possibly reported for various sizes or types of plants) and the most likely effectiveness (e.g., ability of the process to reduce the presence of a particular pathogen by x $\log_{10}$) and, therefore, on their ability to attain a performance standard (S) with a certain probability. Similarly, if S were a food safety objective, then the technique could be used to assess sets of interventions adopted by various companies throughout the supply chain. The horizontal line in Figure 3.5 indicates points associated with the concept that multiple strategies may meet the necessary effectiveness (S) but with different varying costs.

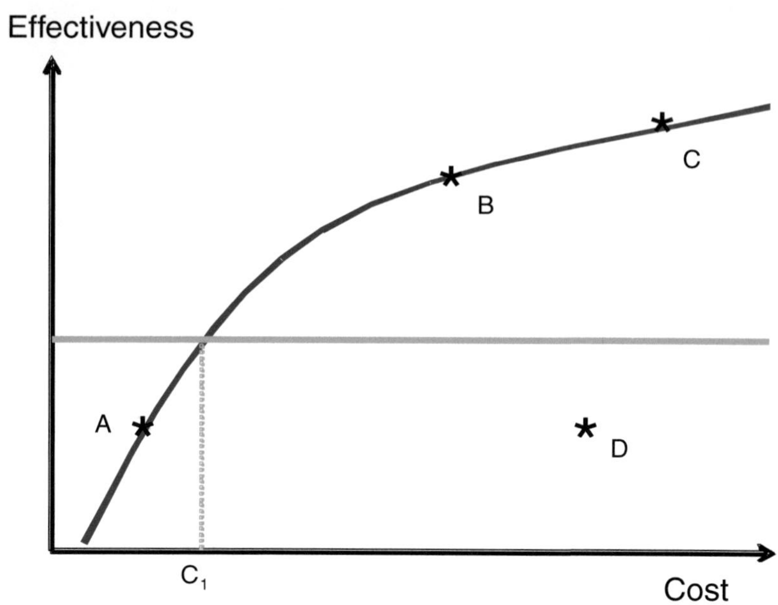

FIGURE 3.5 Relationship between the effectiveness (i.e., pathogen reduction) and cost of hypothetical food safety strategies available to food-processing companies.
SOURCE: Jensen et al. (1998), Markarian et al. (2001).

Strategies such as point D (Figure 3.5) are dominated by each of the other options (A, B, and C) in the figure; these other options have either lower cost (like point A) or higher effectiveness (points B and C), or both. The curved line passing through points A, B, and C links all of the most favorable strategies and therefore provides an optimal path of technical food safety effectiveness. The area to the right of the curved line also suggests that there are marginal costs for various levels of food safety (for example, consider moving from point B to C). The standard S in Figure 3.5 will result in a cost of at least C_1 based on where the optimal curved line and horizontal line intersect. Technical effectiveness (the frontier) is dynamic; innovations shift the curve up, allowing enhanced effectiveness for the same cost. Process criteria essentially dictate the particular strategy that must be followed by the industry (for example, strategy at point D). However, this may not result in the lowest cost (compare A with D). Furthermore, process criteria likely prevent the selection of more effective interventions (like B or C).

The strategies that meet (and in this case exceed) standard S are both B and C. The particular intervention that would be selected by industry is less clear when facing a performance standard (which is considered more flexible, since many options to meet the standard may be available) as opposed to process criteria. This situation illustrates the difficulty in forecasting costs in response to a performance standard. Certain companies may decide to exceed the standard by a long measure, while others may choose to meet the standard and no more. Resulting from these different decisions, an array of potential costs can be established creating a large range (with a well-defined lower bound C_1, Figure 3.5) of estimates for the related economic impact assessment of performance standards. This wide range of impact-assessment estimates would also be related to a broad range for the marginal social cost estimate (recall the marginal social cost curve in Figure 3.4), with the lower bound relating to the minimal cost (C_1 in Figure 3.5) of achieving standard S. This illustrates the difficulty of performing economic impact assessments.

Because of the complicated situation presented above, the committee concluded that uncertainty still exists with respect to the economics of food safety regulations. The following are examples of questions that need to be answered: Has the correct balance of incentives to innovate, benefits, and costs been achieved? From an economic standpoint, are performance standards or process criteria better for food safety? Which economic sector benefits most from performance standards? What about performance criteria? In economic terms, what are the consumer, government, and industry responses to performance standards and performance criteria? Traditional economics suggest that performance standards should lead to a no-higher set of industry (company) costs, yet performance standards may cause the government sector to incur additional costs. Therefore, the specifics of a particular performance standard should be assessed to determine this balance. Further research in these areas is required to better answer the questions above and similar ones not yet raised.

THE IMPACT OF CHANGING TECHNOLOGY: NEW DIAGNOSTIC TOOLS

Any regulatory system is heavily dependent on the technology available to detect deviations from regulatory performance standards. For that matter, the performance standards themselves may be influenced by available diagnostics, with the requirement for nondetectable levels as established by regulations having less meaning when it is possible to detect problems (such as the presence of specific pathogens) with a 10-, 100-, or 1,000-fold increase in sensitivity.

Current regulatory standards for foodborne pathogens, in almost all instances, assume use of traditional culture techniques to determine the presence and number of pathogens or indicator organisms in a product. However, culture techniques tend to be slow, with two or three days often required for initial isolation of a microorganism, followed in many instances by several days of additional testing to confirm that the microorganism isolated is indeed pathogenic or that it carries the necessary virulence genes to represent a hazard to humans. There has been increasing movement toward the use of immunological assays in diagnostics which, when combined with traditional culture techniques, can provide results in less time and with greater accuracy. However, it is genetic techniques that have the greatest potential for revolutionizing these more traditional approaches. There is now increasing experience with PCR, and PCR and probe-based methods are being used with increasing frequency. Examples in work with seafood include the use of DNA probes for *V. vulnificus* (Wright et al., 1996) and pathogenic (*tdh-*, *trh-*, or *tlh*-containing) strains of *V. parahaemolyticus* (DePaola et al., 2000), and use of PCR assays for the *tdh* gene in assessing possible virulence of clinical and environmental *V. parahaemolyticus* strains (Yeung et al., 2002).

Further rapid advances in molecular diagnostics may be anticipated, including the development of some microarray assays for pathogenic microorganisms. Microarrays, as currently formulated, are multiple assay arrays on glass slides on which hundreds or thousands of probes are spotted, permitting a test sample to be screened against all probes simultaneously. Currently, the most common application of microarrays is to measure the presence and quantity of up to 20,000 messenger ribonucleic acid (mRNA) transcripts from mammalian cells (Schena et al., 1996). However, genomic microarrays to distinguish among species of bacteria using the 16S ribosomal RNA gene have also been reported (Bavykin, 2001), with each probe on the microarray selected to identify a species of bacteria. In addition, microarrays have been used to identify genes lost between different strains of *E. coli* (Ochman and Jones, 2000), *Helicobacter* (Salama et al., 2000) and *Staphylococcus* (Fitzgerald et al., 2001). With microarrays it is theoretically possible to immediately and quantitatively identify many, if not all, potential pathogens in a sample; to identify strains carrying specific virulence genes or strain subsets that have been linked with increased transmission potential (i.e., superclones); and to identify other genes of interest, including resistance genes.

While such microarray systems are not currently available commercially, they represent a very promising technology for food safety applications.

The rapid advances being seen in this field of diagnostic technology underscore the need for flexibility in any regulatory approach or development of performance standards. This includes a need for flexibility at several levels.

Currently, there is a perception on the part of regulatory agencies that identification of a pathogen for regulatory purposes is not "real" unless a microorganism is isolated. Regulations need to be changed to recognize that molecular and other rapid methods can produce results of comparable or greater accuracy than those obtained with traditional culture techniques; there must be provisions in regulatory actions for the use of data obtained with such methods.

Any regulatory approaches, including the establishment of performance standards, must have built into them sufficient flexibility to take advantage of the improvements in diagnostics that will almost certainly occur.

THE LIMITS OF SCIENCE

Some portion of the public surely is skeptical about most scientific pronouncements because of the seemingly conflicting advice, over time, from studies conducted in areas such as nutrition and health. However, the committee recognizes that many people believe that science and technology, given time and money, can fix everything. While this expectation may not hold for vexing problems deemed to be natural in origin (e.g., in respect to diseases such as cancer and acquired immune deficiency syndrome), man-made problems seem amenable to man-made solutions. Pathogens in store-bought foods are likely perceived by many as a man-made problem (e.g., *E. coli* in juices). When the committee held an open meeting to hear testimony from families that had suffered tragic losses from foodborne illness, the speakers (on the record as well as in private pleas in hallways after the session) urged committee members to "do something" to prevent others from suffering as they had. Eminent scientists, it was their heartfelt belief, could solve the problem.

Scientists and engineers have developed skills and made discoveries that do enable the solutions to numerous problems of human origin. One example is the carnage done over the years because of vehicle accidents. Technological and legal changes that have made cars and their passengers safer have reduced the vehicular death and disability toll. While increased enforcement could further reduce the problem, this toll could be dramatically reduced through technology by designing all vehicles much like military tanks, but such a drastic step would dramatically increase the costs of vehicular travel and, through greater fuel needs, their environmental impact. Even where science and technology have solutions, their costs may be greater than society is willing to pay to achieve the projected benefits. In these cases, society must determine the trade-off between costs and benefits by tackling the question: What is the optimum level of safety we should seek to achieve? To pick an extreme example, it soon will be possible to test food for all pathogens and toxins of concern; all food could, in theory, be sampled prior to consumption. Such a system would of course be entirely impractical, both financially and logistically, although it would make the food almost thoroughly safe for the consumer.

For our society, ensuring food safety is certainly an important goal that has not yet been adequately achieved. Policymakers who wish to improve the food safety system need to ensure adequate government financial resources for the creation and enforcement of safety rules. Food safety requirements imposed upon the food industry have financial consequences that may result in higher food prices. For example, significant changes could be made in animal husbandry and slaughter practices that would reduce the level of pathogens in food sold to the public. Science might be able to discover better, less expensive means to deal with pathogens in the food supply. Vaccines might be created that prevent food animals from being colonized by pathogens that, while harmless to the animals, are a danger to people. Simple, safe methods to kill pathogens on produce might be developed. Some scientific advances that their proponents claim will lead to a net benefit in food safety—such as food irradiation and changes involving genetic modification—are opposed by some members of the public because of concerns that one set of risks is being exchanged for another, to the frustration of many in the scientific community (Henderson, 2002).

Although there are limits to what science can achieve in consumer protection, a more significant limit in the food safety system may well be the willingness of the public to accept the costs of implementing the measures that are available. Given the high costs to our society of morbidity and mortality that are related to foodborne illness, it would be sensible to require investment in food safety that yields a positive return. That is, to the extent that expenditures to improve food safety overall exceed the costs of the harm, these expenditures should definitely be made (and prices allowed to rise to cover the extra costs). Making such changes might interfere with consumer expectations about the low-cost availability of food. Some of the least-expensive interventions (such as hand washing by food handlers and improving retail worker and consumer compliance with safe food handling and cooking guidelines) are the most difficult to attain because they necessitate changing behaviors of vast numbers of people. However, while everyone must purchase food and eat (and thus everyone has an interest in keeping down the cost of food), the harm from serious foodborne illness falls on a small fraction of the population. Are the many willing to devote resources to prevent serious harm to the few? Those who have lost loved ones (many of whom have been young children) to foodborne illness answer this question loudly in the affirmative; others are far less certain. While science and technology will continue to search for and discover answers to problems involving foodborne illness, inexpensive answers are often unavailable or impractical. Where to draw the line between requirements that should be implemented and that are reasonably cost-effective, and those that would be beneficial but would have too great an impact on food prices, is a question for politics rather than for science.

REFERENCES

ASTM (American Society for Testing and Materials). 1976. *Manual on Presentation of Data and Control Chart Analysis Committee E on Quality and Statistics*. ASTM MNL7. Philadelphia: ASTM.

Bavykin SG, Akowski JP, Zakhariev VM, Barsky VE, Perov AN, Mirzabekov AD. 2001. Portable system for microbial sample preparation and oligonucleotide microarray analysis. *Appl Environ Microbiol* 67:922–928.

Bothe DR. 2001. *Measuring Process Capability*. Cedarburg, WI: Landmark Publishing.

Breyfogle FW, Cupello JM, Meadows B. 2001. *Managing Six Sigma: A Practical Guide to Understanding, Assessing and Implementing the Strategy that Yields Bottom-Line Success*. New York: John Wiley & Sons.

Busta F. 2002. *Application of Science to Food Safety Management*. Presentation to the Institute of Medicine/National Research Council Committee on the Review of the Use of Scientific Criteria and Performance Standards for Safe Food, Washington, DC, April 3.

CAC (Codex Alimentarius Commission). 1997. *Hazard Analysis and Critical Control Point System and Guidelines for its Application*. Annex to CAC/RCP 1-1969, Rev. 3-1997. Rome: Food and Agriculture Organization of the United Nations.

Cassin MH, Lammerding AM, Todd ECD, Ross W, McColl S. 1998. Quantitative risk assessment of *Escherichia coli* O157:H7 in ground beef hamburgers. *Int J Food Microbiol* 41:21–44.

CFSAN/FSIS/CDC (Center for Food Safety and Applied Nutrition/Food Safety and Inspection Service/Centers for Disease Control and Prevention). 2001. *Draft Assessment of the Relative Risk to Public Health from Foodborne* Listeria monocytogenes *among Selected Categories of Ready-to-Eat Foods*. Online. Food and Drug Administration (FDA), U.S. Department of Agriculture (USDA). Available at http://www.cfsan.fda.gov/~dms/lmrisk.html. Accessed May 8, 2003.

Cianfrani CA, Tsiakals JJ, West JE. 2002. *The ASQ ISO 9000:2000 Handbook*. Milwaukee: ASQ Quality Press.

COST Action 920. 2000. *Foodborne Zoonosis: A Co-ordinated Food Chain Approach*. Online. Available at http://www.cost920.com. Accessed December 12, 2002.

CVM (Center for Veterinary Medicine). 2001. *The Human Health Impact of Fluoroquinolone Resistant* Campylobacter *Attributed to the Consumption of Chicken*. Online. FDA. Available at http://www.fda.gov/cvm/antimicrobial/revisedRA.pdf. Accessed August 1, 2002.

DePaola A, Kaysner CA, Bowers J, Cook DW. 2000. Environmental investigation of *Vibrio parahaemolyticus* in oysters after outbreaks in Washington, Texas, and New York (1997 and 1998). *Appl Environ Microbiol* 66:4649–4654.

Dourson ML, Andersen ME, Erdreich LS, MacGregor JA. 2001. Using human data to protect public health. *Reg Toxicol Pharmacol* 33:234–256.

Escherichia coli O157:H7 Risk Assessment Team. 2001. *Draft Risk Assessment of the Public Health Impact of* Escherichia coli *O157:H7 in Ground Beef*. Online. FSIS, USDA. Available at http://www.fsis.usda.gov/OPPDE/rdad/FRPubs/00-023N/00-023NReport.pdf. Accessed September 12, 2001.

FAO/WHO (Food and Agriculture Organization of the United Nations/World Health Organization). 2000. *Hazard Characterization, Exposure Assessment of* Listeria monocytogenes *in Ready-to-Eat Foods (RTE)*. Joint FAO/WHO Expert Consultation on Risk Assessment of Microbiological Hazards in Foods. Rome: FAO

FAO/WHO. 2001. *Hazard Identification, Exposure Assessment, and Hazard Characterization of* Campylobacter *spp. in Broiler Chickens and* Vibrio *spp. in Seafood*. Joint FAO/WHO Expert Consultation on Risk Assessment of Microbiological Hazards in Foods. Geneva: WHO.

FDA. 1999a. Food labeling: Safe handling statements: Labeling of shell eggs; Shell eggs: Refrigeration of shell eggs held for retail distribution; Proposed rule. *Fed Regist* 64:36491–36516.

FDA. 1999b. *Grade "A" Pasteurized Milk Ordinance. 1999 Revision*. Online. Available at http://www.cfsan.fda.gov/~acrobat/pmo99-1.pdf. Accessed July 19, 2002.

FDA. 2001. Hazard Analysis and Critical Control Point (HAACP); Procedures for the safe and sanitary processing and importing of juice; Final rule. *Fed Regist* 66:6137–6202.

FDA. 2002. *FDA Food Code*. Online. Available at http://www.cfsan.fda.gov/~dms/foodcode.html. Accessed December 12, 2002.

FDA/FSIS. 2001. Relative risk to public health from foodborne *Listeria monocytogenes* among selected categories of ready-to-eat food risk assessment document and risk management action plan. *Fed Regist* 66:5515–5517.

Fitzgerald JR, Sturdevant DE, Mackie SM, Gill SR, Musser JM. 2001. Evolutionary genomics of *Staphylococcus aureus*: Insights into the origin of methicillin-resistant strains and the toxic shock syndrome epidemic. *Proc Natl Acad Sci USA* 98:8821–8826.

FSIS. 1996. Pathogen reduction; hazard analysis and critical control point (HACCP) systems; Final rule. *Fed Regist* 61:38805–38855.

FSIS. 1998. *Lethality and Stabilization Performance Standards for Certain Meat and Poultry Products: Technical Paper*. Online. USDA. Available at http://www.fsis.usda.gov/oa/haccp/lethality.pdf. Accessed August 1, 2002.

FSIS. 1999. *1999 National Residue Program: Residue Data*. Online. USDA. Available at http://www.fsis.usda.gov/OPHS/red99/intro.pdf. Accessed August 1, 2002.

FSIS. 2001. *HACCP-Based Inspection Models Project (HIMP): Young Chicken Inspection*. Online. USDA. Available at http://www.fsis.usda.gov/OPPDE/Nis/HIMP/Docs/YNGChk_Drf6.pdf. Accessed July 19, 2002.

Gallagher DL, Ebel ED, Kause JR. 2003. *Draft FSIS Risk Assessment for* Listeria *in Ready-to-eat Meat and Poultry Products*. Online. FSIS, USDA. Available at http://www.fsis.usda.gov/OPHS/lmrisk/DraftLm22603.pdf. Accessed May 5, 2003.

Garthright WE, Chirtel S, Graves Q. 2002. *Derivation of Sampling Plan to Meet the Testing Requirement in the Juice HACCP Final Rule for Citrus Juices that Rely Solely or in Part on Surface Treatments to Achieve the 5-Log Reduction Standard*. Washington, DC: Office of Plant, Dairy Food and Beverages, CFSAN, FDA.

Gavin A, Weddig L. 1995. *Canned Foods: Principles of Thermal Process and Control, Acidification, and Container Closure Evaluation*, 6th ed. Washington, DC: Food Processors Institute.

Golan E. 2002. *Performance Standards and the Economics of Compliance and Innovation*. Presented at the USDA Symposium on Pathogen Reduction—A Scientific Dialogue, Economic Research Service, USDA. Washington, DC, May 6.

Hein I, Klein D, Lehner A, Bubert A, Brandl E, Wagner M. 2001a. Detection and quantification of the iap gene of *Listeria monocytogenes* and *Listeria innocua* by a new real-time quantitative PCR assay. *Res Microbiol* 152:37–46.

Hein I, Lehner A, Rieck P, Klein K, Brandl E, Wagner M. 2001b. Comparison of different approaches to quantify *Staphylococcus aureus* cells by real-time quantitative PCR and application of this technique for examination of cheese. *Appl Environ Microbiol* 67:3122–3126.

Henderson M. 2002, September 9. Public "must allow scientists to take risks." Online. *The Times* (London). Available at http://www.timesonline.co.uk/article/0,,2-408587,00.html. Accessed October 10, 2002.

Holcomb DL, Smith MA, Ware GO, Hung YC, Brackett RE, Doyle MP. 1999. Comparison of six dose-response models for use with food-borne pathogens. *Risk Analysis* 19:1091–1100.

ICMSF (International Commission on Microbiological Specifications for Foods). 1988. *Microorganisms in Foods 4. Application of the Hazard Analysis Critical Control Point (HACCP) System to Ensure Microbiological Safety and Quality.* Oxford: Blackwell Scientific Publications.

ICMSF. 1998. Potential application of risk assessment techniques to microbiological issues related to international trade in food and food products. *J Food Prot* 61:1075–1086.

ICMSF. 2002. *Microorganisms in Foods 7. Microbiological Testing in Food Safety Management.* New York: Kluwer Academic/Plenum Publishers.

IFT (Institute of Food Technologists). 2002. *IFT Expert Report on Emerging Microbiological Food Safety Issues: Implications for Control in the 21st Century.* Chicago: IFT.

IOM (Institute of Medicine). 1990. *Cattle Inspection.* Washington, DC: National Academy Press.

IOM. 1991. *Seafood Safety.* Washington, DC: National Academy Press.

IOM. 2002. Escherichia coli *O157:H7 in Beef. Review of a Draft Risk Assessment.* Washington DC: National Academy Press.

IOM/NRC (National Research Council). 1998. *Ensuring Safe Food from Production to Consumption.* Washington, DC: National Academy Press.

Jensen HH, Unnevehr LJ, Gomez MI. 1998. Costs of improving food safety in the meat sector. *J Agric Appl Econ* 30:83–94.

Kane VE. 1989. *Defect Prevention: Use of Simple Statistical Tool.* Milwaukee, WI: ASQ Quality Press.

Karel M, Fennema OR, Lund DB. 1975. *Physical Principles of Food Preservation.* New York: Marcel Dekker.

Ketola J, Roberts K. 2001. *ISO 9001:2000 Management Responsibility in a Nutshell.* Milwaukee, WI: ASQ Quality Press.

Konz S, Perterson G, Joshi A. 1981. Reducing inspection errors. *Quality Progress* 14:24–27.

Kroes R, Kozianowski G. 2002. Threshold of toxicological concern (TTC) in food safety assessment. *Toxicol Let* 127:43–46.

Kuchler F, Golan E. 1999. *Assigning Values to Life: Comparing Methods for Valuing Health Risks.* Agricultural Economics Report No. 784. Washington, DC: Economic Research Service, USDA.

Kume H. 1985. *Statistical Methods for Quality Improvement.* Tokyo: The Association for Overseas Technical Scholarship.

Lammerding AM, Paoli GM. 1997. Quantitative risk assessment: An emerging tool for emerging foodborne pathogens. *Emerg Infect Dis* 3:483–487.

Law AM, Kelton WD. 2000. *Simulation Modeling and Analysis*, 3rd ed. Boston: McGraw-Hill.

Li WL, Drake MA. 2001. Development of a quantitative competitive PCR assay for detection and quantification of *Escherichia coli* O157:H7 cells. *Appl Environ Microbiol* 67:3291–3294.

LSRO (Life Sciences Research Office). 1995. *Third Report on Nutrition Monitoring in the United States, Appendix III.* Washington, DC: U.S. Government Printing Office.

MacDonald JM, Crutchfield S. 1996. Modeling the costs of food safety regulation. *Am J Agric Econ* 78:1285–1290.

Maijala R, Lyytikainen O, Johansson T, Autio T, Aalto T, Haavisto L, Honkanen-Buzalski T. 2001. Exposure of *Listeria monocytogenes* within an epidemic caused by butter in Finland. *Int J Food Microbiol* 70:97–109.

Markarian V, Hooker NH, Murano EA, Acuff GR, Carroll S. 2001. Comparative costs of pathogen reduction strategies for Australian beef slaughter plants. In: Hooker NH, Murano EA, eds. *Interdisciplinary Food Safety Research.* Boca Raton, FL: CRC Press. Pp. 25–41.

Montgomery DC. 2001. *Introduction to Statistical Quality Control*, 4th ed. New York: John Wiley & Sons.

NACMCF (National Advisory Committee on Microbiological Criteria for Foods). 1997. *Recommendations on Fresh Juice.* Online. FDA. Available at http://cfsan.fad.gov/~mow/nacmcf.html. Accessed January 23, 2003.

NACMCF. 1998. Hazard analysis and critical control point principles and application guidelines. *J Food Prot* 61:1246–1259.

Neubert D. 1999. Risk assessment and preventative hazard minimization. In: Marquardt H, Schäfer SS, McClellan RO, Welsch F, eds. *Toxicology*. New York: Academic Press. Pp. 1153–1190.

NRC (National Research Council). 1985a. *An Evaluation of the Role of Microbiological Criteria for Foods and Food Ingredients*. Washington, DC: National Academy Press.

NRC. 1985b. *Meat and Poultry Inspection: The Scientific Basis of the Nation's Program*. Washington, DC: National Academy Press.

Ochman H, Jones IB. 2000. Evolutionary dynamics of full genome content in *Escherichia coli*. *EMBO J* 19:6637–6643.

Paige JC, Pell F. 1997. Drug residues in food-producing animals. Online. *FDA Veterinarian Newsletter*. Available at http://www.fda.gov/cvm/index/fdavet/1997/july.htm#res. Accessed April 11, 2003.

Paustenbach DJ. 2000. The practice of exposure assessment: A state-of-the-art review. *J Toxicol Environ Health* 3:179–291.

Porter ME, van der Linde C. 1995. Green and competitive: Ending the stalemate. *Harv Bus Rev* 73:120–134.

Posnick L, Burr D, Bowers J, Walderhaug M, Miliotis M. 2001. *Draft Risk Assessment on the Public Health Impact of* Vibrio parahaemolyticus *in Raw Molluscan Shellfish*. Online. CFSAN, FDA. Available at http://www.cfsan.fda.gov/~dms/vprisksu.htm. Accessed August 1, 2002.

President's Council on Food Safety. 1999. *Egg Safety from Production to Consumption: An Action Plan to Eliminate* Salmonella *Enteritidis Illnesses Due to Eggs*. Online. Available at http://www.foodsafety.gov/~fsg/ceggs.htm. Accessed July 19, 2002.

Rose JB, Haas CN, Regli S. 1991. Risk assessment and control of waterborne giardiasis. *Am J Public Health* 81:709–713.

RTI (Research Triangle Institute). 2000. *HACCP-Based Inspection Models Project: Baseline Results for Young Chickens*. Online. FSIS, USDA. Available at http://www.fsis.usda.gov/oa/haccp/base_broilers.pdf. Accessed January 13, 2002.

Salama N, Guillemin K, McDaniel TK, Sherlock G, Tompkins L, Falkow S. 2000. A whole-genome microarray reveals genetic diversity among *Helicobacter pylori* strains. *Proc Natl Acad Sci USA* 97:14668–14673.

Salmonella Enteritidis Risk Assessment Team. 1998. Salmonella *Enteritidis Risk Assessment: Shell Eggs and Egg Products*. Online. FSIS, USDA. Available at http://www.fsis.usda.gov/OPHS/risk/index.htm. Accessed August 1, 2002.

Schena M, Shalon D, Heller R, Chai A, Brown PO, Davis RW. 1996. Parallel human genome analysis: Microarray-based expression monitoring of 1000 genes. *Proc Natl Acad Sci USA* 93:10614–10619.

Singer DL. 2001. *A Laboratory Quality Handbook of Best Practices and Relevant Regulations*. Milwaukee, WI: ASQ Quality Press.

Steel RGD, Torrey JH, Dickey DA. 1997. *Principles and Procedures of Statistics: A Biometrical Approach*, 3rd ed. New York: McGraw-Hill.

Stevenson KE, Bernard DT, eds. 1995. *HACCP. Establishing Hazard Analysis Critical Control Point Programs. A Workshop Manual*, 2nd ed. Washington, DC: Food Processors Institute.

Taylor M. 2002. *Microbiological Performance Standards for Food Safety*. Presentation to the Institute of Medicine/National Research Council Committee on the Review of the Use of Scientific Criteria and Performance Standards for Safe Food, Washington, DC, April 3.

USDA/FDA. 2002. *HACCP Training Programs*. Online. National Agricultural Library. Available at http://www.nal.usda.gov/foodborne/haccp/training.html. Accessed October 16, 2002.

Vose D. 2000. *Risk Analysis: A Quantitative Guide*, 2nd ed. New York: John Wiley & Sons.

Wheeler DJ, Chambers DS. 1992. *Understanding Statistical Process Control*, 2nd ed. Knoxville, TN: SPC Press.

Whiting RC, Buchanan RL. 1997a. Development of a quantitative risk assessment model for *Salmonella* Enteritidis in pasteurized liquid eggs. *Int J Food Microbiol* 36:111–125.

Whiting RC, Buchanan RL. 1997b. Predictive modeling. In: Doyle MP, Beuchat LR, Montville TJ, eds. *Food Microbiology: Fundamentals and Frontiers.* Washington DC: ASM Press. Pp. 728–739.

WHO. 1999. *HACCP Principles and Practice. Teacher's Handbook.* CD-ROM. Geneva: WHO.

Woteki CE. 2000. *Is There a Place for Food Safety Objectives in USDA's Food Safety Program?* Online. FSIS, USDA. Keynote Address to the CERES Forum On Food Safety Objectives, Washington, DC, December 4. Available at http://www.fsis.usda.gov/OA/speeches/2000/cw_ceres.htm. Accessed May 20, 2002.

Wright AC, Hill RT, Johnson JA, Roghman M-C, Colwell RR, Morris JG Jr. 1996. Distribution of *Vibrio vulnificus* in the Chesapeake Bay. *Appl Environ Microbiol* 62:717–724.

Yeung PSM, Hayes MC, DePaola A, Kaysner CA, Kornstein L, Boor KJ. 2002. Comparative phenotypic, molecular, and virulence characterization of *Vibrio parahaemolyticus* O3:K6 isolates. *Appl Environ Microbiol* 68:2901–2909.

4

Scientific Criteria and Performance Standards to Control Hazards in Meat and Poultry Products

DESCRIPTION OF THE MEAT AND POULTRY INDUSTRY

Animal production in the United States has undergone a transformation over the last 50 years from a system mainly comprised of independent animal producers to one mainly comprised of concentrated animal feeding operations. The major production animal species, beef cattle, swine, chickens, and turkeys, are produced under a variety of conditions that may have significance in regard to the presence or absence of potential foodborne pathogens. The following is a brief synopsis of animal production in the United States.

Beef

A major percentage of the world's beef is produced in the United States both for domestic use and for export. The U.S. fed-cattle industry is the largest in the world (ERS, 2000). Most beef produced in and exported from the United States is the grain-finished, high-quality, choice-cut variety, while imported beef is generally grass-fed and is used primarily for processing as ground beef (ERS, 2002).

Red meat production is a concentrated industry. Feedlots and steer and heifer slaughter facilities are geographically concentrated in the Great Plains (MacDonald et al., 2000). Iowa, Kansas, Nebraska, and Texas accounted for over 51 percent of the U.S. commercial red meat production in 2001 (NASS, 2002). Since cows generally move directly to plants from dairy farms and beef cow-calf operations, cow and bull sales and slaughter plants are more widely distributed across the country (MacDonald et al., 2000). In commercial plants, red meat production totaled 45.7 billion pounds in 2001, of which beef production accounted for 26.2 billion pounds (NASS, 2002). Four companies slaughter and process 82 percent of the beef in the United States (MacDonald et al., 2000; REAP, 2001). Twenty percent of beef consumed originates from cull cows of the dairy industry (University of Vermont, 2003; Wallace, 2003).

Over 25 years ago, most beef was sold as whole or half carcasses that were fabricated by other processors or retailers. The advent of boxed meat (i.e., assembly cut and packaged meat) revolutionized the beef industry so that most fresh beef is sold as vacuum-packaged primals (large sections of a carcass cut for wholesale, such as the round, chuck, or rib) and subprimals (retail cuts) (Kinsman, 1994). Case-ready beef (retail cuts packaged and brand labeled) is a new concept currently being embraced by some companies (Eilert and Rathje, 2001). Processed beef products (i.e., those in which the carcass identity is lost or that are subject to some treatment that affects its texture, color, and flavor) accounted for 13.9 percent of beef consumed in 2001 (Nalivka, 2002).

Poultry

The U.S. poultry industry is comprised primarily of three segments: broilers, turkeys, and eggs. Of these three, broilers (i.e., young chickens) dominate with 66 percent of the dollar value of production (Nalivka, 2002). The United States produced more than 8.2 billion chickens, 2.6 billion turkeys, and more than 71 billion table eggs in 2000.

The U.S. broiler and turkey industries are referred to as "vertically integrated." The company or integrator controls all aspects of the process but contracts with individual landowners for growing services. The landowners furnish the poultry houses, energy, and labor, while the companies furnish the animals, feed, and technical support. The basic unit of this arrangement is the "complex," which consists of parent flocks, multiplier flocks, hatchery, feed mill, and processing plant (Figure 4.1).

Breeder farms, also called multiplier flocks, supply all of the eggs that will become the chickens for processing. For each day of processing, the hatchery must hatch enough chicks to account for losses in the field and for a standard amount of weight gain to match sales projections for the time period when these birds will be processed. The feed mill must supply feed for all of the houses within the complex to ensure that no chicken goes hungry.

The complex also usually has water treatment facilities and also may have rendering capabilities for by-products. The typical complex processes over 1 million chickens per week.

A typical young broiler plant can have from one to four processing lines. The maximum speed of each line is determined by the amount of inspection in place from the U.S. Department of Agriculture's (USDA) Food Safety and Inspection Service (FSIS). The categories of inspection are:

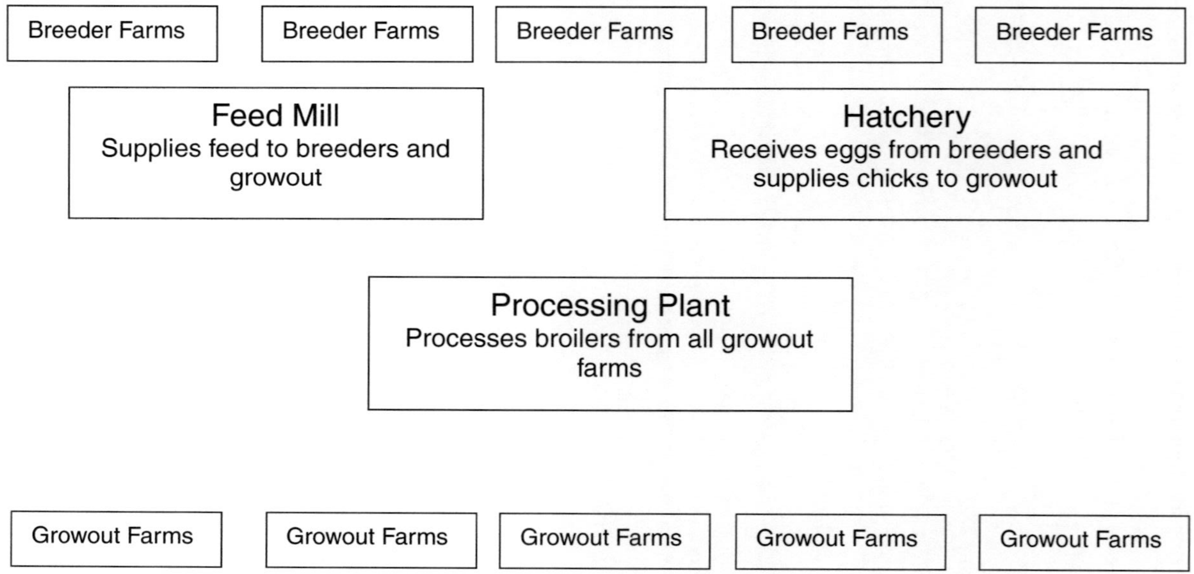

FIGURE 4.1 Poultry production complex.

- The Streamlined Inspection System, which allows 70 birds/min with two inspectors per evisceration line (35 birds/min/inspector)
- The New Enhanced Line Speed, which allows 91 birds/min with three inspectors and additional plant inspection (30.3 birds/min/inspector)
- The New Evisceration Systems: Maestro (Meyn Poultry, Gainesville, GA) and Nu-Tech (Stork Gamco, Gainesville, GA), which allow 140 birds/min with four inspectors per line (35 birds/min/inspector).

Pork

The United States is a major pork producer, second only to China. The U.S. pork industry rapidly expanded during the 1990s; more pork was produced (nearly 19 billion pounds) and more hogs slaughtered (more than 99 million head) in the United States in 1998 than ever before. Previous records in production had been set in 1992, 1994, and 1995.

Approximately 85,000 pork producers are in business today compared with nearly 3 million in 1950. Farms have grown in size; over 80 percent of the hogs are grown on farms producing 1,000 or more hogs per year, while over half are grown on farms producing 2,000 or more hogs per year. These operations, which are often very technically sophisticated, are still predominantly individual family farms.

The geographic location of pork production is shifting as well. While the traditional Corn Belt represents the overwhelming share of production, growth is also occurring in nontraditional hog states such as Texas, Colorado, and Oklahoma. North Carolina, which ranked fourteenth in pork production 30 years ago, now ranks second.

MEAT AND POULTRY INSPECTION

The Federal Inspection System

Under the Federal Meat Inspection Act and the Poultry Products Inspection Act, USDA, through FSIS, inspects all domestic meat and poultry to be sold in interstate commerce in the United States (FSIS, 2001c). Approximately 6,000 meat and poultry processing plants and 130 import establishments are inspected by FSIS (FSIS, 2002c). Products inspected under FSIS authority include all products from cattle, sheep, swine, goats, horses and other equines, chickens, turkeys, ducks, geese, and guinea fowl (FSIS, 1998a). It also applies to ostriches and emus (FSIS, 2001b). Processed products containing 3 percent or more raw meat and poultry or 2 percent or more cooked meat and poultry are also included (FSIS, 2001c), with some exceptions. Products that do not cross state lines may be inspected by state rather than federal inspection agencies; there are approximately 1,500 meat and poultry establishments that are inspected by state programs (GAO, 2001). Twenty-seven states have established inspection systems equivalent to the federal system; however, products that are state-inspected can only enter intrastate commerce.

To ensure the safety of imported meat and poultry products, FSIS maintains a wide-ranging system of inspection and controls. On an annual basis, FSIS evaluates the inspection systems in all foreign countries eligible to export meat and poultry to the United States to ensure that their inspection systems are equivalent to the U.S. system (FSIS, 2001c). This evaluation consists of a document review of the country's laws, regulations, and other written information, and an on-site review of plant facilities and equipment, laboratories, and training programs. In addition, all imported meat and poultry products may be reinspected (including testing) upon entering the United States (FSIS, 2003).

The 1997 implementation of the Pathogen Reduction; Hazard Analysis and Critical Control Point Final Rule (PR/HACCP rule) initiated a significant change in the regulatory philosophy and roles of both inspectors and industry. In the past, some plants relied heavily on USDA inspectors to identify plant and process deficiencies before the company would take action to correct them. The PR/HACCP rule defined the respective roles, tasks, and responsibilities of both industry and FSIS (FSIS, 1996). Businesses that produce the meat and poultry products are now directly accountable for their safety (FSIS, 1998b).

The introduction and implementation of the PR/HACCP rule attempted a significant change in regulatory philosophy and respective roles and responsibilities of industry and inspectors over a relatively short time period. The transition has not been entirely smooth; there have been some inconsistencies and setbacks in the start-up process. In response to reports published by the General Accounting Office, USDA's Office of the Inspector General, and its own self-assessment, FSIS is taking steps to provide supplemental guidance and clarification to assist inspection staff and industry in adapting to these changes (GAO, 2002).

U.S. Department of Agriculture Inspection Models Project Pilot Program

USDA began the HACCP-based Inspection Models Project (HIMP) pilot program in 1997 (FSIS, 1997, 2001a). This program was designed to explore extending HACCP and process controls to the slaughter of young animals to further improve food safety and reduce or eliminate product quality defects. A key component of HIMP includes setting performance standards by FSIS and requiring the meat and poultry processors to use process control techniques to meet the performance standards. However, the collection of the data needed to assess the effectiveness of the program has not been completed, so an evaluation of HIMP at this point would be premature.

The committee supports the conclusion of previous National Academies reports (NRC, 1985b, NRC, 1987) that carcass-by-carcass inspection is ineffective from a food safety perspective. If successful, HIMP may provide a useful model to reduce FSIS dependence on carcass-by-carcass inspection and increase the use of process control techniques to assure the safety of meat and poultry products.

State Inspection Programs with Federal Oversight

Twenty-seven states operate state meat and poultry inspection programs. These state programs, with federal oversight, were established with the passage of the Wholesome Meat Act of 1967 and the Wholesome Poultry Act of 1968. State meat and poultry inspection programs were required to implement the inspection system mandated by USDA in the PR/HACCP rule beginning in 1997. The transition from traditional meat and poultry inspection to the HACCP system represents a major philosophical, cultural, and procedural change for the state inspection programs. USDA provides matching funds to cover 50 percent of state program costs through the administration of renewable federal grants (WI DATCP, 2002).

State meat and poultry inspection programs are required to meet standards at least equal to the federal program, and FSIS is responsible for determining that they do so. In addition to conducting their own internal audits, state meat and poultry inspection programs are audited by USDA on a one-, two-, or four-year basis, with the frequency based on prior performance. Each state submits a state performance plan as part of an annual report for review by USDA. These plans must describe the operating practices and procedures for administering the state meat and poultry inspection programs, including laws and regulations, funding and financial accountability, resource management, staffing and training, program operations, facilities and equipment, labels and standards, in-plant review and enforcement, and laboratories (WI DATCP, 2002).

Meat and poultry plants are divided into three size categories. Large plants have 500 or more employees, small plants have 10 to 499 employees; and very small plants have fewer than 10 employees or annual sales of less than $2.5 million (FSIS, 1996). While plants under federal inspection comprise all three size categories, plants under state meat and poultry inspection programs are currently small and very small plants only (FAIM, 2002). Consequently, the state inspection programs have developed specialized expertise in working with small and very small plants. In a historical context, it was believed that state inspection programs offered economic benefits such as lower ongoing costs of state inspection compared with federal inspection, greater flexibility in the scheduled time of inspection, and the ability to accommodate low-volume slaughter or processing from local livestock markets (WI DATCP, 2002). In addition, state programs inspect and monitor custom plants, which are those that slaughter and process meat and poultry products for personal use by the animals' owners (i.e., not for subsequent sale).

State and Local Government Inspection of Retail Meat Processors

Retailers who process meat and poultry only for direct sales to consumers are subject to different inspection processes and regulations than those whose products are sold wholesale. The Food and Drug Administration Model Food Code (FDA, 2001), implemented in 1993 and updated biennially, is a template for the regulation of retail and food service operations. As of April 2002, 49 states had either adopted or were in the process of adopting one of the biennial versions of FDA's Model Food Code. New Mexico is not pursuing adoption of the Food Code, but the state still utilizes it for guidance and interpretation (CFSAN, 2003; FDA, 2001).

The committee recommends that collaboration among USDA, FDA, and state and local governments continue, to help ensure the production of safe meat and poultry products and consumer protection in the United States.

Laboratory Analysis

Microbiological testing of product samples obtained by the federal and state inspection programs is conducted at USDA-approved laboratories. These are actually lagging indicators in measuring the process performance of meat or poultry plants because samples are taken after the product is prepared and packaged, and even with rapid methods, there is a significant lag time between the collection of the sample and the analysis of the laboratory data. By the time these data become available, the corresponding meat and poultry products often have been in the market for varying periods of time and may already have been consumed. Therefore, although microbiological samples provide both the plant and regulatory agency with a "score card" for plant performance, if further significant gains in the safety of the U.S. meat and poultry supply are to be realized, meat and poultry establishments need to implement more effective process control measures. As mentioned in Chapter 3, these process control measures should be linked to a systematic continuous improvement process to achieve the level of safety demanded by the U.S. consumer.

The Significance of Proper Implementation and Enforcement of the HACCP System

It is important to stress that any HACCP system, including one with scientifically valid microbiological performance standards, must be properly implemented to achieve its intended effect. The Government Accounting Office (GAO) audited HACCP implementation by FSIS (GAO, 2002) and concluded that there were deficiencies in the implementation process.

The GAO report identified three major areas of concern. The first relates to establishment of scientifically valid HACCP plans that properly identify hazards and appropriate Critical Control Points (CCPs). Some establishments have failed the hazard analysis or have omitted some legitimate hazards in it and have consequently not provided for adequate control or interventions of these hazards (e.g., chemical residues or *Salmonella*). Validation of a HACCP plan is the responsibility of industry personnel. FSIS inspectors are charged with verification of the Sanitation Standard Operating Procedures and HACCP plans, which may include reviewing the plan and the records and corrective actions taken—a task that requires training FSIS personnel. To this effect, a recent addition to the FSIS field staff, Consumer Safety Officers, will receive more training on HACCP than the traditional inspection personnel and will be tasked with critical evaluation of HACCP plans as part of HACCP phase-2 implementation, the "Next Steps." This program is being built slowly due to budget constraints.

A second area of concern mentioned in the GAO report, which if not corrected would make it difficult to implement scientifically valid performance standards, is the issue of corrective action if a plant experiences deviations from its HACCP plan and is deemed to be in noncompliance. Audits of these plants suggest that a majority have repetitive incidences of noncompliance without subsequent corrective action. The third concern identified in the GAO report is that if plants fail the *Salmonella* performance standard, regulatory action is not necessarily taken. Regulatory action letters may be delayed up to nine months. The report also indicates that, even when conditions occur that could lead to an order for suspension of inspection, orders are often put into abeyance by USDA.

As shown by GAO's analysis, complex factors appear to have hampered FSIS's ability to effectively enforce HACCP implementation in its initial phases. It is not within the charge of this committee to audit the administrative procedures involved in implementation of performance standards, but rather to comment on the scientific criteria involved in establishing them. However, the committee believes that scientific criteria, including performance standards, may be part of a HACCP program and can only be successful in reducing contamination if they are uniformly implemented, and if this implementation is enforced in a timely fashion by the responsible regulatory agency. Promulgation of new standards and establishment of rigid scientific criteria for safe food are useless if monitoring and enforcement are not ensured. To that effect, the responsibility of meat and poultry inspectors should be redefined to reflect their role within a HACCP food safety assurance system.

Consistency of the Inspection Process

There has been a consolidation of the meat and poultry industries in recent years. Many of the larger meat and poultry companies manage multiple processing plants across the United States that are regulated by both FDA and FSIS. This presents challenges to the plants and corporate management due to the inconsistent interpretation and enforcement of regulations, which in turn hinders implementation of consistent product safety strategies. Anecdotal stories abound in the industry about inconsistencies in the enforcement of rules and regulations between plants and between districts.

The committee recommends that FSIS continue its training program and the development of means to measure and evaluate the performance of its inspection team (i.e., Inspectors-in-Charge, Supervisory Veterinary Medical Officers, and inspectors), and state meat and poultry inspection teams, to ensure that regulations are consistently enforced across the country.

Concurrently, the committee recommends that FDA also continue to develop training programs and various means to measure and evaluate the performance of FDA inspectors and state regulatory agencies that conduct FDA inspections.

REVIEW OF CURRENT STANDARDS FOR MEAT AND POULTRY

Current Criteria and Performance Standards

USDA specifically charged this committee to develop definitions for terms such as "performance criteria" and "performance standard." The definitions of these and other relevant terms are presented in tabular form in Appendix A. The definitions adopted by the committee that are of particular relevance to the remaining sections of this chapter are those of performance standard and microbiological criterion.

Within the last decade, FSIS has established several criteria, including performance standards, as part of the current regulatory and inspection system for meat and poultry. These include criteria for process control and standards for pathogen reduction in raw products, adulteration, standards for cooked products, and general sanitation standards. Among these, criteria for process control and standards for pathogen reduction in raw products involve microbiological sampling and testing programs. The results of these testing programs are used by the agency to determine whether processors receive a "fail" or "pass." In contrast to these microbiological standards and criteria, which apply to a broad range of products, "adulteration" is very narrowly interpreted for a specific bacterium and product, *Escherichia coli* O157:H7 in raw ground beef.

Standards for cooked products differ from the standards for raw meat and poultry in that they require the reduction of a stated number of a specific pathogen, as well as validation of the process used to achieve that reduction, instead of a testing and sampling program.

Sanitation standards (as they are specifically referred to in the *Code of Federal Regulations*) are less prescriptive and contain vague descriptors such as "adequate" and "sufficient." Consequently, these standards are subject to more interpretation than either the cooking process or microbiological criteria or standards. Several types of standards or criteria are summarized and discussed in the following sections.

Contamination with Microorganisms; Process Control Verification Criteria and Testing; Pathogen Reduction Standards for Red Meats (9 Vol 2 C.F.R. §310.25)

These criteria are part of the PR/HACCP rule and include both process control criteria for *E. coli* Biotype I (generic *E. coli*) and performance standards for a specific pathogen (salmonellae). The process control criteria are based on the quantitative level of generic *E. coli* on or in fresh meats. The sampling technique includes a swab or excision method for intact carcasses and a destructive analysis for ground products. The sampling frequency varies both by species and by the relative size of the processing establishment (Table 4.1).

The sampling and testing protocol for the process control criteria are based on a three-class sampling program. In a three-class plan, m is the analytical value that differentiates good quality from marginally acceptable quality, M is defined as the analytical value that differentiates marginally acceptable quality from unacceptable quality, n is the number of samples taken, and c is the maximum number of samples out of n that may exceed the value set for m. For a sample set to pass, no sample may exceed the M value and no more than c samples may exceed the m value. The values for the various species are given in Table 4.2.

TABLE 4.1 Sampling Frequency for Process Control Indicator (Generic *Escherichia coli*) for Fresh Meat

Species or Size of Establishment	Samples per Number of Carcasses
Cattle, sheep, or horses	1 per 300
Swine	1 per 1,000
Very low-volume establishments	At least 1 per week, beginning June 1 of each year, until 13 in-compliance samples are collected in a row

SOURCE: 9 C.F.R. §310.25.

TABLE 4.2 Values for m, M, n, and c for the Process Control Indicator (Generic *Escherichia coli*) for Fresh Meat[a]

Species	m	M	n	c
Cattle	Negative[b]	100	13	3
Swine	10	10,000	13	3

[a] m = the analytical value that differentiates good quality from marginally acceptable quality, M = the analytical value that differentiates marginally acceptable quality from unacceptable quality, n = the number of samples taken, c = is the maximum number of samples out of n that may exceed the value set for m.

[b] Negative is defined by the sensitivity of the method used in the baseline study, with a limit of sensitivity of at least 5 cfu/cm^2 carcass surface area.

SOURCE: 9 C.F.R. §310.25.

TABLE 4.3 Values for *n* and *c* for the Pathogen Reduction Standard (*Salmonella* Performance Standard) for Fresh Meat

Product	Performance Standard (% positive for salmonellae)	Number of Samples Tested (*n*)	Maximum Number of Positives to Achieve Standard (*c*)
Steers/heifers	1.0	82	1
Cows/bulls	2.7	58	2
Ground beef	7.5	53	5
Hogs	8.7	55	6
Fresh pork sausage	NA[a]	NA	NA

[a] NA = not applicable.
SOURCE: 9 C.F.R. §310.25.

The sampling frequency for the pathogen reduction standard for *Salmonella* is identical to that for the process control indicator (Table 4.1). The sampling technique includes a swab or excision method for intact carcasses and a destructive analysis for ground products. In practice, FSIS will take an initial sample set (the A set). If an establishment fails the A set, FSIS will take up to two more sample sets (the B and C sets). Failure of all three sample sets would be grounds for USDA to withdraw inspection from an establishment.

The pathogen reduction standard is based on a two-class sampling plan, in which *n* is the number of samples taken and *c* is the number of samples allowed to fail the specification. The standard is based on a qualitative assay for the presence or absence of *Salmonella*. The values for the various species and products are given in Table 4.3.

Contamination with Microorganisms; Process Control Verification Criteria and Testing; Pathogen Reduction Standards in Raw Poultry (9 Vol 2 C.F.R. §381.94)

The process control criteria and the pathogen reduction standard for raw poultry are structured in an identical manner to those for red meats. The process control criteria are based on the numerical populations of *E. coli* Biotype I (generic *E. coli*) on or in fresh poultry meats. The sampling technique includes a whole-bird rinse for intact carcasses and a destructive analysis for ground product. The sampling frequency varies both by species and by the relative size of the processing establishment (Table 4.4).

The sampling and testing protocols are based on a three-class sampling program, as previously described. The values for the various species are given in Table 4.5.

For the pathogen reduction standard for *Salmonella,* the sampling frequency is identical to that for the process control indicator (Table 4.4). The sampling

TABLE 4.4 Sampling Frequency for Process Control Indicator (Generic *Escherichia coli*) for Raw Poultry

Species or Size of Establishment	Samples per Number of Carcasses
Chicken	1 per 22,000
Turkeys	1 per 3,000
Very low-volume establishments	At least 1 per week, beginning June 1 of each year, until 13 in-compliance samples are collected in a row

SOURCE: 9 C.F.R. §310.25.

TABLE 4.5 Values for *m*, *M*, *n*, and *c* for the Process Control Indicator (Generic *Escherichia coli*) for Raw Poultry[a]

Species	*m*	*M*	*n*	*c*
Chicken	100	1,000	13	3
Turkey	NA[b]	NA	NA	NA

[a] m = the analytical value that differentiates good quality from marginally acceptable quality, M = the analytical value that differentiates marginally acceptable quality from unacceptable quality, n = the number of samples taken, c = is the maximum number of samples out of n that may exceed the value set for m.
[b] NA = not applicable.
SOURCE: 9 C.F.R. §310.25.

technique includes a whole-bird rinse for intact carcasses and a destructive analysis for ground products. In practice, FSIS will take an initial sample set (the A set), and if an establishment fails the A set, FSIS will take up to two more sample sets (the B and C sets). Until recently, failure of all three sample sets would be grounds for USDA to withdraw inspection from an establishment.

The pathogen reduction standard is based on a two-class sampling plan, where n is the number of samples taken and c is the number of samples allowed to fail the specification. The standard is based on a qualitative assay for the presence or absence of salmonellae. The values for the various species and products are given in Table 4.6.

Adulteration of Ground Beef; E. coli O157:H7 (9 C.F.R. §417)

USDA believes that *E. coli* O157:H7 is an adulterant in raw ground beef based on its interpretation of the following section of the Federal Meat Inspection Act:

TABLE 4.6 Values for *n* and *c* for the Pathogen Reduction Standard (*Salmonella* Performance Standard) for Raw Poultry

Product	Performance Standard (% positive for salmonellae)	Number of Samples Tested (*n*)	Maximum Number of Positives to Achieve Standard (*c*)
Broilers	20.0	51	12
Ground chicken	44.6	53	26
Ground turkey	49.9	53	29
Turkeys	NA[a]	NA	NA

[a] NA = not applicable.
SOURCE: 9 C.F.R. §310.25.

> (m) The term ''adulterated'' shall apply to any carcass, part thereof, meat or meat food product under one or more of the following circumstances:
>
> (1) if it bears or contains any poisonous or deleterious substance which may render it injurious to health; but in case the substance is not an added substance, such article shall not be considered adulterated under this clause if the quantity of such substance in or on such article does not ordinarily render it injurious to health.
>
> (4) if it has been prepared, packed, or held under unsanitary conditions whereby it may have become contaminated with filth, or whereby it may have been rendered injurious to health. (21 U.S.C. §601 (m)(1) and (4))

USDA interpreted these statements to mean that the detectable presence of *E. coli* O157:H7 in raw ground beef product, irrespective of the method used to detect it, would meet either of the circumstances above and, therefore, such product would be considered adulterated.

Requirements for the Production of Cooked Beef, Roast Beef, and Cooked Corned Beef Products (9 Vol 2 C.F.R. §318.17)

The previous regulations for the production of cooked meat were modified so that they are now included as performance standards within the specific HACCP plans. Using HACCP terminology, the cooking step would be a CCP and the specific requirements would be the critical limits. The cooked red meat regulation includes two performance standards specifying (1) that the cooking process achieves a certain lethality for salmonellae, and (2) a specific rate of chilling (i.e., stabilization) for control of *Clostridium perfringens*. These requirements differ from the microbiological sampling programs required for raw meat and poultry in that the processor must show that its process is validated and, therefore, that it achieves the stated standard.

The standard for lethality, which must include a cooking step, specifies a 6.5-$\log_{10}$ reduction of *Salmonella* or an alternative lethality that achieves an equivalent probability that no viable *Salmonella* remain in the finished product. The standard for stabilization requires no multiplication of toxigenic microorganisms, such as *C. botulinum,* and no more than a 1-$\log_{10}$ multiplication of *C. perfringens.*

As an alternative, USDA has provided "safe harbor" processes for both lethality and stabilization standards that relieve the processor from having to validate the process. Briefly, a safe harbor process is one that has been established as accomplishing the objective. The safe harbor processes are compiled in FSIS Directives 7370.2 (FSIS, 1995) and 7110.3 (FSIS, 1989).

Requirements for the Production of Fully Cooked Poultry Products and Partially Cooked Poultry Breakfast Strips (9 Vol 2 C.F.R. §381.150)

The cooked poultry meat regulations contain process control requirements similar to the standards for red meats, and these requirements also need to be included in a plant's HACCP plan. The cooking step would be a CCP and the specific requirements would be the critical limits. The standard for lethality is a 7-$\log_{10}$ reduction of salmonellae or an alternative lethality that achieves an equivalent probability that no viable salmonellae remain in the finished product (it must include a cooking step). For stabilization, there can be no multiplication of toxigenic microorganisms such as *C. botulinum* and no more than a 1-$\log_{10}$ growth of *C. perfringens.*

The safe harbor processes are compiled in FSIS Directives 7370.2 (FSIS, 1995) and 7110.3 (FSIS, 1989).

Animal Drug Residues

The Center for Veterinary Medicine (CVM) of FDA is primarily responsible for establishing tolerances and action levels for antibiotics and hormones in the edible tissues of food-producing animals. The setting of such tolerances, and their surveillance by FSIS, was discussed earlier in the chemical risk assessment section of Chapter 3. A complete review of this area can also be found in the report *The Use of Drugs in Food Animals: Benefits and Risks* (NRC, 1999).

There are numerous types of drugs used in food animals. It is generally accepted in the United States that anabolic steroid hormones used to promote weight gain and feed efficiency enjoy a wide safety margin for human health when used at approved rates (21 Vol 6 C.F.R., parts 522, 556, and 558). Antibiotics may be used either to promote growth and feed efficiency (subtherapeutic use) or to treat actual disease (therapeutic use); the latter involves a veterinarian in the diagnosis and management of the disease. Compounds are either available over the counter or only by order of a licensed veterinarian. Veterinarians can prescribe drugs and dosages that are not specifically approved if a medical need arises. In food-producing animals, the veterinarian must also ensure that a substantially extended withdrawal time is allowed to eliminate residues from the edible tissue. Some chemicals are specifically prohibited from off-label use in food-producing animals (e.g., higher dose or for indication or species not on the approved label) (CVM, 2002a). These currently include chloramphenicol, clenbuterol, diethylstilbestrol, dimetridazole, ipronidazole, other nitroimidazoles, furazolidone, nitrofurazone, sulfonamide drugs in lactating dairy cattle (except approved use of sulfadimethoxine, sulfabromomethazine, and sulfaethoxypyridazine), fluoroquinolones, and glycopeptides (21 Vol 1 C.F.R. §530.41).

The use of drugs in food animals continues to undergo regulatory review. CVM recently promulgated a revised definition of the term "no residue" when it appears in new animal drug regulations to mean that no residue is detected using an approved regulatory method (21 Vol 1 C.F.R. §500.84). This term normally occurs in regulations where a drug is purported to be a human carcinogen, which is a toxic class that is regulated differently than other compounds. Also, CVM has issued a draft guidance to evaluate, through use of qualitative risk analysis methods, the safety of new antimicrobial animal drugs with regard to the possibility of eliciting development of resistance by bacteria that are of concern to human health (CVM, 2002). The tolerance that has already been set for some of these chemicals could be used as a performance standard.

Sanitation (9 Vol 2 C.F.R. §416)

The sanitation performance standards were changed from multiple, detailed, prescriptive regulations to standards. The regulations contain specific sections on grounds and facilities; equipment and utensils; sanitary operations; employee hygiene; and tagging of unsanitary equipment, utensils, rooms, or compartments. Although described as standards, the actual language includes numerous references to "adequate," "preventing sources of adulteration," and "sufficient." These regulations provide little in the way of a descriptive and objective standard and are better characterized as "guides." For example, the language of these regulations is sufficiently different from that of the regulations described previously as to question whether they are true standards, as defined by this committee in Appendix A. Appendix B summarizes the details of the sanitation performance standards.

Using a Science-Based Approach to Develop Performance Standards and Other Scientific Criteria

As described in Chapter 3, a science-based approach to developing criteria, including performance standards, entails gathering, analyzing, and utilizing the best available data. The strategy of combining a controlled study and expertise accepts the fact that gaps in the data will always exist and that these data gaps need to be supplemented with the qualitative knowledge of (and assumptions developed by) experts in the particular subject matter. Pilot studies are the preferred method of gathering data because they can be designed with the specific objective of developing performance standards. The qualitative data and assumptions are critical issues that can affect the quality of the performance standard; transparency in describing the assumptions made becomes a critical component in the development of a standard.

For example, the lethality and stabilization standard document for meat and poultry products describes the method USDA prescribed to achieve the 7-D reduction of *Salmonella* in ready-to-eat (RTE) poultry products and the 6.5-D reduction of *Salmonella* in RTE beef products (FSIS, 1998c). In this document, which also describes the scientific basis for the stabilization performance standard, the validity of the data used and the assumptions made are not clear from either a mathematical or microbiological perspective. In addition, the microbiological and technological assumptions may not reflect actual manufacturing conditions. For example, the baseline data used were the FSIS Nationwide Microbiological Baseline Data Collection Programs and the Nationwide Federal Plant Microbiological Surveys, published between 1994 and 1996. Because these data were gathered prior to the implementation of the PR/HACCP rule, they do not reflect improvements that were made as a result of the implementation of the rule. The authors of the performance standard assumed that the rule would not reduce the incidence of *Salmonella* in RTE products.

Regulatory agencies need to properly set performance standards. This is a balancing act between setting a highly conservative performance standard and setting an excessively tolerant one. Although the safety margin approach is valid and useful, developing a standard that uses a safety margin based on a highly conservative worst-case scenario may lead to production of overprocessed products of inferior quality and may place an undue economic burden on the processor, without significantly increasing product safety. Setting performance standards that are too tolerant, on the other hand, may lead to production of unsafe products.

As discussed in Chapter 3, the committee stresses the importance of and recommends an increase in transparency during the development of performance standards. This transparency must include making public—within limits of the Freedom of Information Act and taking into consideration confidentiality and trade secrets—any analytical data used, the method used to analyze the data, and the assumptions that are made to fill in any data or technical gaps. Increasing the transparency of the process to set performance standards provides an opportunity for informed comments and input from the affected public to the regulatory agencies. This transparency is needed to increase the quality of performance standards and to provide appropriate information for conducting better reviews of the standards, either by external agencies such as GAO or by internal teams; to update the performance standard; and to meet future public health objectives.

The committee also stresses the need to use proper assumptions in developing performance standards. When regulatory agencies set performance standards, they need to balance a number of factors, including public health objectives, economic burden, available technologies, and the effect of the interventions on product quality.

The specific standards and the basis and rationale for their implementation are discussed in subsequent sections.

The Scientific Basis of Current Criteria and Performance Standards

USDA discussed the rationale for the introduction and use of process control criteria and pathogen reduction standards for fresh meats in the PR/HACCP rule (FSIS, 1996). The following sections include portions of the rule. They also include the committee's summary and analysis of the scientific basis and rationale for each standard, as argued in the rule. Based on the analyses, the committee presents recommendations for improvements.

Process Control Criteria; Generic E. coli in or on Fresh Meats (9 Vol 2 C.F.R. §310.25)

> In slaughter establishments, fecal contamination of carcasses is the primary avenue for contamination by pathogens. Pathogens may reside in fecal material and ingesta, both within the gastrointestinal tract and on the exterior surfaces of animals going to slaughter. Therefore, without care being taken in handling and dressing procedures during slaughter and processing, the edible portions of the carcass can become contaminated with bacteria capable of causing illness in humans. Additionally, once introduced into the establishment environment, the organisms may be spread from carcass to carcass.
>
> Because the microbial pathogens associated with fecal contamination are the single most likely source of potential food safety hazard in slaughter establishments, preventing and removing fecal contamination and associated bacteria are vital responsibilities of slaughter establishments. Further, because such contamination is largely preventable, controls to address it will be a critical part of any slaughter establishment's HACCP plan. Most slaughter establishments already have in place procedures designed to prevent and remove visible fecal contamination.
>
> There is general agreement within the scientific community that generic *E. coli* is the best single microbial indicator for fecal contamination. FSIS, therefore, is requiring that establishments slaughtering livestock or poultry begin testing for *E. coli* (*E. coli*, biotype I, nonspecific as to species, hereinafter referred to simply as *E. coli*) at the frequency and following the procedures described in 'Process Control Verification; *E. coli* Performance Criteria and Testing' section, . . . , 6 months after publication of the final rule FSIS considers the required testing to be essential for meeting current statutory requirements

> for sanitation and the prevention of adulteration. This testing also will play an integral role in the successful implementation of HACCP in slaughter establishments. In addition, FSIS is establishing process control performance criteria for fecal contamination based on the frequency and levels of contamination of carcasses with *E. coli.* (FSIS, 1996, Pp. 38837–38838)
>
> FSIS is also establishing performance criteria based on national microbiological baseline surveys. The criteria are not regulatory standards but rather provide a benchmark for use by slaughter establishments in evaluating *E. coli* test results. Test results that do not meet the performance criteria will be an indication that the slaughter establishment may not be maintaining adequate process control for fecal contamination and associated bacteria. Such results will be used in conjunction with other information to evaluate and make appropriate adjustments to ensure adequate process control for fecal contamination and associated bacteria. (FSIS, 1996, P. 38811)
>
> FSIS believes that testing for generic *E. coli* is the appropriate and necessary means by which meat and poultry slaughter establishments must verify their process controls. (FSIS, 1996, Pp. 38838–38839)

According to a report by the National Research Council (NRC, 1985b), there are other bacteria or groups of bacteria (fecal streptococci, for example) that may serve equally well as indicators of fecal contamination as generic *E. coli*. However, that report also stated that limits for indicator organisms were impractical because "there is no direct relationship between the presence of these types [indicator organisms] and the presence or absence of pathogens." Although arguable, there is in fact general agreement within the scientific community that generic *E. coli* is perhaps the best indicator of fecal contamination. In spite of this controversy, the FSIS rationale makes reasonable assumptions and proceeds in a logical fashion. The baseline data used to develop the performance standard were collected from 1992 to 1997 as part of the FSIS Nationwide Microbiological Baseline Data Collection Programs and the Nationwide Federal Plant Microbiological Surveys. These programs were intended to give a general microbiological profile of a product for the selected microorganisms as a reference for further investigations and evaluations of new programs. The use of a three-class sampling protocol is appropriate for the intended purpose. The values of m, M, n, and c were established based on the national baseline data for each species and were set at levels that would allow approximately 80 percent of the establishments to pass the criteria.

Because the generic *E. coli* limits are a guideline, industry is not obligated to have a sampling and testing program in place. Although the data collected by the industry are not within the public domain and therefore not available for review, the criteria for generic *E. coli* (Biotypes I and II) have been implemented in essentially all federally and state inspected establishments. The criteria have been used to detect problems and document acceptable control of the process, and anecdotal reports indicate that the criteria have served to document a reduction in the levels of carcass contamination and have led to process improvement. An additional benefit of the generic *E. coli* criteria has been an increased awareness in the meat and poultry industry of the importance and significance of process control on the microbiological status of carcasses. The concept of continuous improvement is central to food safety. In principle, if populations of generic *E. coli* are extremely low, the sampling results from carcass data may not provide sufficient information to enable the processor to detect remaining problems and further improve operations. In situations where the populations of generic *E. coli* are too low to provide valuable information to the processor, the committee recommends that a reevaluation of the criteria be conducted, to identify either an alternate system of testing (i.e., sampling a larger area) or another indicator of carcass hygiene. Because the *E. coli* data collected by industry are not in the public domain, it is currently not possible to determine whether this is in fact a significant limitation to continuous process improvement.

The committee recommends that an anonymous national database be created to collect the available generic *E. coli* data on carcasses so that industry and regulatory and public health agencies have benchmarks available for comparative purposes. The committee further recommends that this database be operated by a nonregulatory government agency or under contract to a university or nonprofit organization. This would allay industry concerns about potential use of such industry-generated data for regulation enforcement purposes.

In addition, the committee recommends the implementation of criteria for generic *E. coli* in ground beef. These criteria should be developed using the generic *E. coli* criteria for carcasses as the model. The data from these criteria should be handled in the same manner as recommended for the *E. coli* criteria for carcasses (i.e., a national, anonymous database).

> FSIS is purposely using the term performance "criteria" rather than performance "standard" in this context because no single set of test results can demonstrate conclusively that adequate process control for fecal contamination is or is not being maintained. As explained below, if test results do not meet the applicable criterion, it raises questions about the adequacy of the process control. FSIS intends to consider the establishment's results and corrective actions, together with other information and inspectional observations, in evaluating whether a problem exists that requires regulatory action or other measures to protect consumers and ensure compliance with the law. (FSIS, 1996, P. 38838)

FSIS has established that a "criterion" is similar to a "microbiological guideline," as defined by the International Commission on the Microbiological Safety of Foods (ICMSF). That is, a microbiological guideline is a criterion to monitor a food process or system (ICMSF, 2002). These criteria are usually considered advisory, but may be mandatory. In the case of criteria for process control, the recommended levels are advisory, although FSIS clearly expects action to be taken if there is routine failure of the criteria.

Pathogen Reduction Standard; Salmonella Performance Standard (9 Vol 2 C.F.R. §310.25)

> FSIS is also establishing pathogen reduction performance standards for *Salmonella* that will require all slaughter establishments to reduce the incidence of *Salmonella* contamination of finished meat and poultry carcasses below the national baseline prevalence as established by the most recent FSIS national microbiological baseline data for each major species. FSIS will conduct *Salmonella* testing in slaughter establishments to detect whether they are meeting the pathogen reduction performance standards, and will require corrective action or take regulatory action, as appropriate, to ensure establishments are meeting the pathogen reduction standards.
>
> Pathogen-specific performance standards for raw products are an essential component of the FSIS food safety strategy because they provide a direct measure of progress in controlling and reducing the most significant hazards associated with raw meat and poultry products. The *Salmonella* standards being established in this final rule, which are based on the current national baseline prevalence of *Salmonella* (expressed as a percentage of contaminated carcasses), are a first step in what FSIS expects to be a broader reliance in the future on pathogen-specific performance standards. FSIS plans to repeat its baseline surveys and collect substantial additional data through other means and, on that basis, adjust the *Salmonella* performance standards and possibly set standards for additional pathogens, as appropriate. Also, FSIS will continue to explore establishing pathogen-specific performance standards based on the levels of contamination (i.e., the number of organisms) on a carcass. Future FSIS efforts on such performance standards will reflect the fact that achieving the food safety goal of reducing foodborne illness to the maximum extent possible will require continuous efforts and improvement over a substantial period. (FSIS, 1996, Pp. 38811–38812)

The stated purpose of the *Salmonella* performance standard is to promote a reduction in the levels of *Salmonella* on raw meat, hence the name Pathogen Reduction Standard. The NRC report (NRC, 1985a) stated that limits for pathogenic microorganisms in microbiological criteria for raw meats are impractical. However, since data from the USDA verification program show that the goal was achieved—a reduction of the incidence of salmonellae in or on meat—the committee concludes that these standards are valid. In some instances, however, if the populations or incidences of salmonellae are extremely low, especially on carcasses of some production animal species, the testing may no longer be providing the information needed by the processor to continue making improvements in the process. Other testing approaches may need to be considered in such cases.

Because of the importance of the baseline data, the committee recommends that a new baseline survey be conducted on a periodic basis to evaluate the microbiological status of carcass, trim, ground product, and RTE products, both at the site of production and at the retail level. This survey should evaluate the same microorganisms that were evaluated in the previous baseline surveys unless evidence for newly established pathogens is presented. The sampling design for the survey should be weighted based on the production of the establishment and account for geographical location and seasonality. Also, it is important that data for this new baseline be collected in such a way as to address two competing concerns. First, it should be possible to compare the results of the new baseline to the old baseline to determine if the situation is improving, worsening, or staying the same. Second, the new baseline should be representative and statistically valid and should correct deficiencies in the sampling plan used for the 1992 to 1997 baseline. The survey should ideally be coordinated with other baseline data collection projects, such as the Animal and Plant Health Inspection Service's National Animal Health Monitoring Survey (NAHMS).

The baseline data used to develop the *Salmonella* performance standard were collected in the same manner as that for the *E. coli* process control criteria. The use of a two-class sampling protocol is appropriate for the intended purpose. The values of n and c were established based on the national baseline data for each species, and set at levels that would allow approximately 80 percent of establishments to pass, based on the baseline data.

USDA's implementation of the PR/HACCP rule in meat and poultry plants is one of several recent control measures credited with decreasing the overall incidence of foodborne illness in the United States from 1996 to 2002 (HHS, 2002). Data obtained from the Foodborne Diseases Active Surveillance Network (FoodNet) reveal an overall decline of 23 percent in bacterial foodborne illnesses during this 6-year period (CDC, 2002). Since the introduction of PR/HACCP, declines in the rate of *Salmonella* infections in the U.S. population have coincided with declines in the prevalence of *Salmonella* detected in FSIS-regulated products (CDC, 2002; USDA, 2002). Rose and colleagues (2002) reported on the prevalence of *Salmonella* in raw meat and poultry, assessed on the basis of the proportion of inspected meat-production facilities passing the *Salmonella* performance standard in 1998, 1999, and 2000, compared with the defining pre-HACCP baseline prevalence data. This study consisted of 98,204 samples and 1,502 completed sample sets collected from large, small, and very small processing plants that produced one of the following: broilers, market hogs, cows, bulls, steers and heifers, or ground beef, chicken, or turkey. The overall conclusion was that greater than 80 percent of the sample sets met the *Salmonella* performance standards of 20.0 percent for broilers, 8.7 percent for market hogs, 2.7 percent for cows and bulls, 1.0 percent for steers and heifers, 7.5 percent for ground beef, 44.6 percent for ground chicken, and 49.9 percent for ground turkey. The percentage of samples positive for *Salmonella* was generally lower than in the pre-HACCP baseline data. Data were also collected on second and third visits to plants that did not meet the performance standards on the first visit. Of the 98,206 samples collected, 6,260 were from second visits and 752 were from third visits.

These results are encouraging despite some significant limitations in the data sets collected relevant to balance of the samples based on establishment size. In addition, the post-HACCP data were not designed to serve as a prevalence survey, but for verification and compliance purposes; thus, direct comparison to the pre-HACCP baseline survey is problematic. For this reason, it may not be statistically valid to compare the two data sets; however, because of the vast number of data sets collected, a decrease in *Salmonella*-positive samples can be clearly observed since the implementation of the *Salmonella* standard.

The committee points out, however, that correlation and causation are two separate and distinct concepts, and while correlated, it may not be scientifically defensible to assume a cause-and-effect relationship between the PR/HACCP rule and the observed decline in the incidence of salmonellosis. The committee, recognizing the importance of measuring the public health impact of pathogen reduction performance standards, addressed this issue in Chapter 2 and recommended expanded foodborne disease surveillance and microbial testing of foods, linked to a comparison of microbial serotypes in isolates from animals, humans, and foods, as a means to enable regulatory and public health agencies to allocate the burden of foodborne disease to specific foods or classes of food.

A number of changes have occurred coincident with HACCP implementation. The positive side of this survey (Rose et al., 2002) is that *Salmonella* meat contamination levels were generally reduced, a finding consistent with improvement through HACCP implementation. As discussed elsewhere in this report, this does not mean that raw meat products are free from *Salmonella*, only that the performance standards based on pre-HACCP baseline prevalence targets have been met. These targets are very different across meat classes. For example, the performance standard for steers and heifers showed only one positive sample out of a sample set of 82. For ground chicken, there were 26 positive samples out of a sample set of 53. The goal of the *Salmonella* performance standards was to reduce the prevalence of *Salmonella* in raw meat and poultry products. The committee recognizes that this goal is apparently being achieved.

Despite the statistical validity and possible contribution to improving public health, the *Salmonella* performance standards have been highly debated, especially for ground products. The stated regulatory purpose of the *Salmonella* performance standard for ground products is to provide an evaluation of the HACCP plan of grinding operations. On October 7, 2002, FSIS issued a *Federal Register* notice informing establishments that produce raw beef product, especially intact and nonintact products in the process categories of raw product ground, raw not ground, and slaughter, about the need to reassess HACCP plans for *E. coli* O157:H7 (FSIS, 2002a). Until October 2002, the raw material used to manufacture ground beef (boneless beef trim) may have passed all parts of the inspection system, and may have been processed under a valid HACCP system, and yet still contain *E. coli* O157:H7. Since there is no required testing of the trim itself, the possible presence of the bacterium is not detected until testing of the final product is conducted. As currently practiced, the testing performed by FSIS often does not result in detection of the bacterium until after the ground beef has been distributed, and is often already in the hands of the consumer. Until the October 2002 *Federal Register* notice, the regulatory burden fell solely on the producer of the ground beef, even though the actual source of the bacterium may not be within the grinding operation, but at the production of the trim. The beef grinding operations do have a responsibility to regulate the quality of the incoming raw materials, but the producers of that raw material also have a responsibility to take active measures to reduce contamination of the trim. This point has been addressed by several large companies in that they now provide purchase specification letters to their customers describing their intervention procedures on carcasses and testing for *E. coli* O157:H7 on trimmings and in ground beef (Shire, 2003).

As a consequence of the weaknesses of the *Salmonella* performance standard for ground beef, enforcement of this standard has been particularly problematic. With ground beef, the pathogen may be an indication of cross-contamination; however, unless testing of the numerous sources of trimmings is performed, the standard alone cannot be appropriately used to judge the sanitary conditions of the grinding plant. The question of who is responsible for the regulatory failure when a grinding plant fails to meet the standard has not been resolved.

In addition, and although the regulations state that failing the *Salmonella* performance standard may result in withdrawal of federal inspectors, recent litigation has raised questions about USDA's statutory authority for such an action. The statutory framework for government enforcement of performance standards created to assure food safety has proven to be inflexible. In *Supreme Beef Processors v. USDA,* 275 F. 3d 432 (5th Cir. 2001), the United States Court of Appeals decided that USDA's *Salmonella* performance standard improperly regulated the *Salmonella* levels of meat entering Supreme Beef's grinding plant and that cross-contamination of ground beef with *Salmonella* could not be considered an unsanitary condition rendering the product "injurious to health." Thus, in the absence of finding unsanitary conditions at the establishment, USDA could not withdraw inspection from a grinding plant that had failed the *Salmonella* performance standard.

The Court's reading of 21 U.S.C. §601(m)(4) was that "it cannot be used to regulate characteristics of the raw materials that exist before the meat product is 'prepared, packed or held'." That is, the USDA *Salmonella* performance standard, as applied to grinding plants, is invalid "because it regulates the procurement of raw materials," not the sanitary conditions of the grinding plant. Also, because ground beef can be cooked to control *Salmonella* and therefore may not be injurious to health, the Court decided that *Salmonella* is not itself considered an "adulterant" subject to the prohibition of 21 U.S.C. §601(m)(1). In addition,

USDA's claim that the *Salmonella* performance standard is a proxy for the presence or absence of pathogen controls was dismissed by the court, which found USDA's motivation for the performance standard to be regulation of *Salmonella* itself. The *Supreme Beef* case clearly illustrates how the legal environment in which food safety regulatory bodies operate is in conflict with the implementation of current performance standards.

In a more recent, high-profile case, USDA entered into a settlement with Nebraska Beef Ltd. that did not result in withdrawal of federal inspection, after issuing numerous citations against the firm for unsanitary conditions linked to the discovery of hamburger contaminated with *E. coli* O157:H7. While this case was not based upon failure of the *Salmonella* performance standard, it sparked considerable discussion and concern, including an editorial in the *New York Times* (Becker, 2003), about whether USDA had adequate authority to protect the public health.

Whether *Salmonella* is an adulterant under existing statutes should not be the issue. The law currently forbids the holding or processing of foods under unsanitary conditions. The law should also ensure that foods that pose an unacceptable risk to consumers (because of either unusually high levels of pathogens or a high incidence of pathogens) are not marketed. The committee, recognizing all of the above, recommends that a *Salmonella* performance standard or other appropriate indicator be developed for beef trim intended for grinding (see Figure 4.2). Such a standard could be defined as either the presence/absence of the indicator or a quantitative measurement whenever possible. In addition, the committee recommends that the *Salmonella* performance standard for ground beef be reevaluated after appropriate interventions and the trim performance standard are in place. Further research should be conducted to determine an appropriate performance standard for ground beef at the grinding operation.

Furthermore, the committee recommends that all meat intended for trim for ground products, especially ground beef, be exposed to some form of verified intervention. This also applies to meat derived from heads, which currently may not be subjected to any intervention.

Adulteration of Ground Beef; Escherichia coli O157:H7 (21 U.S.C. §§601, 608, 621)

FSIS interpreted the statements in the above sections of the U.S. Code to mean that the detectable presence of *E. coli* O157:H7 in ground beef, irrespective of the method used, would meet either of the circumstances that would qualify this pathogen as an adulterant in ground beef. The rationale for this interpretation appears to be that ground beef contains meat from multiple carcasses, and that grinding incorporates the bacteria throughout the meat. In contrast, intact muscle cuts originate from a single carcass, and therefore, any microbial contamination that is present is only on the external surfaces of the meat. The significance of this

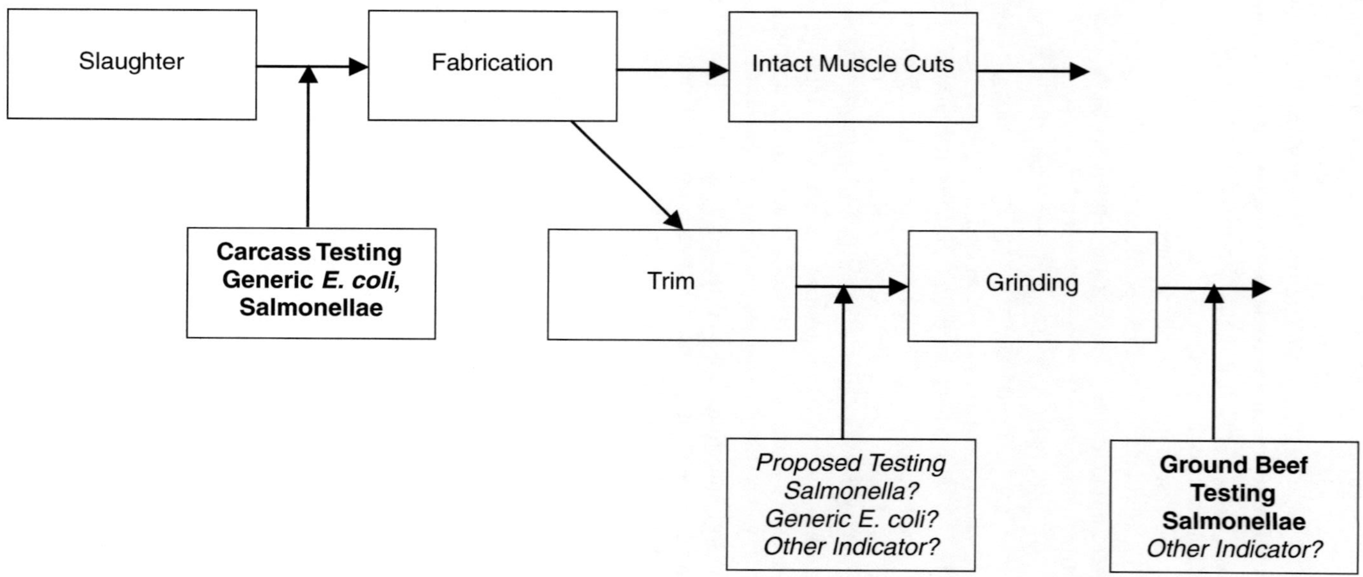

FIGURE 4.2 Current and proposed microbiological testing of ground beef. Text in **bold** indicates existing testing; text in *italics* indicates proposed testing.

is that with intact muscle cuts, cooking will destroy the bacteria on the surface—and therefore any *E. coli* O157:H7 present—even if the internal temperature of the cut does not reach a temperature sufficiently high to destroy this pathogen. In contrast, ground product does contain bacteria throughout the meat, and if the internal temperature does not reach a temperature sufficiently high to destroy *E. coli* O157:H7, a health hazard may exist (FSIS, 1999a).

This interpretation results in a situation where beef trim, if contaminated with *E. coli* O157:H7, is still considered acceptable under FSIS regulations, but is considered adulterated if that trim is ground. In the United States, it is common to blend beef carcass trim from a variety of domestic and foreign sources to achieve a specific ratio of lean muscle tissue to fat, and then grind the blended trim to produce ground beef. Many independent establishments produce ground beef for both the retail and foodservice markets, and to do this they buy beef trim from various suppliers. For these independent establishments, the burden of enforcement falls entirely upon them. That is, an independent grinding establishment may buy beef trim that is inspected and passed by FSIS, but may be classified as adulterated after grinding if it is contaminated with *E. coli* O157:H7. The grinding process in and of itself may not introduce the bacterium into the product; however, if the bacterium is present, it is redistributed throughout the ground meat.

Because of the low infectious dose attributed to *E. coli* O157:H7 and the potential severity of the disease it causes, the presence of this pathogen in foods is a serious human health hazard. However, even though *E. coli* O157:H7 has been declared an adulterant in ground beef (i.e., there is a zero tolerance policy), the regulation has been insufficient to reduce the rate of human illness attributable to this microorganism. Thus, the corresponding human health data have shown no significant change in disease rates since 1996 (CDC, 2002). (A reported increase in the incidence of the pathogen in ground beef since 1999, as indicated by FSIS testing, is most likely the result of a change to a more sensitive analytical methodology in 1998.)

It is difficult to rely on zero tolerance to achieve significant public health improvements. While it is impossible to guarantee the absence of *E. coli* O157:H7 or any pathogen in food through a zero tolerance policy, the evidence indicates that either cooking to at least 160°F or irradiating to a high enough dose are reliable means of reducing the levels of *E. coli* O157:H7. Irradiation, however, does not replace the need for proper cooking.

The advice to cook hamburger to the recommended internal temperature of 160°F often goes unheeded by those who prepare it. Considerably more education of the public and particularly of food service managers and workers is needed. Ground beef products should bear clear and concise labels warning of the potential for harm if the product is not properly cooked.

Irradiation occurs as part of the process, before distribution, so that the meat that reaches the consumer has a reduced risk of contamination. When the contamination is reduced before distribution, the potential for cross-contamination is significantly reduced at the level of preparation and consumption. Irradiation is applied to meats that have already passed all existing federal regulatory requirements and is used as an additional intervention to assure the microbiological safety of the meat. The committee believes that when used, irradiation must be incorporated into the overall HACCP system; it must not be used as a substitute for existing CCPs and other interventions.

Microbial contaminants have to be prevented from entering the food supply or eliminated by applying an effective intervention measure to the food. Within the HACCP concept, if there are no CCPs for a hazard, then, in the literal sense, there is no way for HACCP to control the pathogen. This is the situation with *E. coli* O157:H7 in raw ground beef, for which CCPs are yet to be defined. To define CCPs, in turn, it is essential that the ecology and mode of transmission of this pathogen, from the farm to the slaughter, carcass decontamination stage, and into the trims, be understood. The assumption has been that *E. coli* O157:H7 is transmitted through feces. However, recent research has suggested that the bacterium may also be transmitted by other means such as the oral cavity of animals (Keen and Elder, 2002).

Therefore, the committee points to the urgent need for research on the ecology of *E. coli* O157:H7 and other close serotypes in beef, from the farm through transportation, lairage, slaughter, decontamination treatments, and into the trim, and recommends that USDA promptly undertake or fund such research. Parallel research to develop better interventions to prevent contaminated trim destined for ground product, especially ground beef, should be urgently conducted as well.

In the meantime, until such information on the ecology and mode of transmission of this pathogen is available and effective preventive or corrective controls can be applied at the identified CCPs so that HACCP can be put into practice for ground beef, the committee urges regulatory and health authorities to (1) advise those members of the public who would prefer to minimize the risk of this product to cook irradiated and nonirradiated ground beef products to the appropriate temperature, (2) require the products to be clearly labeled with a warning of the potential for harm if not properly cooked, and (3) expand educational efforts to the public and to target commercial and noncommercial food service managers and workers.

Once the ecology of *E. coli* O157:H7 is better understood, other technologies may prove effective to control it. For example, the concept of selective use for contaminated trim discussed in Chapter 2 (e.g., for irradiation or cooking only) could then be contemplated as an additional tool to protect consumers.

As mentioned previously, FoodNet data (CDC, 2002) suggest that the occurrence of illness due to *E. coli* O157:H7 has not declined during the past five years, raising questions as to whether the current testing of ground beef for *E. coli* O157:H7 is achieving its desired goal. The committee felt that it was important to emphasize the need for testing and interventions prior to the grinding operation. If the contamination of the trim used for ground beef could be reduced, or if contaminated trim could be diverted to other processes, then the potential for contaminated fresh ground beef reaching the consumer would be reduced. The current survey testing at the retail level serves a purpose as a means of monitoring progress on this issue. However, there is also a need for more effective monitoring of the process itself.

Adulteration of Ready-to-Eat Meats (9 Vol 2 C.F.R. §§301, 303, 317, 318, 319, 320, 325, 331, 381, 417, 430)

FSIS also applies the interpretation of adulteration to the presence of any human pathogen in RTE products. RTE meats, even though some may be labeled with instructions to reheat before consumption, are generally considered adulterated if they contain organisms or toxins that are hazardous to the public health. As an example, the detectable presence of *L. monocytogenes* in RTE processed meats, such as hot dogs, would be considered adulteration.

The regulations on lethality and stabilization were based on the incidence of salmonellae in precooked, ready-to-serve roast beef (FSIS, 1999b). The present concerns with *L. monocytogenes* in RTE meats are also based on this interpretation of adulteration, and the current tolerance for *L. monocytogenes* in RTE meats is "none detectable" within the analytical unit (FSIS, 1999b).

It is difficult to rely on zero tolerance to achieve significant public health improvements. This is even more evident with *L. monocytogenes* than with *E. coli* O157:H7, because *L. monocytogenes* does not survive the thermal process applied in the processing of RTE meats and contaminates the meat after processing and either before or during packaging. Since *L. monocytogenes* is a common environmental bacterium, there are many potential sources of contamination, including the packaging environment and the employees themselves (FSIS, 1999b).

The incidence of *L. monocytogenes* in RTE meats in the United States is low (overall 1.82 percent [Gombas et al., 2003]) and the incidence of human listeriosis is apparently declining (CDC, 2002); however, the incidence of *L. monocytogenes* in these products has not been reduced to zero. Canada, as well as other countries, has recognized that zero tolerance is not practically achievable and has established numerical standards for the presence of *L. monocytogenes* in cheeses that do not support the growth of *L. monocytogenes*. Unless a terminal process can be applied after RTE meat has been sealed in its final packaging, the absence of *L. monocytogenes* in any randomly selected package of any specific RTE meat cannot be ensured.

Lethality; Standards for the Production of Certain Meat and Poultry Products (9 Vol 2 C.F.R . §§318.17, 381.150)

The *Lethality and Stabilization Performance Standards for Certain Meat and Poultry Products: Technical Paper* (FSIS, 1998c) describe the method FSIS issued to achieve the 7-D reduction of *Salmonella* in RTE poultry products and the 6.5-D reduction of *Salmonella* in RTE beef products.

The rationale given by FSIS for the lethality guidelines was based on the establishment of a worst-case population of salmonellae, by animal species, then the probability of salmonellae survival in 100 g of finished product after the specific lethality processes was calculated. Specifically, the worst case was defined as an approximate 97.5 percent upper bound for the number of salmonellae in a sample with the highest density of salmonellae from each baseline survey. Considering estimates of 2,300 salmonellae/g in raw poultry, a 30 percent recovery rate of salmonellae after processing, and the 97.5 percent defined upper bound, a worst-case value of 37,500 organisms/g was calculated. In a serving size of 143 g of raw product (assuming a serving size of 100 g of the cooked product), there would be approximately 5,362,500 (6.7 $\log_{10}$) salmonellae. Thus, to minimize the risk to the consumers, a process that results in a 7-D reduction of salmonellae would be necessary.

From the statistical standpoint, this approach of determining a worst-case scenario is more appropriate than using an arbitrary safety factor in that it allows FSIS to better address any uncertainty associated with the worst-case value. However, the committee believes that several of the estimates were incorrectly assumed, which resulted in an excessively conservative performance standard. For example, the worst-case definition and lethality for RTE poultry products were determined using the raw ground poultry surveys. These surveys had certain limitations, including that they did not cover all of the summer months, and therefore did not completely represent possible seasonal variations in the prevalence and levels of salmonellae. In addition, the decimal reduction value (the D_{10} value) was applied on the total population instead of on a per-gram basis. A 7-D reduction would be sufficient to bring the salmonellae population from 10,000,000 to a theoretical 1 cell/g. In fact, when using the highly improbable FSIS worst-case figure of 37,500 salmonellae cells/g, the regulation should require only a 4.5-$\log_{10}$ reduction or 4.5-D process.

Stabilization; Performance Standards for the Production of Certain Meat and Poultry Products (9 Vol 2 C.F.R. §§318.17, 381.150)

The standard for stabilization requires no multiplication of toxigenic microorganisms, such as *C. botulinum,* and no more than 1-$\log_{10}$ multiplication of *C. perfringens*. The stabilization guidelines were derived by assuming a worst-case population for *C. perfringens* and assuming that at least 1 million cells are necessary to result in illness in most cases. The worst-case population was assumed to be 10,000 for both beef and poultry, and therefore, a 1-$\log_{10}$ increase in population would still maintain a level below the 1 million/g population necessary to cause illness. This is a valid approach and provides an ample margin of safety. However, this margin may be too conservative and may force the meat processor to overprocess products, thus reducing quality.

FSIS proposed to codify the chilling recommendations in FSIS Directive 7110.3 (FSIS, 1989) as safe harbors. FSIS determined that this chilling directive would constitute a safe harbor because compliance would yield cooked poultry products that would meet the stabilization performance standard and because most, if not all, establishments were already following this directive.

From the statistical and the microbiological perspectives, the paper on the scientific basis for the stabilization standards (FSIS, 1998c) is very confusing and hard to use to determine the validity of either the data or the assumptions. Therefore, it is difficult to critically review this performance standard and assess the validity of the assumptions made during its development. This again illustrates the need for greater transparency in the development of food safety criteria.

Cured meat products are not included in this directive and, therefore, the lethality and stabilization standards should not be applied to these products.

APPLICATION OF PERFORMANCE STANDARDS WITHIN THE HACCP SYSTEM

Beef and Pork

The HACCP-based regulatory system is a good example of a regulatory approach that includes government, industry, and the public sector. Various companies throughout the food industry have been using HACCP principles since their inception to manage the risk of unsafe products entering commerce, especially for foods that have a terminal process, such as commercially sterile low-acid canned foods. FDA used HACCP principles when promulgating the low-acid canned food regulations (21 C.F.R. Part 114).

The use of performance standards is different from establishing specific microbiological criteria for foods. The National Research Council Subcommittee on Microbiological Criteria addressed the subject of microbiological criteria in raw meats (NRC, 1985a). One of its summary statements was:

> Microbiological standards for raw meats will prevent neither spoilage nor foodborne illness and thus do not appear warranted. Instead, application of the HACCP system to the entire processing and distribution chain including the meat-processing plant, retail units, foodservice establishment, and home should be used to produce a product with satisfactory shelf-life and public health safety. (NRC, 1985a, P. 198)

The validity of this conclusion is under scrutiny. At the time of the 1985 report, only three outbreaks of *E. coli* O157:H7 had been documented and much was yet to be learned about this microorganism from both a scientific and a societal perspective. The failure of a microbiological criterion to achieve its public health goal is illustrated by the zero tolerance for *E. coli* O157:H7 in ground beef; outbreaks still occur. However, due to the potential severity of the resulting illness, especially in children, it may now be inappropriate to establish a level of tolerance other than zero.

The PR/HACCP rule established three mandatory provisions (FSIS, 1996). One provision mandates HACCP systems as a means of preventing or controlling contamination from pathogens. Two other provisions mandate testing for either *E. coli* biotype I or *Salmonella*. The *E. coli* criteria attempt to evaluate the processing efficacy at slaughter in preventing or removing fecal contamination of the carcasses. The stated purpose of the *Salmonella* performance standards for slaughter and for grinding operations is to verify that HACCP systems are working.

The question of whether *Salmonella* or other microorganisms should be used to evaluate control of the slaughter process is controversial. USDA held three technical meetings between the time of the proposed rule (February 1995) and publishing the final rule (July 1996). One of these meetings dealt with the role of microbiological testing in verifying food safety (FSIS, 1996). Several of the presenters at this meeting advocated the use of *E. coli* instead of *Salmonella* as the organism of choice to make evaluations on control of the slaughter process. Arguments made for using *E. coli* were based upon (1) quantitative results as compared with qualitative results for *Salmonella*, (2) a much higher association with fecal contamination than *Salmonella,* and (3) the ability of plants to have results within 24 hours. In contrast, other speakers supported using *Salmonella* instead of *E. coli*, primarily because they believed that it would be established that HACCP was indeed reducing microorganisms of concern. It was also argued that the qualitative test for *Salmonella* was more appropriate because mishandling of the sample after collection would not result in a false positive, whereas mishandling of a quantitative sample could cause the data to be much higher than at the point of sample collection.

Of primary concern is the *Salmonella* performance standard and its link to HACCP. Within red meats, *Salmonella* incidence was and continues to be much lower than in poultry. The primary reason is that poultry is produced with its skin on and the skin is the main harbor for bacteria, including *Salmonella*. In addition, sampling for *Salmonella* in poultry is done on a whole-carcass rinse rather than on a comparable area of beef.

Poultry

The PR/HACCP rule indicated that the HACCP principles adopted by the National Advisory Committee for Microbiological Criteria for Food (NACMCF) in 1992 would be utilized. However, many poultry companies had not identified fecal contamination as a hazard in their hazard analyses as late as January 1998 because feces did not appear to fit the definitions given by NACMCF for a biological, chemical, or physical hazard. FSIS published a *Federal Register* notice stating that it considered feces to be a hazard and that HACCP plans would have to have a CCP to deal with visible fecal contamination (FSIS, 1997). Plants were also sent letters giving them 72 hours to respond to this notice in writing to establishment Inspectors-in-Charge, showing that their HACCP plans included feces in the hazard analysis and that at least one CCP had been identified to control the hazard. This notice did make a direct regulatory connection between fecal contamination and the HACCP plan, which may not have been there otherwise. It also created a regulatory connection between the *Salmonella* performance standard and fecal contamination because the HACCP plan must address fecal contamination and the *Salmonella* performance standard is to evaluate the HACCP plan. The measures taken to control fecal contamination have resulted in reduced *Salmonella* incidence.

The post-PR/HACCP directive (FSIS, 1997) where FSIS considers fecal material in prechilled carcasses to be a CCP led to significant changes in broiler processing lines. Primarily, water usage nearly doubled due to the addition of washers, which may have resulted in a dilution of pathogens. Also, continuous on-line reprocessing emerged where antimicrobial rinses were used. Therefore, although published scientific studies have failed to establish a correlation between visible fecal contamination and presence of *Salmonella* in raw poultry carcasses, the measures taken to control fecal contamination have resulted in reduced *Salmonella* incidence. Many poultry plants also did not have an identifiable CCP within their process designated to reduce *Salmonella* to an acceptable level because no point in the slaughter process was designed to control *Salmonella* incidence on poultry and, therefore, no point met the definition of a CCP (i.e., points where the identified hazard may be prevented from entering the food, eliminated from it, or reduced to acceptable levels; see Chapter 3). This situation may not have been anticipated by FSIS because the pathogen reduction component of the rule established procedures for failing to meet the *Salmonella* performance standard that included evaluation of the HACCP plan on the first failure, reevaluation and an in-depth verification audit process on the second consecutive failure, and withdrawal of marks of inspection on the third consecutive failure (CDC, 2002).

A concern in poultry processing is the possibility of cross-contamination. The process of preparing broilers for consumption is highly automated and there is much opportunity for the cross-contamination and spread of pathogenic microorganisms among carcasses. This was demonstrated by Lillard (1989), who documented that 3 to 5 percent of the birds were positive for *Salmonella* when flocks entered the process, which increased to 35 percent positive for carcasses at the end of the process. However, since that study, changes in industry practices may have improved this scenario. For example, use of counter-current scalders and chillers, as well as chlorination, have been reported as having a dramatic effect on cross-contamination (Waldroup et al., 1992). In the USDA baseline study covering 200 broiler processing plants, the national average was down to 20 percent *Salmonella*-positive carcasses, with an average population of *Salmonella* of only 38 cfu per positive broiler carcass (Conner et al., 2001).

Another concern is that, whereas ground beef comes from using large quantities of lean and fat trims blended to achieve the desired fat level, ground poultry comes from either legs and drumsticks with the skin on, or from backs, necks, and frames after deboning, which may also include the skin. The skin is important to the overall product palatability as well as to the profitability, but it may add *Salmonella* into the system.

Since HACCP implementation, several antimicrobial treatments have been approved in poultry; however, the only treatments that significantly reduce *Salmonella* are proper cooking or irradiation to a high enough dose.

Ground Products

In the production of ground products, the PR/HACCP rule acknowledges that grinding establishments cannot use the same technologies for reducing pathogens that are used by slaughter plants, and that the establishments may have to use raw material contractual specifications to meet the performance standard (FSIS, 1996). This, in essence, is a confirmation that the process of producing raw ground products does not reduce pathogens and that whatever pathogens are present in the raw material will remain in the finished product. While the *Salmonella* performance standard for ground products provides a guide to overall performance through the slaughter and processing continuum, it may not be appropriate to verify either the HACCP plan or the actual performance of the grinding process.

ECONOMIC COSTS AND BENEFITS OF THE PR/HACCP RULE

A large share of the recent food safety economics literature has attempted to assess impacts of the PR/HACCP rule (Unnevehr, 2000). Discussions of the cost of compliance in firms of various sizes and on the potential for changing market structure due to the rule have led this research.

This literature is based on the cost–benefit analysis accompanying the PR/HACCP rule (FSIS, 1996), a document that received criticism for its cost assumptions and hypothesized pathogen reductions. The cumulative and speculative nature of the cost data is inevitable and correct for the purpose of comparison against similarly aggregated and forecasted benefits of the regulation. However, no study has been able to use actual cost data linked to true plant-level hazard reductions associated with identifiable strategies adopted by firms in response to the PR/HACCP rule—including interventions targeting microbial, chemical, and physical food safety concerns—to address such criticisms retrospectively. As mentioned in Chapter 2 and earlier in this chapter, the link between quantifiable reductions in foodborne illness and the direct actions of firms is not clear, and thus it is not yet possible to directly relate benefits and costs (Kuchler and Golan, 1999). The data requirements to accurately assess the societal impacts, even for one pathogen (e.g., *Salmonella*), would include enumeration of each plant's reduction in prevalence following the policy linked to fixed and variable costs of the particular strategy or intervention under analysis. For example, if a plant purchased a lactic acid carcass decontamination unit only because of the performance standard, economists would need information of initial cost of $\$x$ and annual recurring costs of $\$y$, as well as the z percent $\log_{10}$ reduction in the incidence of *Salmonella* to correctly assess the impact of the standard. This information would be required of each plant and pathogen and would then still need to be linked to impacts on public health and changes in the relationships between firms at various stages of the supply chain.

The most contentious cost issue in USDA's regulatory impact assessment focused on the details of process modifications required by firms to ensure compliance with the pathogen reduction standards. The rule established performance standards for *Salmonella* for all plants that slaughter and that process raw ground product. Further, all slaughter establishments are to employ a generic *E. coli* testing program to validate their process. Debate has centered on the additional equipment costs required by plants of various sizes, the potential structural implications of the standards, and the relationship between the recurring and nonrecurring elements of such process modification and other related PR/HACCP costs.

The in-house review of costs of current pathogen reduction strategies performed by FSIS based on plant size suggests that manual hot water spraying was the most cost-effective intervention for small slaughter facilities (8¢ per carcass). Alternative strategies that were considered included a pre-evisceration acid-spray system with both a prewash spray cabinet and a sanitizing cabinet at a cost of 79¢ per carcass for low volume use, and a trisodium phosphate-based system at a cost of 85¢ per carcass. The use of steam vacuum systems, with a nonrecurring cost of $10,000 and a recurring cost of around $4,500, was also discussed. The poultry data were based on the use of trisodium phosphate rinses, estimated to cost $40,000 per line. (Large poultry establishments average two lines, small ones average one and one-half.) This translates to a cost of 0.3¢ per broiler and 1.4¢ per turkey.

The use of both high and low scenarios of the costs of process modification in the final regulatory impact assessment is indicative of the methodological problem within the analysis. The low-cost scenario was based on the assumption that 10 percent of the 66 large hog and beef slaughter plants would need to install a steam vacuum system to ensure compliance with the *Salmonella* performance standard. Further, "half of the 376 small establishments must install a hot water rinse at $.08 per carcass" (FSIS, 1996). Conversely, the high-cost scenario suggested that 100 percent of the small and very small plants and as many as half (33) of the large plants (implying that the other plants already have such systems in place) would need to incur these costs. For facilities that do not slaughter (i.e., grinders), however, process modification costs for compliance with the *Salmonella* performance standard were not calculated; this approach suggests that these plants "must depend on the *Salmonella* levels of their incoming product to meet the performance standards" (FSIS, 1996). This one clear statement made by FSIS meant that no additional costs were included or anticipated for compliance with the performance standard for grinders (which include the Supreme Beef plant). Thus, the cost–benefit analysis contained in the final rule assumed that compliance with the other portions of the PR/HACCP rule would lead to higher costs, but that the PR portion would not. An analysis of neither the marginal impact of the performance standard, nor its potential as a dynamic policy tool, has been attempted.

A similar exercise in process modification costs for poultry suggests that the low-cost scenario would have 36 large establishments installing a trisodium phosphate-based system, with the high-cost scenario increasing this number to 182 (100 large and 82 small plants). Finally, the process modification costs for the generic *E. coli* sampling standard were related to the *Salmonella* performance standard. FSIS concluded that

> . . . if the low cost scenario for compliance with *Salmonella* standards proves to be more accurate, there will likely be more separate compliance costs for generic *E. coli*. As the costs for *Salmonella* compliance go up, the likelihood of separate *E. coli* costs goes down. It is important to note that under the high cost scenario, all cattle and swine slaughter establishments are using the steam vacuum system or hot water rinse and half of all poultry slaughter establishments are using TSP systems. Under this scenario, it is difficult to imagine that any establishments would still be failing to meet the performance criteria for generic *E. coli*. (FSIS, 1996, Pp. 38981–38982)

Little consideration was given to the unique costs related to compliance with the performance standards other than to suggest the adoption of equipment that appears to have become standard in most large slaughter operations.

In order to assess these estimates, Jensen and Unnevehr (2000) calculated the minimal costs of attaining a range of pathogen standards for large pork slaughter plants. Among the strategies selected were water rinses at three temperatures, with and without the application of a sanitizing spray. The per carcass costs of the wash and spray systems were found to be below the 79¢ and 85¢ estimates discussed above. Even when the most restrictive pathogen standard was simulated, costs were still under 50¢ per carcass, suggesting that the regulatory impact assessment may have overestimated the costs. The authors also attempted to test which of the two FSIS cost scenarios is more appropriate. They suggested that if the selection of an intervention strategy is made on a least-cost basis, then actual process modification costs may be higher than suggested in the regulatory impact assessment for large pork-slaughter plants.

Jensen and Unnevehr (2000) present a clear framework for incorporating pathogen reduction data into their assessment of least-cost interventions. However, care must be taken in applying these microbiological results. As the authors admit, their data come from two separate (although small) sources. One study tested interventions in a plant environment; the other did not. One used inoculated samples; the other did not. The inoculation procedure effectively elevates pathogen populations to an observable level, thus implying that although real-world reductions (the results of interventions) will not be of the same magnitude, they will be of the same relative order. This remains an untested hypothesis for most interventions.

Without further analysis, it cannot be presumed that a certain $\log_{10}$ reduction due to an intervention will be an improvement over current strategies; that it will be achieved in all plants at all times, regardless of the "cleanliness" of animals being presented for slaughter; or that it will lead to a risk reduction downstream at the point of consumption. Therefore, it may be more appropriate to presume that this analysis overestimated the benefits to the consumer.

Broader Economic Impacts: What Needs to Be Assessed?

Several potential indirect impacts should be considered in the broader economic analysis of the PR/HACCP rule. First are scale effects or implementation costs, which differ significantly by plant size. As HACCP-based regulations expand in their coverage (e.g., to the retail sector with many small and very small firms), it is argued that scale effects will be of paramount importance.

The food safety system put in place by a plant can also impact nonsafety quality attributes, thus increasing overall efficiency (Unnevehr and Roberts, 1997). That HACCP can help limit product rejection or rework, thus reducing the variability inherent to all production processes, also deserves more attention. This benefit allows for increased customer and consumer satisfaction (e.g., reduced complaints and product return); and may increase, although it is often difficult to quantify, measures of consumer confidence. Also, international trade is clearly facilitated when harmonized HACCP-based regulations are adopted (Caswell and Hooker, 1996).

Potential legal liability and insurance cost savings can arise from the use of innovative food safety controls. An advantage can be achieved by those plants and firms that are first to adopt a proven intervention. This can improve the overall company image, potentially providing a competitive and marketing advantage. Such innovation offset dynamics are discussed by Cockbill (1991) and Hobbs and Kerr (1992) and may or may not be candidates for inclusion in future regulatory impact assessments, depending upon the details of the HACCP-based regulation under consideration.

Difficulties in Forecasting Costs and Benefits for Novel Innovations

The PR/HACCP rule has an admirable degree of flexibility (i.e., minimal process criteria). Further, the performance standard elements of the rule seem to have provided some incentive to promote innovation in the pathogen reduction strategies employed. However, in part due to such success in regulatory design, ex post costs may differ significantly from ex ante estimates as more plants adopt validated pathogen reduction strategies that differ from those that USDA presumed would be used. This is further confounded when the selection of such strategies is not made on a least-cost basis.

Limited economic research exists to provide reliable estimates of costs and resultant benefits of many food safety interventions. Several pathogen reduction strategies, particularly multiple-hurdle techniques, incorporate novel approaches for which only limited commercial applications exist, thus requiring a cautious approach to forecasting potential costs. Further, plant-level pathogen reduction benefits of multiple-hurdle interventions are not always simply additive.

The potential use of novel individual interventions, as well as innovative combinations of traditional interventions, clearly make the prerule estimation of costs and benefits extremely difficult. It seems likely that in future regulatory impact assessments, the role of pilot programs to forecast real-world impacts will be expanded.

Hopefully, these studies will utilize representative firms' experiences with HACCP (or whatever food safety controls are being considered) and consider all state-of-the-art interventions. Special care must be taken in estimating the impact of any novel intervention not widely adopted in the industry based on plant-level experiences and not just on laboratory or theoretical assessments. At all times, the effectiveness of novel interventions should be compared with current systems on a microbiological as well as a cost basis.

THE NEED FOR ADDITIONAL APPROACHES TO REDUCE MICROBIAL HAZARDS

Preventing Pathogen Contamination and Amplification Before Slaughter

Pathogens, including *E. coli* O157:H7, *Salmonella*, and *Campylobacter,* on hides and in internal organs of live animals arriving for slaughter are important sources of contamination of meat. Substantial surveys of pathogen prevalence in dairy herds, feedlot populations, and culled dairy cattle have been conducted. Surveys of dairy farms show that a small percentage of farms or animal feces are positive for *E. coli* O157:H7 at a single point in time but, with repeated sampling, the organism is likely to be detected on most farms (Hancock et al., 1998). In a survey of 36 dairy herds, with repeated sampling over six months, the pathogen was ultimately detected on 75 percent of the herds, probably because carriage lasts no more than a few weeks in any animal (Hancock et al., 1997a, 1997b). The prevalence of fecal shedding of *E. coli* O157:H7 was 0.9 percent among dairy cows and 2.9 percent among dairy cows about to be culled; these data suggest that culling either selects for animals likely to be contaminated or contributes to their contamination. On average, 24.2 percent of dairy operations had at least one positive animal; this prevalence was seasonal, increasing in the summer months. Surveys of beef cattle in feedlots show a similar pattern, though the prevalence of contamination is generally higher (Veterinary Services, 2001a). Lately, methods based on immunomagnetic separation have allowed better detection of animals shedding low levels of *E. coli* O157:H7 (Besser et al., 2001). Due to the higher sensitivity methods, it is currently believed that the prevalence of *E. coli* O157:H7 is higher than previously thought.

Given that about 23 percent of the nation's dairy herd is culled and sent for slaughter annually (APHIS, 1996) and that much of it becomes ground beef (Troutt et al., 2001), the committee concludes that prevalence data on *E. coli* O157:H7 in culled animals is needed. Better understanding of the circumstances associated with the presence of pathogens could lead to targeted efforts to mitigate or prevent their circulation among live animals.

E. coli O157:H7 is a hardy pathogen, able to survive in damp cattle manure for up to 70 days, to survive and multiply in the sediment of cattle water troughs for months, to rapidly grow in moist cattle ration, and to be carried by wild deer (Keene et al., 1997; LeJeune et al., 2001; Lynn et al., 1998; Wang et al., 1996). Epidemiological studies that link the presence or absence of the organism in a herd to various management practices have suggested stronger association with using corn-based feed or feeding barley than with feeding soy meal or spreading fresh manure on forage crops (Dargatz et al., 1997; Hancock et al., 1997b; Herriott et al., 1998). The rumen of a fasted animal may be more hospitable to growth of *Salmonella* and *E. coli* O157, and it has been suggested that the common practice of fasting animals preslaughter may increase the shedding and spread of *E. coli* O157:H7 (Hancock et al., 1998; Rasmussen et al., 1993).

Salmonella are also commonly present among dairy herds and feedlots. The 1996 NAHMS survey of dairy cattle reported a prevalence of 5.4 percent among animals and 27 percent among dairy operations sampled a single time (Wells et al., 1998). As with *E. coli* O157:H7, the data also suggest that the level is higher in culled animals. Among feedlot cattle, the prevalence of *Salmonella* was 6.3 percent in animals, 22.3 percent in pens, and 51 percent in feedlots (Veterinary Services, 2001b). Factors associated with the presence of *Salmonella* on farms have not been examined as thoroughly as for *E. coli* O157:H7. Nevertheless, some general principles of control of *Salmonella* among cattle herds have been defined and are also applicable to the control of *Salmonella* Typhimurium DT104 (Dargatz et al., 1998) and other important animal-borne illnesses such as Johne's Disease (Groenendaal and Galligan, 1999; Wells et al., 1999).

In addition to the prevalence on the farm, other factors that may increase the risk of pathogens in meat relate to the transportation of herds in trucks from a pasture or barn through auction yards, feedlots, and holding pens, where they are exposed to fecal or other means of contamination from animals previously or currently there.

The 1996 NAHMS survey of dairy cattle reported that 15 percent of feces from individual culled dairy cattle were positive for *Salmonella* at market and that 67 percent of markets had at least one animal shedding *Salmonella* (Wells et al., 1998). Furthermore, a recent systematic national survey of 5,000 culled dairy cattle reported that 23 percent of animals carried *Salmonella* at the point of slaughter, with a range of 0 to 93 percent on a given day at a given establishment (Troutt et al., 2001).

Similarly, the prevalence of *E. coli* O157:H7 among culled dairy cattle at market in the NAHMS study was 1.8 percent, twice that on the farm, and, when tested a single time, 31 percent of the markets had a positive animal (Wells et al., 1998). In a recent survey of cattle in 29 pens in 5 major feedlots, and based on a single fecal sample from each animal, 23 percent of individual animals and 100 percent of feedlot pens were positive for *E. coli* O157:H7 (Smith et al., 2001). The environmental conditions in the pen (e.g., muddy grounds after a rain) were associated with the likelihood of finding the pathogen.

The final point of potential introduction and amplification of live-animal contamination with pathogens is the holding pens immediately before slaughtering. Two recent studies suggest that, for swine and cattle, the abattoir terminal holding pen is a significant point of contamination with *E. coli* O157:H7 and that, therefore, sanitation of the terminal holding pen is likely to be an important control point for this pathogen (Avery et al., 2002; Hurd et al., 2001).

In summary, the committee concludes that efforts to reduce preslaughter contamination are likely to be an important part of a farm-to-table food safety strategy, not only to reduce pathogen load at the slaughter plant, but also to prevent the hazard from direct contact with infected animals, from runoff on feedlots and farms, and from contaminated water supplies (Crump et al., 2002; Hilborn et al., 1999; Kassenborg et al., 1998; Martin et al., 1986; O'Brien and Adak, 2002; PPHB, 2000). This prevention process, beneficial to both animal and human health, comprises on-farm management practices that may reduce the spread and amplification of pathogens, as may sanitation practices during transportation and in feedlots, final holding pens, and slaughter boxes. Moreover, measures that increase the resistance of animals to intestinal contamination in the last days of their lives should be examined and evaluated through formal intervention trials.

Therefore, the committee recommends that USDA conduct or fund research on the role of nonfecal carriage and commingling prior to and after slaughter to elucidate the factors that contribute to the microbial pathogen contamination of live animals, carcasses, and products. The committee also recommends a research focus on intervention trials at all stages of the production process of meat and poultry products.

The committee further concludes that the level of contamination of animals coming to slaughter is likely to be associated with the contamination of the meat; therefore, monitoring levels of contamination on and in the incoming animals is likely an important measurement of the level of risk and could help determine or require the use of mitigation steps. More importantly, measures that may reduce such contamination, such as changing what animals are fed in the last week of life, reducing fecal contamination on hides in the muddy seasons, or sanitizing the terminal holding pen and kill box, should be rapidly evaluated so that the level of contamination at the slaughter plant may be reduced.

Consequently, the committee recommends that industry and regulatory agencies continue to place greater emphasis on contamination prevention rather than rely on inspection and end-product testing to ensure the safety of meat.

Monitoring Pathogen Contamination of Herds and Flocks to Assign Raw Foods to Further Processing

The nature of foodborne hazards has changed dramatically over the last century since the first federal meat inspection system was created. The hazard posed by diseased and dying animals has been replaced by hazards that are more difficult to detect. Common zoonotic pathogens such as *Campylobacter* in broilers, *S.* Enteritidis in layers, *E. coli* O157:H7 in cattle, and *Yersinia enterocolitica* in pork cause no apparent illness in the food animals that harbor them, yet can contaminate the foods produced from these animals. Public health surveillance and investigations have attempted to measure the human illness burden that these and other foodborne pathogens cause, and have traced them back to food animal reservoirs. In the absence of grossly visible markers for contamination of live animals with microbial pathogens, the effectiveness of new systems for control may depend on such measures as accurate separation of higher-risk flocks or herds from others. The Pennsylvania Egg Quality Assurance Program, for example, is an *S.* Enteritidis control program in layer flocks that began in 1992 (FSIS, 2002b). Routine monitoring of flocks for the presence of *S.* Enteritidis is part of this program and is linked to vigorous efforts to prevent contamination of the next generation of birds that will enter the farm, as well as to the diversion to pasteurization of eggs from contaminated flocks. The result has been a slow but steady decline in the proportion of egg-producing facilities that have *S.* Enteritidis, from 25.7 percent in 1994 to 7.3 percent in 1998 (PFMA, 2000).

A review of the change in prevalence of the four most common *Salmonella* serotypes found in broiler chickens in the United States indicated that all four declined substantially and significantly after the PR/HACCP rule was implemented (RTI, 2002). In other countries, even more dramatic declines have been achieved by using microbial monitoring to drive farm- or flock-based control efforts. Sweden has largely controlled *S.* Enteritidis in chicken-rearing operations (Wierup et al., 1995). This achievement, however, has come at a high cost derived from destruction of contaminated flocks. The European Union, in turn, issued a directive in 1992 mandating the screening of flocks and herds for *S.* Enteritidis and *S.* Typhimurium with a view to subsidized destruction of those found to be contaminated (EC, 1992); Denmark, Finland, Sweden, and Ireland joined the program by 1999 (Mulder and Schlundt, 1999). However, given the vast difference in the scale of poultry production between the United States and European countries, such an approach would need to be structured differently in the United States. In 2001, Norway launched a national control program for *Campylobacter* based on the testing of chicken flocks and of finished carcasses; chickens from positive flocks are slaughtered after the negative flocks to minimize cross-contamination, and the carcasses are either sent for supervised cooking or are frozen (Norwegian Zoonosis Centre, 2002). It is too soon to tell whether carcass contamination with *Campylobacter* has actually been reduced as a result of this program.

DO MEAT AND POULTRY PERFORMANCE STANDARDS IMPROVE PUBLIC HEALTH?

The committee recognizes that substantial declines in four bacterial foodborne diseases observed in the United States via FoodNet surveillance since 1996 indicate that the collective efforts to improve food safety are having an effect (CDC, 2002). As the most prominent declines are in infections caused by the meat-associated pathogens *Campylobacter*, *Listeria,* and *Y. enterocolitica*—27, 35, and 49 percent declines, respectively—it is likely that the PR/HACCP rule is contributing to this effect, although concurrent changes in distribution, retail, and consumer behavior could also be important in decreasing infections due to such pathogens (CDC, 2002). The fact that no sustained decline has been observed yet in infections caused by *E. coli* O157:H7 may mean that the established zero tolerance for this pathogen does not offer added protection, perhaps because the principal determinants of contamination are preslaughter, or perhaps because it was effective and blunted what otherwise would have been an increase. The data needed to distinguish between these possibilities are lacking. The decline in listeriosis is particularly noteworthy. Listeriosis declined between 1988 and 1995 and had appeared to reach a plateau. Further industry efforts, including formulation and process changes, stimulated by a large outbreak associated with hot dogs in 1999, as well as efforts to educate high-risk populations, may have resulted in an additional 35 percent decline (CDC, 2002) in human cases.

A persistent challenge is that attributing such changes to any one factor is difficult because many food safety measures may be taking place at the same time, and because a given infection may have multiple possible food and nonfood sources. As was recommended in Chapter 2, measuring changes in consumer behavior, as well as microbial subtyping of pathogen strains from different food sources and comparison with isolates from human infections, could help conquer this challenge.

REFERENCES

APHIS (Animal and Plant Health Inspection Service). 1996. *Dairy '96. Part 1: Reference of 1996 Dairy Management Practices*. Online. U.S. Department of Agriculture (USDA). Available at http://www.aphis.usda.gov/vs/ceah/cahm/Dairy_Cattle/dr96des1.pdf. Accessed July 19, 2002.

Avery S, Small A, Reid CA, Buncic S. 2002. Pulsed field gel electrophoresis characterization of Shiga-toxin producing *Escherichia coli* O157:H7 from hides of cattle at slaughter. *J Food Prot* 65: 1172–1176.

Becker E. 2003, January 23. Government in showdown in bid to shut beef processor. *New York Times*. P. A16.

Besser TE, Richards BL, Rice DH, Hancock DD. 2001. *Escherichia coli* O157:H7 infection of calves: Infectious dose and direct contact transmission. *Epidemiol Infect* 127:555–560.

Caswell JA, Hooker NH. 1996. HACCP as an International Trade Standard. *Am J Agric Econ* 78:775–779.

CDC (Centers for Disease Control and Prevention). 2002. Preliminary FoodNet Data on the incidence of foodborne illnesses—Selected sites, United States, 2001. *Morb Mortal Wkly Rep* 51:325–329.

CFSAN (Center for Food Safety and Applied Nutrition). 2003. *Real Progress in Food Code Adoptions*. Online. Food and Drug Administration (FDA). Available at http://vm.cfsan.fda.gov/~ear/fcadopt.html. Accessed April 10, 2003.

Cockbill C. 1991. The Food Safety Act: An introduction. *Br Food J* 93:4–7.

Conner DE, Davis MA, Zhang L. 2001 Poultry-borne pathogens: Plant considerations in poultry meat processing. In: Sams AR, ed. *Poultry Meat Processing*. Boca Raton, FL: CRC Press. Pp. 137–158.

Crump J, Sulka A, Angulo FJ. 2002. An outbreak of *Escherichia coli* O157:H7 infections among visitors to a dairy farm. *N Engl J Med* 347:555–560.

CVM (Center for Veterinary Medicine). 2002a. *Animal Medicinal Drug Use Clarification Act of 1994 (AMDUCA)*. Online. FDA. Available at http://www.fda.gov/cvm/index/amducca/amducatoc.htm. Accessed February 14, 2003.

CVM. 2002b. *Guidance for Industry. Evaluating the Safety of Antimicrobial New Animal Drugs with Regard to Their Microbial Effects on Bacteria of Human Health Concern*. Online. FDA. Available at http://www.fda.gov/OHRMS/DOCKETS/98fr/80040a56.pdf. Accessed May 13, 2003.

Dargatz D, Scott W, Thomas LA, Hancock D, Garber L. 1997. Factors associated with the presence of *Escherichia coli* in feces of feedlot cattle. *J Food Prot* 60:466–470.

Dargatz D, Wells S, Fedorka-Cray P, Akkina, J. 1998. The veterinarian's role in diagnosis, treatment, and prevention of multidrug resistant *Salmonella* Typhimurium DT104. *Bovine Practitioner* 32:1–6.

EC (European Commission). 1992. Council Directive 92/117/EEC of 17 December, 1992 concerning measures for protection against specified zoonoses and specified zoonotic agents in animals and products of animal origin in order to prevent outbreaks of food-borne infections and intoxications. *Off J Eur Communities* L062:38–48.

Eilert SJ, Rathje NM. 2001. Case ready red meat: Demand and technology. *Proc Recip Meat Conf* 54:59–61.

ERS (Economic Research Service). 2000. *Cattle: Background.* Online. USDA. Available at http://www.ers.usda.gov/Briefing/Cattle/Background.htm. Accessed June 25, 2002.

ERS. 2002. *Cattle: Trade.* Online. USDA. Available at http://www.ers.usda.gov/Briefing/Cattle/Trade.htm. Accessed June 25, 2002.

FAIM (Field Automation and Information Management Division). 2002. *FAIM Division Home Page.* Online. Food Safety and Inspection Service, USDA. Available at http://www.fsis.usda.gov/OFO/FAIM/fainmain.htm. Accessed May 15, 2002.

FDA (Food and Drug Administration). 2001. *Food Code 2001.* Online. Available at http://www.cfsan.fda.gov/~dms/foodcode.html#get01. Accessed January 21, 2002.

FSIS (Food Safety and Inspection Service). 1989. *Time/Temperature Guidelines for Cooling Heated Products.* Online. USDA. Available at http://www.fsis.usda.gov/OPPDE/rdad/FSISDirectives/FSISDir7110-3Rev1.pdf. Accessed February 3, 2002.

FSIS. 1995. *Compilation of Issuances on Cooked Meat and Poultry Product Temperatures.* Online. USDA. Available at http://www.fsis.usda.gov/OPPDE/rdad/FSISDirectives/FSISDir7370.2.pdf. Accessed February 3, 2002.

FSIS. 1996. Pathogen reduction; Hazard analysis and critical control point (HACCP) systems; Final rule. *Fed Regist* 61:38805–38855.

FSIS. 1997. Livestock carcasses and poultry carcasses contaminated with visible fecal material. *Fed Regist* 62:63254–63255.

FSIS. 1998a. *Importing Meat and Poultry to the United States.* Online. USDA. Available at http://www.fsis.usda.gov/oa/programs/import.htm. Accessed June 26, 2002.

FSIS. 1998b. *Key Facts: Role of the Inspector Under HACCP.* Online. USDA. Available at http://www.fsis.usda.gov/oa/background/keyrole.htm. Accessed February 3, 2002.

FSIS. 1998c. *Lethality and Stabilization Performance Standards for Certain Meat and Poultry Products: Technical Paper.* Online. USDA. Available at http://www.fsis.usda.gov/OPPDE/rdad/FRPubs/95-033F_tech%20paper.pdf. Accessed June 26, 2002.

FSIS. 1999a. Beef products contaminated with *Escherichia coli* O157:H7. *Fed Regist* 64:2803–2805.

FSIS. 1999b. Performance standards for the production of certain meat and poultry products. *Fed Regist* 64:732–749.

FSIS. 2001a. *HACCP-Based Inspection Models Project (HIMP): Young Chicken Inspection.* Online. USDA. Available at http://www.fsis.usda.gov/OPPDE/Nis/HIMP/Docs/YNGChk_Drf6.pdf. Accessed July 19, 2002.

FSIS. 2001b. *Mandatory Inspection of Ratites and Squabs.* Online. USDA. Available at http://www.fsis.usda.gov/OPPDE/rdad/FRPubs/01-045IF.htm. Accessed May 23, 2003.

FSIS. 2001c. *Protecting the Public From Foodborne Illness: The Food Safety and Inspection Service.* Online. USDA. Available at http://www.fsis.usda.gov/oa/background/fsisgeneral.htm. Accessed June 26, 2002.

FSIS. 2002a. *E. coli* O157:H7 contamination of beef products. *Fed Regist* 67:62325–62334.

FSIS. 2002b. *Egg Quality Assurance.* Online. USDA. Available at http://www.fsis.usda.gov/OPPDE/animalprod/Publications/overview/qa/a84.htm. Accessed July 19, 2002.

FSIS, 2002c. *FAIM Division Home Page.* Online. USDA. Available at http://www.fsis.usda.gov/OFO/faim/faimmain.htm. Accessed May 15, 2002.

FSIS. 2003. *FSIS Import Reinspection.* Online. USDA. Available at http://www.fsis.usda.gov/OPPDE/IPS/Importing.htm#Reinspection. Accessed May 10, 2003.

GAO (General Accounting Office). 2001. *Food Safety: Overview of Federal and State Expenditures.* GAO-01-177. Washington, DC: GAO.

GAO. 2002. *Meat and Poultry: Better USDA Oversight and Enforcement of Safety Rules Needed to Reduce Risk of Foodborne Illnesses. Appendix II: Comments from the U.S. Department of Agriculture.* GAO-02-902. Washington, DC: GAO.

Gombas DE, Chen Y, Clavero RS, Scotta VN. 2003. Survey of *Listeria monocytogenes* in ready-to-eat foods. *J Food Prot* 559–569.

Groenendaal H, Galligan D. 1999. *Economical Consequences of Johne's Disease Control Programs.* Kennet Square, PA: Center for Animal Health and Productivity, University of Pennsylvania.

Hancock D, Besser T, Rice DH, Herriott DE, Tarr PI. 1997a. A longitudinal study of *Escherichia coli* O157 in fourteen cattle herds. *Epidemiol Infect* 118:193–195.

Hancock DD, Rice DH, Herriot DE, Besser TE, Ebel ED. 1997b. Effects of farm manure-handling practices on *Escherichia coli* O157 prevalence in cattle. *J Food Prot* 60:363–366.

Hancock D, Besser T, Rice DH. 1998. Ecology of *Escherichia coli* O157:H7 in cattle and impact of management practices. In: Kaper J, O'Brien A, eds. Escherichia coli *and other Shiga toxin-producing* E. coli *Strains.* Washington, DC: ASM Press. Pp. 85–91.

Herriott D, Hancock D, Ebel ED, Carpenter LV, Rice DH, Besser TE. 1998. Association of herd management factors with colonization of dairy cattle by Shiga toxin-positive *Escherichia coli* O157. *J Food Prot* 61:802–807.

HHS (U.S. Department of Health and Human Services). 2002. *Foodborne Illnesses Post Dramatic Six-Year Decline.* Online. HHS Press Release 4/18/2002. Available at http://www.hhs.gov/news/press/2002pres/200204189.html. Accessed December 15, 2002.

Hilborn E, Mermin J, Mshar PA, Hadler JL, Voetsch A, Wojtkunski C, Swartz M, Mshar R, Lambert-Fair MA, Farrar JA, Glynn MK, Slutsker L. 1999. A multistate outbreak of *Escherichia coli* O157:H7 infections associated with consumption of mesclun lettuce. *Arch Intern Med* 159:1758–1764.

Hobbs JE, Kerr WA. 1992. Costs of monitoring food safety and vertical coordination in agribusiness: What can be learned from the British Food Safety Act 1990? *Agribus Internat J* 8:575–584.

Hurd H, McKean J, Wesley IV, Karriker LA. 2001. The effect of lairage on *Salmonella* isolation from market swine. *J Food Prot* 64:939–944.

ICMSF (International Commission on Microbiological Specifications for Foods). 2002. *Microorganisms in Foods 7. Microbiological Testing in Food Safety Management.* New York: Kluwer Academic/Plenum Publishers.

Jensen HH, Unnevehr LJ. 2000. HACCP in pork processing: Costs and benefits. In: Unnevehr LJ, ed. *Economics of HACCP: Costs and Benefits.* St. Paul, MN: Eagen Press. Pp. 29–44.

Kassenborg H, Hedberg C, Evans M, Chin G, Fiorentino T, Vugia D, Bardsley M, Slutsker L, Griffin P. 1998. Case-control study of sporadic *Escherichia coli* O157:H7 infections in 5 FoodNet sites. In: *Proceedings of the International Conference on Emerging Infectious Diseases.* Atlanta: CDC. P. 50.

Keen JE, Elder RO. 2002. Isolation of shiga-toxigenic *Escherichia coli O157* from hide surfaces and the oral cavity of finished beef feedlot cattle. *J Am Vet Med Assoc* 220:756–763.

Keene W, Sazie E, Kok J, Rice DH, Hancock DD, Balan VK, Zhao T, Doyle MP. 1997. An outbreak of *Escherichia coli* O157:H7 infections traced to jerky made from deer meat. *JAMA* 227:1229–1231.

Kinsman DM. 1994. Historical perspective and current status. In: Kinsman DM, Kotula AW, Breidenstrin BC, eds. *Muscle Foods: Meat, Poultry and Seafood Technology.* New York: Chapman and Hall. Pp. 1–24.

Kuchler F, Golan E. 1999. *Assigning Values to Life: Comparing Methods for Valuing Health Risks.* Agricultural Economics Report No. 784. Washington, DC: ERS, USDA.

LeJeune J, Besser T, Hancock DD. 2001. Cattle water troughs as reservoirs of *Escherichia coli* O157. *Appl Environ Microbiol* 67:3053–3057.

Lillard HS. 1989. Factors affecting persistence of *Salmonella* during the processing of poultry. *J Food Prot* 52:829–832.

Lynn TV, Hancock DD, Besser TE, Harrison JH, Rice DH, Stewart NT, Rowan LL. 1998. The occurrence and replication of *Escherichia coli* in cattle feeds. *J Dairy Sci* 81:1102–1108.

MacDonald JM, Ollinger ME, Nelson KE, Handy GR. 2000. *Consolidation in U.S. Meatpacking*. Agricultural Economics Report No. 785. Washington, DC: Agricultural Research Service, USDA.

Martin DL, Shipman LD, Wells JG, Potter ME, Hedberg K, Wachsmuth IK, Tauxe RV, Davis JP, Arnoldi J, Tilleli J. 1986. Isolation of *Escherichia coli* O157:H7 from dairy cattle associated with two cases of haemolytic uraemic syndrome. *Lancet* 2:1043.

Mulder RWA, Schlundt J. 1999. Safety of poultry meat: From farm to table. In: Molins RA, Corry J, eds. *International Consultative Group on Food Irradiation (ICGFI)*. Vienna: International Atomic Energy Agency.

Nalivka J. 2002. *Meat and Poultry Facts Book 2002*. Mt. Morris, IL: Watt Publishing.

NASS (National Agriculture Statistics Service). 2002. *Livestock Slaughter: 2001 Summary*. Online. USDA. Available at http://usda.mannlib.cornell.edu/reports/nassr/livestock/pls-bban/lsan0302.txt. Accessed October 9, 2002.

Norwegian Zoonosis Centre. 2002. *Action plan—Campylobacter sp. in Norwegian broilers. Summary of results from the surveillance of broiler flocks 2002; Survey of broiler meat products 2002.* Online. Available at http://www.vetinst.no/Zoonosesenteret/campyl-report-action-2002.pdf. Accessed September, 11, 2002.

NRC (National Research Council). 1985a. *An Evaluation of the Role of Microbiological Criteria for Foods and Food Ingredients*. Washington, DC: National Academy Press.

NRC. 1985b. *Meat and Poultry Inspection: The Scientific Basis of the Nation's Program*. Washington, DC: National Academy Press.

NRC. 1987. *Poultry Inspection: The Basis for a Risk-Assessment Approach*. Washington, DC: National Academy Press.

NRC. 1999. *The Use of Drugs in Food Animals: Benefits and Risks*. Washington, DC: National Academy Press.

O'Brien S, Adak G. 2002. *Escherichia coli* O157:H7—Piecing together the jigsaw puzzle. *N Engl J Med* 347:608–609.

PFMA (Pennsylvania Food Merchants Association). 2000. *Pennsylvania Presents Results of Egg Quality Assurance, January 2000*. Online. Available at http://www.pfma.org/media/advisor/JAN00/peqap.html. Accessed January 23, 2003.

PPHB (Population and Public Health Branch). 2000. Waterborne outbreak of gastroenteritis associated with a contaminated municipal water supply, Walkerton , Ontario, May–June 2000. *Can Commun Dis Rep* 26-20:170–173.

Rasmussen M, Cray W, Casey TA, Whipp SC. 1993. Rumen contents as a reservoir of enterohemorrhagic *Escherichia coli*. *FEMS Microbiol Lett* 114:79–84.

REAP (Research-Education-Advocacy-People). 2001. *REAP General 2001 Report on the Meat Packing Industry*. Online. Available at http://www.reapinc.org/REAP%202001%20REPORT%20ON%20MEAT%20PACKING.html. Accessed June 26, 2002.

Rose BE, Hill WE, Umholtz R, Ramnsom GM, James WO. 2002. Testing for *Salmonella* in raw meat and poultry products collected at federally inspected establishments in the United States, 1998 through 2000. *J Food Prot* 65:937–947.

RTI (Research Triangle Institute). 2002. *Revised Final Draft: PR/HACCP Rule Evaluation Report. Effect of the 1996 PR/HACCP Rule on Foodborne Illness: Young Chicken* Salmonella *Study*. Research Triangle Park, NC: RTI.

Shire B. 2003. *Do You Own/Operate a Raw Beef Plant? Here's How to Reassess Your HACCP Plan for* E. coli *O157:H7*. AAMP Special Report. Elizabethtown, PA: American Association of Meat Processors.

Smith D, Blackford M, Younts S, Moxley R, Gray J, Hungerford L, Milton T, Klopfenstein T. 2001. Ecological relationships between the prevalence of cattle shedding *Escherichia coli* O157:H7 and characteristics of the cattle or conditions of the feedlot pen. *J Food Prot* 64:1899–1903.

Troutt H, Galland J, Osburn BI, Brewer RL, Braun RK, Schmitz JA, Sears P, Childers AB, Richey E, Mather E, Gibson M, Murthy K, Hogue A. 2001. Prevalence of *Salmonella* spp. in cull (market) dairy cows at slaughter. *J Am Vet Med Assoc* 219:1212–1215.

University of Vermont. 2003. *Beef Cattle*. Online. Available at http://asci.uvm.edu/course/asci001/beef.html. Accessed January 15, 2003.

Unnevehr LJ, ed. 2000. *The Economics of HACCP: Studies of Costs and Benefits, 2000.* St. Paul, MN: Eagan Press.

Unnevehr L, Roberts T. 1997. Improving cost/benefit analysis for HACCP and microbial food safety: An economist's overview. In: Caswell JA, Cotterill RW, eds. *Strategy and Policy in the Food System: Emerging Issues.* Amherst, MA: University of Massachusetts. Pp. 225–229.

USDA (U.S. Department of Agriculture). 2002. *USDA Data Show a Reduction of Salmonella in Raw Meat and Poultry*. Online. Available at http://www.usda.gov/news/releases/2002/04/0154.htm. Accessed June 11, 2002.

Veterinary Services. 2001a. *Info Sheet: Escherichia coli O157 in United States Feedlots*. Online. APHIS, USDA. Available at http://www.aphis.usda.gov/vs/ceah/cahm/Beef_Feedlot/coli.PDF. Accessed May 14, 2002.

Veterinary Services. 2001b. *Info Sheet:* Salmonella *in United States Feedlots*. Online. APHIS, USDA. Available at http://www.aphis.usda.gov/vs/ceah/cahm/Beef_feedlot/99sal.PDF. Accessed May 14, 2002.

Waldroup AL, Rathgeber BM, Forsythe RH. 1992. Effects of six modifications on the incidence and levels of spoilage and pathogenic organisms on commercially processed postchill broilers. *J Appl Poult Res* 2:111–116.

Wallace RL. 2003. *Market Cows: A Potential Profit Center. Illini Dairy Net*. Online. Available at http://traill.outreach.uiuc.edu/dairynet/paperDisplay.cfm?DyanBizInfoID=984. Accessed January 15, 2003.

Wang G, Zhao T, Doyle MP. 1996. Fate of enterohemorrhagic *Escherichia coli* O157:H7 in bovine feces. *Appl Environ Microbiol* 62:2567–2570.

Wells J, Wagner A, Dargatz A. 1999. Factors associated with Johne's disease on U.S. dairy operations. In: Manning EJB, Collins MT, eds. *Proceedings of the 6th International Collegium of Paratuberculosis*. Madison, WI: International Association for Paratuberculosis. P. 13.

Wells SJ, Fedorka-Cray PJ, Russell R, Besser T, McDonough P, Smith B. 1998. E. coli *O157 and* Salmonella—*Status on U.S. Dairy Operations.* Center for Epidemiology and Animal Health, Veterinary Service, APHIS, USDA. Online. Available at http://www.aphis.usda.gov/vs/ceah/cahm/Dairy_Cattle/ecosalm98.htm. Accessed July 19, 2002.

WI DATCP (Wisconsin Department of Agriculture, Trade and Consumer Protection). 2002. *Wisconsin's Meat Safety & Inspection Program: Analysis and Evaluation*. Madison, WI: WI DATCP.

Wierup M, Engstrom B, Engwall A, Wahlstrom H. 1995. Control of *Salmonella* Enteritidis in Sweden. *Int J Food Microbiol* 25:219–226.

5

Scientific Criteria and Performance Standards to Control Hazards in Seafood

The word "seafood" encompasses a vast array of animals that include not only various genera and species, but also various phylla such as mollusca (e.g., clams and oysters), arthropoda (e.g., crabs and crayfish), and chordata (e.g., finfish). This diversity manifests itself in life forms of different sizes, shapes, and functions, each adapted to unique environments and roles within the ecosystem. More than 350 species of fish are commonly consumed (FAO, 2002). In a culinary sense, this diversity is expressed as a broad spectrum of sensory attributes, product forms, and preparations that are particular to seafood. Whether from traditional harvest or aquaculture production, seafood presents some unique safety concerns that arise from both the intrinsic characteristics of the animals and the environmental conditions from which they are harvested. For example, for some species, food safety issues are dependent on the harvest location and season. In addition, as is the case with meat and poultry products, conditions and handling at harvest and processing, as well as through distribution and final preparation, constitute significant factors that enhance or reduce the risk of seafood-borne disease.

Because of these unique features, certain seafood may present a hazard to public health. First, given the diversity of aquatic animals and environmental conditions within the aquatic environment—saltwater, freshwater, estuarine water, tropical, polar, in-shore, off-shore, pristine, polluted—it is not surprising that specific animals and environmental conditions may result in products unsafe for consumption. Interestingly, most seafood safety problems are present prior to harvesting and are a consequence of the accumulation of natural contaminants in the aquatic environment, such as the presence of *Vibrio vulnificus* in raw molluscan shellfish or methyl mercury in various fish from certain waters (IOM, 1991).

Second, although the expansion of aquaculture production would seem to offer opportunities for greater environmental control, concerns similar to those of land-based muscle foods have emerged; such is the case with the presence of therapeutic agents and human pathogens in seafood as a consequence of the production environment and practices. Third, all these concerns are further complicated by an increasing dependence on seafood products from some international waters, which are subject to less surveillance by domestic authorities than are American waters.

Additional factors that increase the risk of seafood as foodborne disease vehicles relate to handling, distribution, and preparation. For example, unique and notable characteristics of seafood consumption are that a significant portion is consumed live (e.g., oysters, mussels, and clams), raw (e.g., sushi), or cooked to a rare state (e.g., cod and mahi-mahi). Also, many recipes include consumption of nonmuscle components such as eyes, eggs, and viscera (raw and cooked), some of which may pose unique risks. In addition, the fact that seafood is the largest commodity group with an extensive recreational element can have serious public health implications. For example, recreational fishermen can thermally abuse scombroid-susceptible species, leading to scombroid fish poisoning, an acute illness associated with the consumption of certain fish having elevated levels of biogenic amines. These elevated levels are a result of growth of certain bacteria when temperature abuse of fish occurs during or after harvesting (CFSAN, 2001). Furthermore, vacationers have been known to ignore or misunderstand posted advisories prohibiting the harvest of molluscan shellfish from nonapproved waters, thus exposing themselves and their families to potentially contaminated toxic shellfish. It is believed that some recreationally harvested seafood enters commercial channels (e.g., when sold directly to restaurants), which could also contribute to outbreaks attributed to commercially produced seafood. The true extent to which this practice occurs is not known, but recent undercover investigations have revealed illegal fish sales from recreational harvest exceeding six figure incomes for the culprits (Waters, 2002). Bootlegging, which is the sale of molluscan shellfish illegally harvested from closed areas, is another issue with significant food safety implications, but the true extent of the problem is not known.

Listeria monocytogenes and the debate over zero tolerance have not escaped the seafood industry. As with other muscle protein foods, the concern with seafood is focused on ready-to-eat products. Especially problematic are products such as fresh crabmeat and cold-smoked fish. The processes involved are traditional for the respective products, but are relatively uncommon for most meat-type products. Fresh crabmeat, for instance, does have a terminal heat step that destroys most foodborne pathogens, including *Listeria*, but it precedes the meat removal step, which is traditionally done by hand. With respect to cold-smoked fish, this product does not have a lethal heating step, therefore other parameters, such as salt concentration, become important risk minimization steps.

DESCRIPTION OF THE SEAFOOD INDUSTRY

Although the United States seafood-processing sector includes approximately 5,000 firms (Fisheries Statistics and Economics, 2002), fewer than 20 percent of these firms produce over 80 percent of the products. When the Food and Drug Administration (FDA) issued the Procedures for the Safe and Sanitary Processing and Importing of Fish and Fishery Products; Final Rule (the seafood HACCP rule) (FDA, 1995), a significant objective was to apply it primarily to the processing sector, even though many factors outside the processing plant contribute to risks from seafood consumption. The processing sector is more identifiable, accessible, and controllable than the harvesting, distribution, and transportation sectors; moreover, it is more concentrated than retail or food service operations. However, although the processing sector can be better monitored, the abundance of small processing operations has added complexity to the implementation of, and compliance with, the seafood HACCP rule. These smaller firms—which are a majority in the processing sector—often have limited financial resources and operations that are significantly influenced by seasonal fluctuations in supply and demand. This situation has discouraged long-term investments and has created a specialized industry that is dependent on imported products.

Current trends in international seafood commerce further add to the complexity of the food safety aspects derived from seafood diversity and the uniqueness of the industry. In 2000, the estimated total international trade in fishery commodities, by volume (live weight equivalents) and including aquaculture, was approximately 37 percent of the total world production (FAO, 2000). In terms of value, exports from developing countries in 2000 represented over 50 percent of total exports of fishery products (FAO, 2000). International trade is expected to increase in response to efforts by various industrialized nations to supplement their dwindling domestic seafood resources. Supply is becoming the most significant issue in the world of seafood commerce. The anticipated significant shortfalls for the next decade may result in the reduced availability of seafood and elevated prices in industrialized countries, while serious shortages could occur in regions of the world that are dependent on subsistence fisheries.

This situation could influence international decisions relative to seafood safety, and because over 50 percent of domestic seafood consumption involves imported products (Figure 5.1), it should be thoroughly considered when developing food safety regulations in the United States. Imports to the United States exceed 80 percent for certain popular seafood products. FDA recently estimated that over 8,500 importing firms are subject to surveillance in accordance with the seafood HACCP rule.

A relatively recent additional development in world fisheries production is an increase in dependence on aquaculture products, illustrated by the growth in the volume of cultured shrimp, one of the most prominent aquaculture products in the world (Figures 5.2 and 5.3). There is a need to develop specific strategies to

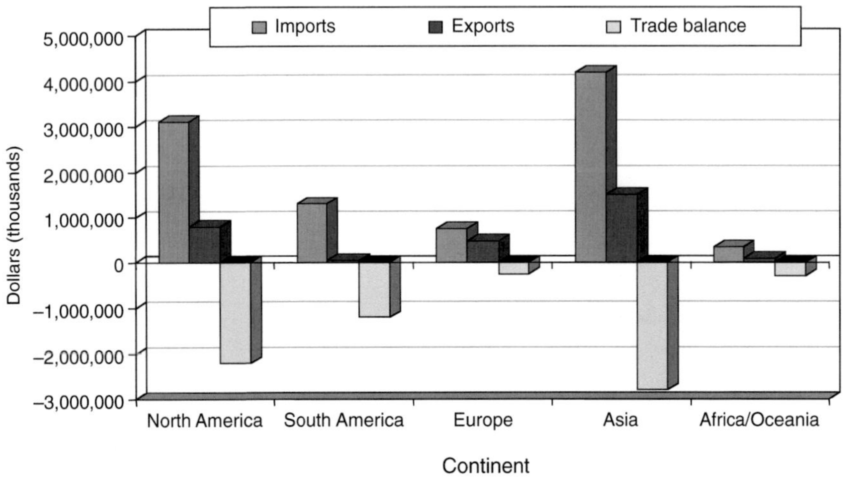

FIGURE 5.1 United States trade in edible fishery products during 2000.
SOURCE: Fisheries Statistics and Economics Division (2001a, 2001b).

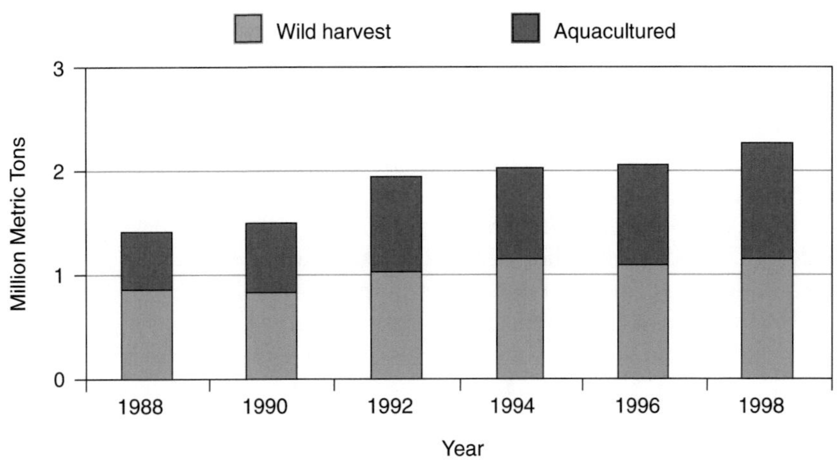

FIGURE 5.2 World shrimp production, 1988–1998: wild vs. aquaculture.
SOURCE: FAO (2000).

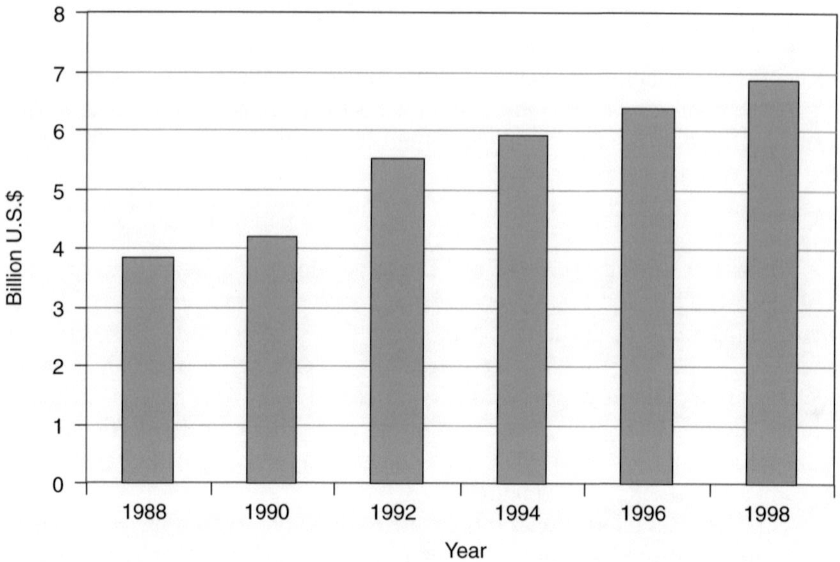

FIGURE 5.3 World volume and value of aquaculture production of shrimp, 1988–1998. SOURCE: FAO (2000).

address the unique challenges presented by aquaculture production of seafood (e.g., indigenous levels of *Salmonella* and use of unapproved antibiotics). For example, recent evidence for residual chloramphenicol (an illegal antibiotic) in aquaculture shrimp from various Asian farms and processing plants in China, Vietnam, and Thailand resulted in major product recalls involving numerous retail operations in the United States and Europe (Louisiana Department of Agriculture and Forestry, 2002; NFI, 2002a, 2002b). At one point the European Union banned the import of cultured shrimp from China and neighboring countries with shrimp aquaculture. Regulatory response in the United States was initiated by state agencies and there was general confusion concerning the proper sampling methods and analytical procedures for residual detection in the parts per billion range.

REVIEW OF CURRENT FOOD SAFETY CRITERIA FOR SEAFOOD

Current Food Safety Criteria

FDA and the U.S. Environmental Protection Agency (EPA) have established various food safety criteria that address the intrinsic nature of seafood (e.g., scombrotoxicity) or characteristics of the environment from which it was harvested (e.g., paralytic shellfish toxin, methyl mercury, fecal coliforms). The current list of regulations intended to ensure the safety of seafood that is harvested or cultured domestically or is imported reflects the extreme and unique diversity of this food group. Among these regulations are microbiological criteria associated with specific microorganisms, such as *Salmonella* and *Clostridium botulinum*, and with product categories, such as ready-to-eat products and molluscan shellfish.

The traditional approach used by FDA to develop performance standards for food safety can be a somewhat slow and lengthy process or it can be a precipitous one resulting from the agency's need to react to a sudden crisis. Irrespective of how they are developed, once seafood safety criteria are in place, there is no mechanism for periodic review to modify or rescind them. This poses a challenge because the previously mentioned increasing dependence on international seafood sources and aquaculture products is introducing new regulatory challenges not fully anticipated in prior regulations.

As reliance on international supply and demand for seafood items continues to increase in terms of both product volume and diversity, food safety issues will become more challenging and varied. Therefore, the committee concludes that food safety regulations will need periodic review by the regulatory agencies to remain up-to-date (i.e., to be aligned with current science, commercial practice, and public health objectives) in such an evolving situation. These reviews should be conducted by the regulatory agencies and include discussions that address not only the safety issues associated with the products and their sources, but also the capacity of regulators to communicate the food safety risks and to enforce compliance within the existing regulatory frameworks in both the domestic and international settings. The reviews must prioritize the issues in need of more immediate attention, based on the application of risk assessment.

The HACCP System for Seafood Safety Control

Concerns within industry, government, and consumer groups about the need to improve seafood safety began in the 1980s and eventually culminated in the federally mandated seafood HACCP rule. This rule was initially proposed on January 28, 1994 (FDA, 1994) and published in final form on December 18, 1995 (FDA, 1995), with an implementation date of December 18, 1997. As a regulation based on HACCP, the seafood HACCP rule was based on identification and implementation of preventive critical control points (CCPs), with processors responsible for development and maintenance of the program. (Processor is defined in the HACCP rule as any person engaged in commercial, custom, or institutional processing of fish or fishery products, either in the United States or in a foreign country; persons engaged in the production of foods that are to be used in market or consumer tests are also included. Persons who only harvest or transport seafood, without otherwise engaging in processing, are not covered by these regulations [FDA, 1994].)

The seafood HACCP system differs from that in the meat and poultry industry in that government inspections are not performed on a continuous, on-site basis. One reason for this is that such a program is difficult to justify due to the wide variety of species, variable sources, and diverse product forms characteristic of the seafood industry. Most importantly, however, organoleptic inspections of freshly harvested marine species would be of little significance in terms of product safety. Moreover, because such performance standards as specific pathogen reductions are not included in the seafood HACCP rule, verification testing is not part of the FDA inspection. Seafood safety concerns are not dominated by any single pathogen or contaminant. Data reported by the Centers for Disease Control and Prevention (CDC, 2000) indicate that from 1993 through 1997, seafood was the vehicle of transmission in 6.8 percent of the total foodborne disease outbreaks during this period, but involved less than 3 percent of the total cases. The percentage of outbreaks associated with shellfish was 1.7 percent, and fish (species other than shellfish) were associated with 5.1 percent of the outbreaks. Most of the outbreaks associated with fish were the result of chemical hazards such as ciguatoxin and scombrotoxin (CDC, 2000). It is important to note that the seafood HACCP rule did not replace existing regulations and that, therefore, it must be implemented along with Good Manufacturing Practices (GMP) (21 C.F.R. part 110) as foundational prerequisites. Required monitoring and recording of sanitation control procedures (21 C.F.R. part 123) are also prerequisites for implementing a HACCP plan.

Although the National Marine Fisheries Service of the U.S. Department of Commerce conducts a fee-for-service National Seafood Inspection Program derived from the Agricultural Marketing Act of 1946, the inspection is voluntary. In addition, these inspections are designed to ensure compliance with minimum sanitation practices and product-grade standards, not with the HACCP rule. Inspections, whether of domestic or imported products, are carried out for quality purposes, not for safety.

Application of Food Safety Criteria in HACCP

FDA has been responsible for developing an extensive list of seafood regulations (see Appendix C). Many of these regulations consist of food safety criteria—categorized as tolerances, action levels, and guidelines—with the underlying purpose of protecting public health through adherence to GMPs and the prevention of product adulteration and misbranding. While public health is a common goal for all criteria, the specific scientific basis for each of them differs, depending mainly on the availability of data about a hazard. As examples, the tolerance for methyl mercury content in fish (1.0 ppm) is based on the level necessary for consumer safety, the labeling requirement for sulfite residues (10 ppm) is based on the lower limit of analytical capability, and the fecal coliform standard for shellfish harvesting waters is based on the potential presence of microbial and viral pathogens. Apart from scientific data, there are other factors that have been considered when establishing seafood safety criteria, such as the perception of risk by the public or the availability of technologies that reduce the hazard to a level of public protection deemed appropriate by FDA. Although the final decision regarding development or modification of a food safety criterion resides with FDA, the rule-making process requires periods of review by and comment from the various stakeholders, which unavoidably make it a slow process.

As mentioned previously, all food safety criteria established prior to the seafood HACCP rule remain in place within the current regulatory system; thus, in addition to HACCP, processors are obligated to produce seafood that comply with all relevant food safety criteria. In most cases these criteria are not useful for inclusion as critical limits for CCPs in HACCP plans; however, they can be used as verification criteria in situations where end-product testing may be warranted. The National Advisory Committee on Microbiological Criteria for Foods (NACMCF), an advisory body to federal food safety agencies, specifically addressed the issue of microbial criteria with the following statement: ". . . the use of microbiological testing is seldom an effective means of monitoring CCPs because of the time required to obtain results. In most instances, monitoring of CCPs can best be accomplished through the use of physical and chemical tests and through visual observations. Microbiological criteria do, however, play a role in verifying that the overall HACCP system is working" (NACMCF, 1998).

Although the NACMCF statement is focused specifically on microbiological criteria, the same rationale could apply for many of the food safety criteria the regulatory agencies have developed for chemical hazards. Although EPA and FDA have established limits for some chemical contaminants, direct monitoring with analytical tests for chemical contaminants in seafood is often impractical as a CCP because the variability in concentration for some of these contaminants among geographic areas is significant and required sampling would be impractical. As an alternative, the geographical variability in contaminant concentration indicates that the potential exists for reducing exposure through restrictions of harvesting sites (IOM, 1991). As the FDA *Fish and Fisheries Products Hazards and Controls Guide* states, such a CCP could be described as follows: "No fish may be harvested from an area that is closed to commercial fishing by foreign, federal, state, or local authorities; and no fish may be harvested from an area that is under a consumption advisory by federal, state, or local regulatory authority based on a determination by the authority that fish harvested from the waters are reasonably likely to contain contaminants above the federal tolerances, action levels, or guidance levels" (CFSAN, 2001).

Chemical hazards that are not of environmental origin (i.e., biogenic amines, such as histamine) require a different control strategy. Elevated biogenic amine levels, a potential food safety hazard in some finfish such as tuna, mackerel, and mahi-mahi, are produced as a result of the growth in fish of certain indigenous bacteria during improper cooling or storage conditions. FDA has established an action level of 50 ppm histamine in any edible portion of the fish (CFSAN, 2001). Monitoring of histamine levels in each fish received at a processing plant is impractical, expensive, and not a viable method of control by seafood processors. In contrast, review of the harvest records—time and temperature—associated with each lot of fish is deemed an acceptable alternative. If this control alternative is used, harvest vessel records for each lot must include the following information: "1) Icing on-board the harvest vessel was performed in accordance with the vessel's cooling rate study that validates cooling to 50°F [10°C] or below within 6 hrs of death regardless of maximum exposure temperature, or placement in ice within 12 hrs of death if the maximum exposure temperature does not exceed 83°F [28.3°C]; 2) method of capture; 3) date and time of landing; 4) estimated time of death; 5) method of cooling; 6) date and time cooling began; 7) sea and air temperature if exposure temperatures exceeds 83°F [28.3°C]; 8) adequacy of ice during on-board holding" (CFSAN, 2001).

As noted before, the option to apply the current standard on histamine (i.e., a histamine limit of 50 ppm) in the HACCP plan does exist; however, this is seldom practical. If a concentration of 50 ppm of histamine were used as the critical limit in tuna processing operations, an argument could be made that all histamine-susceptible fish would have to be tested to ensure compliance with the HACCP plan. Given the current analytical methods for histamine determination, this would require excessive time and additional product handling that could further jeopardize product quality and safety. Even if more rapid or less expensive histamine analytical methods for use in a commercial setting were forthcoming, the utility of such tests would be limited by the viability of the sampling plan parameters (number and size of samples) required to obtain statistically meaningful data. Consequently, in keeping with the preventive character of HACCP, the processor will customarily choose preventive options that are the least costly and disruptive to plant operations and will thus avoid after-the-fact analyses or end-product testing as verification tools for a particular hazard. In the case of histamine, therefore, processors will typically opt for preventing high histamine levels through the already described option: control of abusive handling conditions that lead to histamine formation in fish and recording of time and temperature parameters in the vessel and at the plant. These records can be further supplemented with sensory screening for early signs of temperature abuse and evidence of adequate refrigeration. When appropriate, specific analytical tests are performed as part of HACCP verification; in this case, verification may include the periodic analysis of histamine concentrations in fish showing signs of temperature abuse. If the process is under control, the expectation is that such histamine analyses would indicate levels of less than 50 ppm.

The Scientific Basis, Public Health Impact, and Economic Feasibility of Safety Criteria

HACCP has been acclaimed as an appropriate, science-based, food safety assurance system by the food science community (IOM, 1991; NRC, 1985a, 1985b), although it has not yet been universally applied in the food industry. For some groups, implementation of HACCP raises concerns about reduced government oversight of food processing. For example, a report issued by the General Accounting Office (GAO, 2001) suggested that FDA's oversight of seafood firms did not sufficiently protect consumers against foodborne disease. Despite these controversies, recent reports suggest that HACCP has played a role in reducing some of the nation's notifiable foodborne illnesses (CDC, 2002). As described in Chapters 2 and 4, and because of the many confounding factors, a relationship between HACCP implementation and reduction of illness attributable to specific food groups cannot be fully established from the available data. However, HACCP has had a very distinct impact on the seafood industry, primarily through enhanced awareness and understanding of potential seafood safety hazards from production and processing through preparation and consumption. Since enactment of the seafood HACCP rule, extensive education and training programs for industry personnel have been made available through the Seafood HACCP Alliance (SHA, 2001) and other programs. This training has been among the most beneficial developments in assisting industry managers to recognize food safety as an integral aspect of their operations in promoting change (Gall, 1999). A recent FDA progress report for 2002 reveals that the continuing increase in compliance with seafood HACCP programs has increased the margins of safety for American consumers, and that areas of concern are better identified for further government oversight and for emphasis by education programs (Office of Seafood, 2002).

Further benefits from mandatory HACCP will depend not only on continuing education, but also on continuing technical innovations. An example that clearly illustrates this point is the attempt to reduce illness caused by consumption of raw oysters. Despite the impact of HACCP, foodborne illness from consumption of raw oysters remains a major and serious seafood safety concern. The principal culprit is the pathogenic bacterium *V. vulnificus.* Infections caused by this microorganism are relatively rare (approximately 40 reported cases of primary septicemia per year) and usually involve consumers with preexisting liver diseases or immunodeficient conditions, but the fatality rate is high—approximately 50 percent of total reported cases (Mead et al., 1999; Personal communication, M. Glatzer, FDA, December 2002). The oyster industry and the respective regulatory authorities, working through the Interstate Shellfish Sanitation Conference (ISSC), have determined that in addition to consumer education programs, alternative processing technologies such as high hydrostatic pressure are needed to reduce the recurrent illnesses due to *V. vulnificus* and the related species *V. parahaemolyticus* (ISSC, 2002a).

The ISSC is modeled after the Interstate Milk Shippers Conference, which allows participation of state and federal regulatory authorities as well as consumer and industry representatives. The combined expertise and interests of the ISCC participants result in a unique approach, detailed in their Model Ordinance for oyster processing. Among other requirements, this Model Ordinance requires implementation of new postharvest treatments that hopefully will progressively reduce the average annual reported illnesses attributed to raw oysters (ISSC, 2002a). The reduction goals, 40 percent by 2005 and 60 percent by 2007, were considered reasonable based on the decisions of the ISSC committees and board, which involved industry and state and federal agencies. Certain states that do not meet the required reductions in *V. vulnificus* illnesses stipulated in a mandated schedule of annual declines face regulatory consequences that include reduced production and seasonal closure of harvestable waters (Table 5.1).

This unique approach requires adequate industry performance without mandating a specific process or performance standard, but by establishing a public health objective. The flexibility of this approach reflects a regulatory shift from establishing a specific standard to requiring that processors choose and validate technologies appropriate to their specific operations. In fact, their choice of strategy must result in a measurable and improved performance through an increase

TABLE 5.1 Abbreviated Table of Compliance for Source States as Specified in the Interstate Shellfish Sanitation Conference's *Vibrio vulnificus* Management Plan

Deadline	Postharvest Treatment[a]	Illness Reductions[b]
December 2004	25% capacity	
2005–2006		40% (average)
December 2006	50% capacity	
2007–2008		60% (average)
>2008	If the 60% illness reduction rate is not collectively achieved by 2008, additional controls can be imposed including harvest restrictions or closures relative to water temperatures and special labels designating product to be shucked by a certified oyster dealer.	

[a] Postharvest treatment "capacity" will be based on all oysters intended for raw, half-shelled market during the months of May through September harvested from source states, to include the capacity of all operational plants and the capacity of plants under construction.
[b] Illness reductions will be based on the average illnesses rate for years 1995–1999 of 0.306/million persons, using data from California, Florida, Louisiana, and Texas. Adjustments in methodology can be adopted based on further reviews.

in the capacity to implement processing alternatives and through a reduction in illnesses. The capacity is defined as the actual documented ability to perform in terms of having appropriate procedures and facilities for the implementation of a particular processing alternative to reduce *V. vulnificus* in raw oysters. The reduction in illnesses, in turn, is determined using an annual average based on reported illnesses. This is a unique and challenging approach that focuses on encouraging innovation within a mandated HACCP format.

In the absence of an initial risk assessment, FDA and state regulatory agencies have used a nondetectable level (i.e., essentially zero tolerance) as the benchmark for performance (performance standard) for *V. vulnificus* in oysters intended for raw consumption (ISSC, 2002b). This measure currently recognizes the fact that some postharvest treatments can be applied to raw oysters for food safety purposes. Oysters thus treated may not only be exempt from a public advisory or warning statement, but may also be accompanied with a product declaration such as "processed for added safety" (ISSC, 2002b). The decision to allow or mandate the use of specific product labels or statements rests with individual state authorities. In time, use of recent *Vibrio* risk assessments (FAO, 2001; FAO/WHO, 2002) might support the establishment of science-based microbiological performance standards for *V. vulnificus* that ensure a reasonable level of public health protection while allowing flexibility and innovation in the application of post-harvest treatments. For example, a risk assessment may conclude that the use of treatments resulting in levels and types of *V. vulnificus* equivalent to those found in oysters during the less problematic winter season reduces this hazard to a tolerable level of risk.

As another alternative to zero tolerance, FDA may consider use of risk assessments to establish food safety objectives that specify the level of this hazard at the point of consumption; however, as discussed extensively in Chapter 3, the use of food safety objectives is a new concept that has not been fully explored and, in some cases, may encounter opposition.

One of the attractive elements of the current HACCP-based system is the increased involvement of industry in determining appropriate food safety control strategies for hazards associated with specific commodities and processes. While there is opportunity for a greater level of industry participation, most seafood processors still request advice from FDA to direct their decisions and practice.

Given the diversity within the seafood industry, FDA determined that specific guidance would be necessary to assist industry to productively focus its HACCP plan development and implementation efforts. Anticipating this need, FDA issued a special guide, the *Fish and Fisheries Products Hazards and Control Guide*, commonly referred to as "the Guide," to help implement HACCP in the seafood industry (CFSAN, 2001). The Guide contains all FDA performance standards for food safety that are relevant to seafood, as well as guidance in process controls for seafood-borne safety hazards.

The Guide was complemented with a national education program, the Seafood HACCP Alliance, which involved academic and regulatory expertise in every state, plus numerous international training efforts based on a cadre of qualified trainers (SHA, 2001). This Alliance also developed a "Compendium of Fish and Fishery Processes, Hazards, and Controls" that can be accessed via the Internet for detailed information on HACCP programs for various seafood commodities, processes, and hazards (SHA, 1997).

The Guide (CFSAN, 2001) provides recommendations for identifying CCPs, setting critical limits, monitoring CCPs, and setting corrective actions for various seafood species and processes. The Guide is a significant and innovative contribution that benefits field inspectors, the seafood industry, and consumers. However, in many cases, in the absence of other guidance, the recommendations made in the Guide are interpreted by industry and field inspectors as legal requirements, despite the fact that the introduction in the Guide specifically states, "The controls and practices provided in this guidance are recommendations and guidance to the fish and fishery products industry. This guidance provides information that would likely result in a HACCP plan that is acceptable to FDA. However, it is not a binding set of requirements" (CFSAN, 2001).

The recommendations and general guidance provided by the Guide (in addition to established and specified standards) do not limit its utility and impact, except in some instances when the scientific basis for the recommendations contained therein is not readily evident. For example, FDA recommendations to use packaging film with elevated oxygen transmission rates (i.e., breathable film) to avert potential germination and growth of *C. botulinum* in reduced-oxygen packaging of fresh, refrigerated fishery products may be based on the best currently available science (CFSAN, 2001). However, the description of and accessibility to such packaging materials is not readily evident or well communicated.

Likewise, the Guide does not consider the commercial and regulatory implications of some of the recommendations it contains. For example, in some cases, while the recommendations for recording the details on harvesting conditions, such as time of fish death and duration of handling until iced storage, are science-based (CFSAN, 2001), documenting these details can pose impractical situations for the fishermen. In another example, avoidance of potentially toxic fish is based on excluding designated ciguatoxic-prone waters. (Certain tropical reef waters support food chains that progressively accumulate toxins generated by plankton along the food chain; large predator fish at the top of the food chain, in turn, become toxic to humans.) While this approach appears reasonable and scientifically valid, designated waters are often not properly mapped, and many fish are highly mobile so that geographic limits may be meaningless. Such problems do not indicate a weakness in the regulatory approach, but rather a need for continuous attention to advance and improve the Guide for use by both the inspectors and the commercial sector.

The committee recognizes that the Guide is an innovative and useful document that effectively assists seafood processors with the development of their HACCP plans. To improve its utility, the committee recommends that FDA consider introducing a more transparent and collaborative process (i.e., one that allows routine and structured involvement by the respective users and beneficiaries) in further developing the Guide. In keeping with its recommendations about flexibility of the regulatory process made in Chapter 3, the committee further recommends that the progress, utility, and impact of the Guide be enhanced through the addition of programs and actions to better communicate relevant changes in science, commerce, and public health objectives and to facilitate their incorporation into the Guide.

In addition, the committee recommends that general guidance for all products and processes in the Guide be complemented by FDA with more transparent and detailed scientific justification, citing reasons, sources, and limitations for the respective seafood safety criteria, in an accessible format. The intent should be to offer explanations that can support decisions in accordance with the best available science and to help focus appropriate responses to the needs for scientific research, technical innovations, and modifications of regulatory requirements.

To attain the above, and in accordance with the Federal Advisory Committee Act, the committee further recommends that FDA appoint a Hazards and Controls Guide Advisory Committee that has balanced and qualified representation from third-party expertise. This committee should routinely convene to critique the Guide and prepare submissions for changes and interpretations based on current science and commercial practices, and suggest priorities for scientific, commercial, and regulatory attention.

When situations involving questionable seafood safety issues have emerged, some processors have sought assistance from a third party or processing authority to help validate or verify specific seafood-processing methods or variances from traditional methods. The term "processing authority" may refer to private consultants, academics, or other experts. However, there are no current FDA guidelines for establishing the credentials of processing authorities, or for conducting process validations or verifications required for a HACCP plan to be accepted by FDA. In particular, the validation of modern, rapid microbiological methods and the design of appropriate sampling plans need adequate FDA guidance.

The committee recognizes that the use of processing authorities is consistent with the seafood HACCP rule (FDA, 1995). However, the committee recommends that the issues of expert capability and process confidentiality be further addressed by FDA in the light of food safety considerations. A transparent and structured protocol must also be developed by FDA to guide process validations. This protocol must address criteria for distinguishing the creditability of processing authorities, sampling plans, experimental designs, and appropriate methodologies. Validation and verification guidelines, including recommendations for adequate analytical methods and sampling plans, should accompany the recommended controls in the Guide. Similarly, a regulatory protocol is necessary to recognize the application of analytical methodologies such as new rapid test procedures that can be utilized in process validation and in routine verification.

In addition, the committee recommends more timely and continuous communications to ensure awareness, understanding, and consistent application of the Guide. The intent of this recommendation is broad and includes FDA's intraprogram activities, state and federal partnerships, individual firms, and the responsible authorities in countries exporting to the United States. Efforts to enhance communications should include any reports and recommendations from the recommended Hazards and Controls Guide Advisory Committee.

The magnitude of concerns about current HACCP governance for seafood safety is further compounded in international commerce. The regulatory response to the volume and diversity of seafood trade could set the tone for international commerce and regulation of other foods. FDA's new approach regarding international commerce considers all seafood processors equal and challenges each nation to demonstrate the capability of its respective authority for seafood safety. A similar approach has been introduced by Canada (CFIA, 2002) and the European Union (EEC, 1991). Although these regulations require recognition of "competent authorities" and responsible criteria and standards, some nations' efforts to scrutinize other nations' competence and commercial performance appear to be defensive and have been perceived as trade barriers (Cham Prasidh, 1999). The Codex Alimentarius offers some cooperation among national authorities, but its recommendations often lack the necessary details to address the issues raised by specific countries or products. As mentioned earlier, this situation must be addressed by FDA in anticipation of the increasing U.S. dependence on seafood imports.

The committee recommends that FDA give immediate attention to the application of the Guide to ensure food safety equivalence in international seafood commerce. Moreover, the committee recommends that FDA clarify the intent of the Guide and its content to U.S. trading partners. In addition, the committee recognizes that screening limited quantities of seafood products at points of entry is not consistent with the preventive concept of HACCP; therefore, FDA should establish more regulatory oversight prior to receiving foreign seafood products at points of entry into the United States.

Also, with a continuing reliance on a science-based approach, there is a need for more scientific collaboration among nations and for more extensive sharing of information on seafood safety issues applicable in the respective nations. The committee suggests that a scientific program with international participation and support could incorporate the concerns of the authorities regarding specific products, so that agreements regarding appropriate seafood safety standards are reached. This approach could be driven by collaborative research in support of the Codex Alimentarius. Similar efforts have already been made in the area of joint Food and Agriculture Organization of the United Nations (FAO)/World

Health Organization (WHO) microbiological risk assessments (FAO/WHO, 2002). The United States, through EPA and FDA, and using the Guide as a model, could initiate an international seafood safety exchange program. This international program could include research and training to address common concerns about such hazards as *Salmonella* and *Listeria* in fresh seafood and methyl mercury tolerances, and develop recommendations for best practices such as Best Aquaculture Practices. The Best Aquaculture Practices could be similar to Good Agricultural Practices for produce and other land-based crops (CFSAN, 1998), and consistent with Good Manufacturing Practices. The Best Aquaculture Practices could be developed collaboratively and could be recognized as the international prerequisite for the expanding aquaculture production around the world.

In summary, the committee recognizes that limitations in supply are becoming one of the most significant issues in the world of seafood commerce, and that trends in the United States reflect a growing dependence on international sources, particularly with regard to aquaculture products. Regulatory decisions and priorities to address seafood safety must account for this situation.

Therefore, with an awareness of existing international seafood safety programs and efforts (e.g., within Codex Alimentarius, FAO/WHO, and others), the committee recommends that FDA initiate an International Seafood Safety Exchange Program to foster and generate support for international collaboration in seafood safety research and training. A common topic for initial consideration could be the development of Best Aquaculture Practices. The existing FDA *Fish and Fishery Products Hazards and Controls Guide* could be used as a proven format.

REFERENCES

CDC (Centers for Disease Control and Prevention). 2000. Surveillance for foodborne disease outbreaks—United States, 1993–1997. *Morb Mortal Wkly Rep* 49:1–51.

CDC. 2002. Preliminary FoodNet data on the incidence of foodborne illnesses—selected sites, United States, 2001. *Morb Mortal Wkly Rep* 51:325–329.

CFIA (Canadian Food Inspection Agency). 2002. *Food Safety Enhancement Program.* Online. Available at http://www.inspection.gc.ca/english/ppc/psps/haccp/haccpe.shtml. Accessed December 30, 2002.

CFSAN (Center for Food Safety and Applied Nutrition). 1998. *Guide to Minimize Microbial Food Safety Hazards from Fresh Fruits and Vegetables.* Online. Food and Drug Administration (FDA). Available at http://www.cfsan.fda.gov/~dms/prodguid.html. Accessed December 30, 2002.

CFSAN. 2001. *Fish and Fisheries Products Hazards and Controls Guidance*, 3rd ed. Online. FDA. Available at http://www.cfsan.fda.gov/~comm/haccp4.html. Accessed December 27, 2002.

Cham Prasidh HE. 1999. *Food Trade and Implementation of the SPS and TBT Agreements: Challenges for Developing Countries in Meeting the Obligations of the SPS and TBT Agreements and the Codex Alimentarius.* Online. Food and Agriculture Organization of the United Nations. Available at http://www.fao.org/docrep/meeting/X2666E.htm. Accessed December 30, 2002.

EEC (European Economic Community). 1991. Laying down the health conditions for the production and the placing on the market of fishery products. Council Directive 91/493/EEC. *Off J Eur Communities* L268:15.

FAO (Food and Agriculture Organization of the United Nations). 2000. *FAO Yearbook, Fishery Statistics: Commodities 2000, Vol 91*. Online. Available at http://www.fao.org/fi/statist/FISOFT/FishPLUS.asp. Accessed December 27, 2002.

FAO. 2001. *Hazard Identification, Exposure Assessment and Hazard Characterization of Campylobacter spp. in Broiler Chickens and* Vibrio *spp. in Seafood*. Joint FAO/WHO Activities on Risk Assessment of Microbiological Hazards in Foods. Geneva: WHO.

FAO. 2002. *Fisheries*. Online. Available at http://www.fao.org/fi. Accessed December 26, 2002.

FAO/WHO (World Health Organization). 2002. *Risk Assessment of* Campylobacter *spp. in Broiler Chickens and* Vibrio *spp. in Seafood*. Report of a Joint FAO/WHO Expert Consultation. Online. Available at http://www.who.int/fsf/Micro/Reportcv02english.pdf. Accessed December 20, 2002. .

FDA (Food and Drug Administration). 1994. Proposal to establish procedures for the safe processing and importing of fish and fishery products; Proposed rule. *Fed Regist* 59:4142–4214.

FDA. 1995. Procedures for the safe and sanitary processing and importing of fish and fishery products; Final rule. *Fed Regist* 60:65095–65202.

Fisheries Statistics and Economics Division. 2001a. *Foreign Trade*. Online. National Marine Fisheries Service (NMFS), National Oceanic and Atmospheric Administration (NOAA). Available at http://www.st.nmfs.gov/fus/fus01/07_trade2001.pdf. . Accessed December 27, 2002.

Fisheries Statistics and Economics Division. 2001b. *World Fisheries*. Online. NMFS, NOAA. Available at http://www.st.nmfs.gov/fus/fus01/04_world2001.pdf. Accessed December 27, 2002.

Fisheries Statistics and Economics Division. 2002. *Commercial Fisheries: Summary*. Online. NMFS, NOAA. Available at http://www.st.nmfs.gov/st1/commercial. Accessed December 27, 2002.

Gall K. 1999. *Seafood HACCP Implementation Survey Evaluation Report*. Stony Brook, NY: State University of New York.

GAO (General Accounting Office). 2001. *Federal Oversight of Seafood Does Not Sufficiently Protect Consumers*. GAO-01-204. Washington, DC: U.S. Government Printing Office.

IOM (Institute of Medicine). 1991. *Seafood Safety*. Washington, DC: National Academy Press.

ISSC (Interstate Shellfish Sanitation Conference). 2002a. *II. Model Ordinance. Chapter II—Risk Assessment and Risk Management*. Online. FDA. In: Guide for the Control of Molluscan Shellfish. Pp. 29–36. Available at http://issc.org/On-Line_docs/onlinedocs.htm. Accessed May 9, 2003.

ISSC. 2002b. *II. Model Ordinance. Chapter XVI—Post-Harvest Processing*. Online. FDA. In: Guide for the Control of Molluscan Shellfish. Pp. 167–168. Available at http://issc.org/On-Line_docs/onlinedocs.htm. Accessed May 9, 2003.

Louisiana Department of Agriculture and Forestry. 2002. Declaration of Emergency. Chloramphenicol in Crabs: Testing and Sale. LAC 7:XXXV, Chapter 1. *La Regis* 28:1133–1136.

Mead PS, Slutsker L, Dietz V, McGaig LF, Bresee JS, Shapiro C, Griffin PM, Tauxe RV. 1999. Food-related illness and death in the United States. *Emerg Infect Dis* 5:607–625.

NACMCF (National Advisory Committee on Microbiological Criteria for Foods). 1998. Hazard analysis and critical control point principles and application guidelines. *J Food Prot* 61:1246–1259.

NFI (National Fisheries Institute). 2002a. Chloramphenicol residue controls discussed and tightened. *NFI Insider* 1:1.

NFI. 2002b. NFI obtains Louisiana drug sampling regulations, and enforcement details. *NFI Insider* 1:1–2.

NRC (National Research Council). 1985a. *An Evaluation of the Role of Microbiological Criteria for Foods and Food Ingredients*. Washington, DC: National Academy Press.

NRC. 1985b. *Meat and Poultry Inspection: The Scientific Basis of the Nation's Program.* Washington, DC: National Academy Press.

Office of Seafood. 2002. *FDA's Evaluation of the Seafood HACCP Program for Fiscal Years 2000/2001.* Online. CFSAN, FDA. Available at http://www.cfsan.fda.gov/~comm/seaeval2.html. Accessed December 27, 2002.

SHA (Seafood HACCP Alliance). 1997. *Compendium of Fish and Fishery Product Processes, Hazards, and Controls.* Online. National Seafood HACCP Alliance for Training and Education, University of California, Davis. Available at http://seafood.ucdavis.edu/haccp/compendium/compend.htm. Accessed December 28, 2002.

SHA. 2001. *HACCP: Hazard Analysis and Critical Control Point Training Curriculum,* 4th ed. Florida Sea Grant Report No. 120. Gainesville, FL: University of Florida.

Waters S. 2002, Feb 26. Illegal fish deals reportedly yield 6-figure income. *South Florida Sun-Sentinel.* P. C4.

6

Scientific Criteria and Performance Standards to Control Hazards in Produce and Related Products

FRESH FRUITS AND VEGETABLES AND FRESH-CUT PRODUCTS

Background

Fruits and vegetables provide many health benefits and are an important component of the American diet. People interested in lowering their consumption of total calories, fats, and cholesterol, as well as in protecting against certain types of cancer, are incorporating more fruits and vegetables into their diets.

The fresh fruit and vegetable industry experienced solid growth in the late 1990s, as evidenced by the increasing space devoted to these products in supermarkets and on restaurant menus throughout the United States (IFT, 2001). This growth is expected to increase in the future. As many industry and government programs have promoted increased consumption of produce, consumers have responded to these messages by increasing their consumption of fruits and vegetables from 284 pounds per capita in 1987 to 319 pounds in 1997 (Kaufman et al., 2000). Growers, in turn, have responded by producing a wide variety of traditional and new fruits and vegetables. Because of advances in agronomic practices, preservation technologies, shipping practices, and improved cold-chain management, global production and distribution of fresh fruits and vegetables have increased. Through innovative packaging systems and improved marketing and merchandising strategies, consumers can choose from an average of 345 different produce items in a typical retail food store (Litwak, 1998).

Imports of fresh fruits and vegetables also increased significantly as U.S. food preferences and consumption patterns shifted. In 2001, U.S. imports of fresh fruits and vegetables were 38.3 percent and 13.3 percent, respectively, of the total national consumption of these products (Personal communication, G. Lucier and S.L. Pollack, U.S. Department of Agriculture, December 2002). Increases in global food trade have made produce from over 130 countries around the world available to U.S. consumers and provide year-round availability of fresh produce (Rangarajan et al., 1999). Mexico is now the source of 27 percent of U.S. fruit imports and 38 percent of vegetable imports (Jerardo, 2002). Off-season fruit imports from Chile and Argentina and vegetable imports from Peru, Ecuador, and other South American countries are also driving up the overall U.S. import shares of these commodities. Excluding Mexico, Latin American countries supply an additional 40 percent share of U.S. imported fruits, the largest share being bananas, grapes, and melons. It is not surprising that there is a seasonal pattern to fresh vegetable imports, with two-thirds of the import volume arriving between December and April when U.S. production is low and limited to the southern growing regions of the country (ERS, 2002).

A niche for fresh-cut fruits and vegetables was established in the 1980s and its market has increased exponentially since then because of the demand for convenience and value-added products by consumers, food retailers, and the foodservice industry (IFT, 2001). Fresh-cut produce is "any fresh fruit or vegetable, or any combination thereof that has been physically altered from its original form, but remains in the fresh state" (IFPA, 2001).

While providing many health benefits, raw fruits and vegetables have also been known for at least a century to be potential vehicles for human disease (Beuchat, 1998). In the late 1800s, one of the first reports of produce-associated foodborne illness linked typhoid infection to eating celery (Morse, 1899). Another outbreak of typhoid fever was attributed to eating watercress grown in soil fertilized with sewage (Warry, 1903), and two cases were attributed to eating uncooked rhubarb grown in soil fertilized with typhoid excreta (Pixley, 1913). These and other early reports of microorganisms surviving on vegetables and plant tissues (Creel, 1912; Melnick, 1917) demonstrated that raw fruits and vegetables could serve as vehicles for the transmission of human pathogens. While fresh produce can serve as a source of all classes of foodborne pathogens (i.e., bacteria, viruses, protozoa, fungi, and helminths), pathogenic bacteria raise the greatest concerns because the risk of illness they pose may be amplified by potential growth prior to consumption (NACMCF, 1999a).

Although fresh fruits and vegetables have recently been associated with foodborne disease outbreaks, these products were not thought to be common causes of foodborne illnesses in the United States; instead, they were considered to be relatively safe foods (NRC, 1985). The acidity of many fruits was believed to inhibit the growth and to decrease populations of human pathogens, while the edible portions, protected from contamination by a skin or thick rind, were considered safe as well (NRC, 1985). It was recognized, however, that produce imported from countries where polluted water or raw sewage was used for irrigation, fertilization, washing, cooling, or icing could be contaminated with enteric pathogens and might be a potential source of foodborne illness. A report issued in 1985, *An Evaluation of the Role of Microbiological Criteria for Foods and Food Ingredients* (NRC, 1985), addressed the need for microbiological criteria for various food groups. With regard to fresh fruits and vegetables, this report made the following statement: "there is little use for microbiological criteria for fresh fruits and vegetables at the present time. However, future changes in irrigation and fertilization practices in this country or changes in the source of imported produce could mandate testing for certain pathogens or indicator organisms" (NRC, 1985).

In the past two decades, as consumers have increased their consumption of fresh fruits and vegetables, there has also been a significant increase in the number of foodborne disease outbreaks and cases associated with these foods. According to the Centers for Disease Control and Prevention (CDC), foodborne disease surveillance reports for the periods 1983 to 1987 and 1988 to 1992 suggest that the annual number of reported produce-associated disease outbreaks, the number of persons affected annually in those outbreaks, and the proportion of outbreaks due to fresh produce among those illnesses with an identified food vehicle has at least doubled (NACMCF, 1999a). Outbreaks of foodborne illness associated with produce in the United States for the period 1973 to 1997 are shown in Figure 6.1.

An in-depth analysis of published outbreak investigations by a panel of experts (IFT, 2001) revealed that outbreak data has linked the following pathogenic organisms with the consumption of specific produce commodities: *Clostridium botulinum* with cabbage salad; *Campylobacter jejuni* with salad and lettuce; *Escherichia coli* O157:H7 with spring mix, lettuce, seed sprouts, and cantaloupe; *Listeria monocytogenes* with cabbage salad; *Shigella* spp. with shredded lettuce, parsley, and scallions; *Salmonella* spp. with seed sprouts, green onions, tomatoes, melons, and mangoes; hepatitis A virus with tomatoes, lettuce, watercress, and frozen raspberries and strawberries; calicivirus with salad and frozen raspberries; Norwalk virus with cut fruits; *Cyclospora* with raspberries, mesculun lettuce, and basil and basil-containing products; and *Giardia* with lettuce and onions (see Table 6.1). There have also been outbreaks linking *Cryptosporidium* and *E. coli* O157:H7 with nonpasteurized apple cider, and *Salmonella* with nonpasteurized orange juice (IFT 2001; NACMCF, 1999a).

Most of the identified fresh produce-associated disease outbreaks in the United States from 1988 to 1998 were caused by bacteria, especially *Salmonella* spp. and *E. coli* O157:H7, and from 1990 to 1998, three-fourths of the reported outbreaks were attributed to domestic produce (Personal communication, A. Liang, CDC, 1999). In addition to the produce-associated foodborne disease outbreak statistics compiled and reported by CDC, the Center for Science in the Public Interest (CSPI) also developed a database of foodborne outbreaks that occurred in the United States between 1990 and 2001. CSPI (2001) reported that 148 outbreaks consisting of 10,504 cases (an average of 71 cases per outbreak)

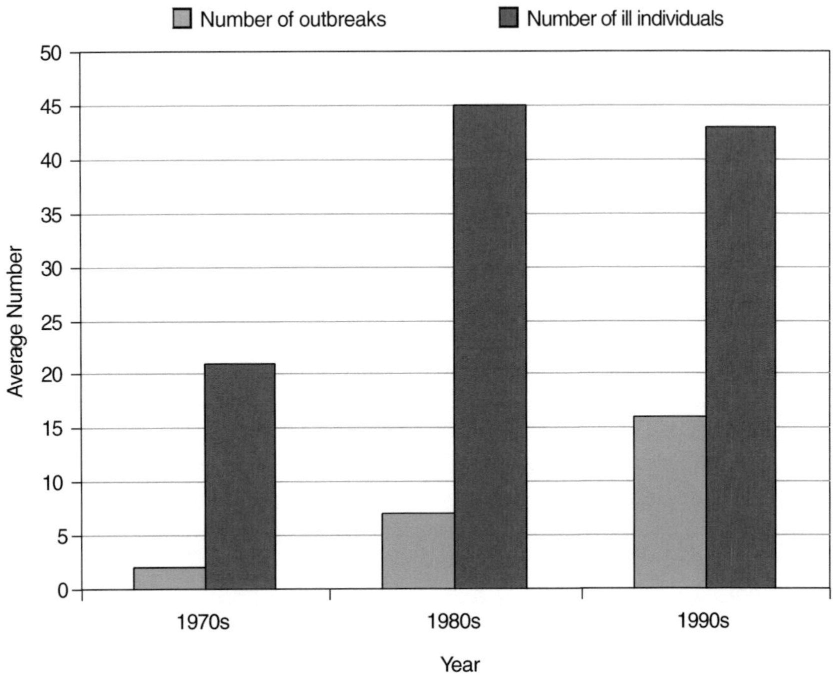

FIGURE 6.1 Outbreaks of foodborne illness associated with fresh produce in the United States, 1973–1997.

were associated with produce; vegetables were associated with 78 percent of these outbreaks and fruits were associated with 18 percent. Five percent were associated with both fruits and vegetables (CSPI, 2001).

Fresh produce safety is of special concern to the public health community because fruits and vegetables do not receive any treatment specifically designed to kill all microbial pathogens prior to consumption. Although the incidence of foodborne illness linked to produce is still low, produce-associated illnesses erode consumer confidence in the safety of fresh fruits and vegetables and cause concern about the risk attributable to the consumption of these foods. There are still many questions about the transmission of microorganisms from their potential reservoirs to fruits and vegetables, including knowledge about any vectors that may be involved in this process. While all produce items have risk factors in common, it is important to recognize that each fruit and vegetable has a unique combination of composition and physical characteristics, as well as growing and harvesting practices, cooling techniques, and optimal storage temperatures under which it is managed. Because of the lack of lethal treatments between farm

TABLE 6.1 Some Multistate Foodborne Disease Outbreaks Involving Produce in the United States, 1994–2001

Year	Pathogen	Number of States	Food Source
1994	*Shigella flexneri*	2	Green onions, probably contaminated in Mexico
1996	*Cyclospora cayetanesis*	20	Raspberries from Guatemala (mode of contamination unclear); cases were also reported in the District of Columbia and two Canadian provinces
1996	*Salmonella* Infantis	2	Alfalfa sprouts, probably contaminated during sprouting
1996	*Escherichia coli O157:H7*	2	The implicated lettuce was traced to a single grower processor; cattle was found near the lettuce fields
1996	*E. coli O157:H7*	4	U.S.-grown apples were phosphoric acid washed, brushed, and rinsed; however, phosphoric acid-based solutions may have been used incorrectly (not intended for produce/waxed produce) or sometimes used at low concentrations; possibly poor quality apples, some dropped apples used, apple orchard near cattle/deer
1997	*C. cayetanesis*	18	Raspberries imported from Guatemala, mesculun lettuce, and products containing basil; cases were also reported in the District of Columbia and two Canadian provinces
1997	Hepatitis A	4	Strawberries from Mexico distributed through the U.S. Department of Agriculture Commodity Program for use in school lunches
1998–1999	*S.* Baildon	Multistate	Tomatoes traced to two packers in Florida; possible field contamination by domestic or wild animals
1998	*S. sonnei*	4	Imported parsley, probably contaminated during washing after harvest
1999	*S.* Muenchen	20	Unpasteurized orange juice produced in Mexico and bottled in the United States
1999	*S.* Mbandaka	4	Sprout seeds were believed to come from the same lot and distributed to various growers in California, Florida, and Washington
2000	*S.* Enteriditis	Multistate	Gallon-sized containers of domestic citrus juices were implicated in the outbreak
2000	*S.* Newport	10	Imported mangoes, likely contaminated during treatment to kill fruit flies
2001	*S.* Poona	16	Imported cantaloupe, probably contaminated in the field or shortly after harvest
2002	*S.* Javiana	50	Tomatoes
2002	*S.* Newport	18	Tomatoes

SOURCE: IFT (2001).

production and consumption, microbial pathogens introduced on fresh produce at any point in the production and distribution chain may be present at the point of consumption. Moreover, anything in the production environment that comes in contact with the plant has the potential for being a source of pathogens. Although the ultimate source of fresh produce contamination with most enteric pathogens is animal or human fecal material, potential direct and indirect sources of contamination from farm to table include soil; manure; irrigation water; wild and domestic animals; farm, packinghouse, and terminal market workers; contaminated equipment; wash and rinse water; ice; cooling units; transportation vehicles; cross-contamination from other food products; and improper storage, packaging, and display (Beuchat, 1998; FDA/USDA/CDC, 1998; Rangarajan et al., 1999).

The growth, survival, and inactivation of microorganisms on fresh fruits and vegetables is dependent on the interaction of many factors; therefore, preventing contamination of produce with microbial pathogens—rather than removing them at a later point—is considered to be the most effective strategy in assuring the safety of these foods (FDA/USDA/CDC, 1998; IFT, 2001). Many effective intervention strategies have been developed and implemented on farms and in packinghouses but, as mentioned above, they cannot completely eliminate microbial hazards potentially present on or in raw produce (IFT, 2001). For these reasons, to reduce the risk of produce-borne disease, the focus of intervention strategies must be on preventing the introduction of biological, chemical, and physical hazards into these products.

Current Criteria and Standards

Unlike the dairy and seafood industry where microbial criteria and standards have been in use for many years, there are virtually no criteria or standards for microbiological safety currently being applied to fresh or fresh-cut produce by U.S. federal government agencies other than those pertaining to sprouts and fruit juices (discussed later in this chapter).

To minimize foodborne disease from being transmitted through fresh produce, it is necessary to prevent initial contamination of these products and to control the potential amplification of pathogens in them throughout the production and distribution chain. Intervention strategies currently being applied in the fresh produce industry are Good Agricultural Practices (GAPs) in the field and packinghouses (FDA/USDA/CDC, 1998) and Good Manufacturing Practices (GMPs) in fresh-cut operations (21 C.F.R. part 110). GAPs are similar to the GMPs used by food processors, but GAPs address agricultural activities, including preplanting, planting, harvest, and postharvest practices that are designed to reduce microbial risks.

Several guidance documents that address GAPs have been developed and widely disseminated by government agencies, growers, shippers, processor trade associations, and academia (IFPA, 2001). Some of these publications include the *Voluntary Food Safety Guidelines for Fresh Produce*, published by the International Fresh Cut Produce Association (IFPA) and the Western Growers Association (IFPA, 1997); the *Quality Assurance Program* of the California Strawberry Commission (1998); the Food and Drug Administration (FDA) guidance document, *Guide to Minimize Microbial Food Safety Hazards for Fresh Fruits and Vegetables* (FDA/USDA/CDC, 1998); and *Food Safety Begins on the Farm*, from Cornell University (Rangarajan et al., 1999). The FDA guidance document describes eight areas in the growing and handling of produce where microbial contamination may occur; it also urges growers to be aware of the potential for contamination and to manage their operations in ways that minimize that potential (FDA/USDA/CDC, 1998). This document sets forth eight principles of microbial food safety that can be applied to the growing, harvesting, packing, and transportation of fresh fruits and vegetables, as follows:

1. The prevention of microbial contamination of fresh produce is favored over reliance on corrective actions once contamination has occurred.
2. To minimize microbial food safety hazards in fresh produce, growers or packers should use GAPs in those areas over which they have a degree of control while not increasing other risks to the food supply or the environment.
3. Anything that comes in contact with fresh produce has the potential of contaminating it. For most foodborne pathogens associated with produce, the major source of contamination is human or animal feces.
4. Whenever water comes in contact with fresh produce, its source and quality dictate the potential for contamination.
5. Agricultural practices using manure or municipal biosolid wastes should be closely managed to minimize the potential for microbial contamination of fresh produce.
6. Worker hygiene and sanitation practices during production, harvesting, sorting, packing, and transportation play a critical role in minimizing the potential for microbial contamination of fresh produce.
7. Follow all applicable local, state, and federal laws and regulations, or corresponding or similar laws, regulations, or standards for agricultural practices for operators outside the United States.
8. Accountability at all levels of the agricultural environment (farms, packing facility, distribution center, and transport operation) is important to a successful food safety program. There must be qualified personnel and effective supervision to ensure that all elements of the program function correctly and to help track produce back through the distribution channels to the producer.

The committee recognizes that the principles that make up the current GAP recommendations are necessarily general given the broad range of fruits and vegetables and their growing conditions and, like GMPs, they focus on minimizing the potential for microbial contamination. In the case of GAPs, these principles focus on prevention of contamination primarily from fecal material, water sources, application of manure or biosolids, or poor personal hygiene.

The committee also recognizes that data on risks associated with many specific practices in the fresh produce sector are lacking, so it is difficult to assess which intervention strategies are necessary and which will provide the greatest reduction in risk. Research in this area has been very active in recent years; therefore, it is expected that data from such research will provide the necessary information to supplement the basic guidelines.

In addition to the use of GAPs to minimize the probability of microbial contamination of fruits and vegetables, some produce buyers have introduced purchasing specifications; letters of guarantee; vendor certification programs; and independent, third-party audits to provide assurance that growers are following GAPs (IFPA, 2001; IFT, 2001).

A unique feature of fruits and vegetables is that although microbial contamination is most often associated with their surfaces, the interior tissues of solid produce have been traditionally considered to be sterile. However, an early study reported that the application of bacteria to the surface of fruits could result in their internalization over time (Samish and Etinger-Tulczynska, 1963). Later, a number of researchers reported isolating low levels of bacteria from internal tissues of intact vegetables or radish sprouts (Lund, 1992; Robbs et al., 1996). Other research findings suggest that *E. coli* O157:H7 in irrigation water and manure can be internalized into lettuce plant tissue (Solomon et al., 2002), but the design of this study did not reflect typical lettuce growing conditions.

The committee, aware of the importance of the issue of internalization of pathogenic bacteria during growth or processing of produce, recommends that FDA conduct or support additional studies to determine whether the internalization of bacteria represents a significant safety hazard in fruits and vegetables.

A more widely recognized fact is that if flume or dump-tank water is cold and contaminated with pathogens and warm fruit (e.g., apples or tomatoes) is immersed in it, the pathogens can be internalized (Buchanan et al., 1999; Rushing et al., 1996; Zhuang et al., 1995). This led to the recommendation that flume water for certain commodities be treated with an appropriate antimicrobial agent such as chlorine, and that it be warmer than the incoming product (FDA/USDA/CDC, 1998).

Although the Hazard Analysis and Critical Control Point (HACCP) system has long been recognized as the most effective and flexible system for assuring the microbiological safety of a variety of foods, there have been few attempts to integrate the various steps associated with the production and processing of fresh produce into a farm-to-table HACCP system. Several HACCP plans have been developed for sprouted seeds, shredded lettuce, and tomatoes (Rushing et al., 1996), but complete validation of these plans has not yet been accomplished (NACMCF, 1999b). Available data are insufficient to develop validated HACCP plans for most fresh produce items. Also, prerequisite programs, such as GAPs and GMPs, which provide the foundation for HACCP systems, are still being defined and evaluated for their effectiveness on farms and in orchards.

As the trend toward greater importation of fruits and vegetables into the United States increases, there are concerns about the harmonization of food safety standards for imported produce (IFT, 2001). Several efforts are currently underway to harmonize these standards. In addition to the FDA guidance document (FDA/USDA/CDC, 1998), the Codex Alimentarius—a joint program of the Food and Agriculture Organization of the United Nations (FAO) and the World Health Organization (WHO)—through its Committee on Food Hygiene, is developing standards for the production of fresh produce, fresh-cut produce, and sprouts (CAC, 2000). This code of practice, similar to the FDA guidance document in that it stresses prevention strategies for growers, is undergoing the Codex Alimentarius comment process for approval.

Recently, FDA collected and analyzed selected samples of imported and domestic produce to determine the incidence of microbial contamination on these commodities. This project was undertaken to gather more data on the incidence and extent of pathogen contamination of fresh produce and to assist the agency in the development of policy for the Produce Safety Initiative (OPDFB, 2001). A total of 1,003 imported fruit and vegetable samples from 21 countries were collected and analyzed. Of these, 4.4 percent tested positive for either *Salmonella* or *Shigella*, whereas no products were positive for *E. coli* O157:H7 (OPDFB, 2001). In the domestic survey, FDA sampled and analyzed 767 commodities of which 1.6 percent tested positive for pathogens; specifically, 0.8 percent (6 samples) were positive for *Salmonella* and an equal percentage were positive for *Shigella* (CFSAN, 2001).

In addition to FDA's surveillance efforts, the U.S. Department of Agriculture, through its Agricultural Marketing Service (AMS), began a cooperative federal/state effort in 2000 to establish a microbiological baseline to assess the risk of contamination in the domestic food supply. As part of this Microbiological Data Program, AMS is collecting retail samples of selected domestic and imported fruits and vegetables to assess the incidence, number, and species of important foodborne pathogens and indicator organisms present in them (AMS, 2001). The information obtained from the data program will be used to establish "benchmarks" for evaluating the efficacy of procedures to prevent or reduce contamination of fresh fruits and vegetables with harmful microorganisms (AMS, 2001).

FRUIT AND VEGETABLE JUICES

Background

Similar to whole fruits, fruit juices were historically considered to present minimal risks to health. This belief was derived from the expected inhibitory

TABLE 6.2 Foodborne Disease Outbreaks Associated with Consumption of Reconstituted Frozen Orange Juice Prior to 1990

Pathogen	Year	Location	Venue	Cases	Reference
Salmonella Typhi	1944	Ohio	Residential hotel	18, 1 death	Duncan et al., 1946
Hepatitis A	1962	Missouri	Hospital	24	Eisenstein et al., 1963
Unknown	1965	California	Football game	563	Tabershaw et al., 1967
S. Typhi	1989	New York	Resort hotel	46 confirmed, 24 suspected	Birkhead et al., 1993

properties of high organic acid levels, and consequent low pH, on bacterial growth, and from the fact that most juices undergo a thermal process. In fact, documented foodborne illnesses were rare (NRC, 1985). In the early 1990s, increased interest in raw fruit juices and improvements in cold distribution systems led to an increase in the processing and distribution of raw, nonpasteurized fruit juices. Many of the foodborne disease outbreaks attributable to juices that had occurred in the United States prior to 1990 were caused by asymptomatic human handlers (workers shedding pathogens in their feces without showing signs of illness) who contaminated orange juice with hepatitis A or *Salmonella* Typhi as the juice was being reconstituted at a food service establishment (see Table 6.2). In one outbreak, the source of contamination was thought to have been the water used to dilute the concentrate (Tabershaw et al., 1967). Outbreaks associated with single-strength raw citrus juices prepared in large commercial processing facilities were identified in the mid 1990s. In one outbreak implicating orange juice, toads in the orange groves were thought to be the source of *Salmonella*, while a general lack of sanitation in the plant was thought to have contributed to the extent of the outbreak (Cook et al., 1998; Parish, 1998). Likewise, foodborne disease outbreaks implicating raw apple juice were uncommon prior to the 1990s. However, beginning in 1991, several outbreaks associated with *E. coli* O157:H7 or with the protozoan parasite, *C. parvum,* were identified (IFT, 2001). Table 6.3 describes some outbreaks of foodborne disease associated with raw juices. Although early outbreaks were associated with small cider mills, an outbreak was associated with a large commercial juice processor in 1996. Lack of sanitation, coupled with the use of wind-fallen or dropped apples, improper or no washing of the fruit prior to pressing, and proximity of cattle or deer (reservoirs for the pathogens) were thought to have contributed to these outbreaks.

TABLE 6.3 Selected Outbreaks of Foodborne Disease Associated with Raw Apple or Orange Juices

Pathogen	Juice	Year	Location	Cases	Reference
Salmonella Typhimurium	Apple	1974	New Jersey	296	CDC, 1975
Escherichia coli O157:H7	Apple	1991	Massachusetts	23	Besser et al., 1993
Cryptosporidium parvum	Apple	1993	Maine	160 primary, 53 secondary	Millard et al., 1994
S. Gaminera, *S.* Hartford, and *S.* Rubislaw	Orange	1995	Florida	63 ill, 7 hospitalized	CDC, 1995; Cook et al., 1998; Parish, 1998
C. parvum	Apple	1996	New York	20 confirmed, 11 suspected	CDC, 1997
E. coli O157:H7	Apple	1996	Connecticut	14	CDC, 1997
E. coli O157:H7	Apple	1996	British Columbia, California, Colorado, and Washington	70, 1 death	CDC, 1996; Cody et al., 1999
S. Muenchen	Orange	1999	United States and Canada	207 confirmed, 91 suspected, 1 death	CDC, 1999
S. Enteriditis	Orange	2000	Multistate	14	Butler, 2000

Current Criteria and Standards for Juices

Pathogen Reduction

As a consequence of larger outbreaks associated with raw juices processed at commercial facilities, FDA introduced regulations in 1998 and 2001 for all juices produced for inter- or intrastate sale (CFSAN, 1998; FDA, 2001). Subpart A of the regulation (21 C.F.R. part 120) mandates that juice be produced under a HACCP plan that has supporting GMPs and Sanitation Standard Operating Procedures. The sanitation procedures must, at a minimum, address monitoring and record-keeping for eight specific points: (1) water safety, (2) cleanliness of food contact surfaces, (3) cross-contamination, (4) hand washing and toilet facilities, (5) adulteration, (6) labeling and use of toxic compounds, (7) employee health, and (8) pest control.

Subpart B of the regulation requires that juice processors achieve at least a 5-D reduction (referred to as a 5-D process) of the pertinent microorganism, which is defined as "the most resistant microorganism of public health significance that is likely to occur in the juice." The identification of this microorganism may be based on disease outbreak data as well as on any other appropriate information available. Currently, *Salmonella* is generally accepted as the pertinent pathogen in citrus juices, whereas *E. coli* O157:H7 and *C. parvum* need to be taken into consideration for apple juice (FDA, 2001).

Although most juice processors currently use thermal treatments to ensure the required 99.999 percent kill, other nonthermal 5-D processes will be accepted if they are appropriately validated. The *Juice HACCP Hazards and Controls Guidance* document provides some background on validating these alternative processes (OPDFB, 2002a). This document was complemented with an educational program developed by the Juice HACCP Alliance (OPDFB, 2002b), modeled after a similar Seafood HACCP Alliance comprised of academic, regulatory, and industry representatives. The training manuals developed for seafood were adapted to juices by the Juice HACCP Alliance.

Processors of raw citrus juices are allowed to use surface decontamination methods to achieve part of the 5-D pathogen reduction requirement if they exclusively use undamaged, tree-picked fruit to prepare the juice. The 5-D pathogen reduction must start after initial culling and cleaning and must take place in a single facility. Processors must also conduct end-product testing to ensure that generic *E. coli* and *E. coli* Biotype I are absent (< 1 cfu/20 mL) from the juice. One 20-mL sample for each 1,000 gal of juice produced must be sampled, except when a processor produces less than 1,000 gal/wk, in which case one sample must be collected and analyzed per week. When two out of seven consecutive samples are positive for *E. coli*, the process is considered inadequate, and the processor must follow one of a number of corrective actions. Until corrective actions are complete, any juice processed at the facility must be subjected to an alternative processing method that achieves a 5-D pathogen reduction in the expressed juice.

Producers of shelf-stable (canned) juices that fall under 21 C.F.R. part 113 or part 114 are exempt from demonstrating a 5-D reduction. However, these processors must have a HACCP plan in place that includes the scheduled thermal process with their hazard analysis. Similarly, juice processors who only sell directly to consumers (e.g., food service or retailers) are also exempt from the 5-D pathogen reduction rule; however, when such processors do not process the juice to achieve a 5-D pathogen reduction, they are required to place a warning label on the product. The warning label must read as follows: "WARNING: This product has not been pasteurized and, therefore, may contain harmful bacteria that can cause serious illness in children, the elderly, and persons with weakened immune systems" (FDA, 1998).

Patulin

Patulin is a mycotoxin produced by various molds (*Penicillium, Aspergillus, Byssochlamys*) commonly present in the environment; these molds cause the brown rot of various fruits. Damage to apples promotes mold growth and patulin production; thus, presence of patulin in apple juice is a general indicator of the quality of fruit used. Levels of patulin in contaminated apple juice may vary widely; it is also a frequent contaminant of purees and unfermented ciders (Stoloff, 1975). Patulin levels can be substantially reduced in the juice by trimming decayed tissue (Lovett et al., 1975). FDA believes that processors can control the levels of patulin in apple products by removing spoiled and visibly damaged apples from the product stream used for the production process (CAST, 2003).

The FDA HACCP document on apple juice (OPDFB, 2000) and its accompanying compliance policy guide (Office of Regulatory Affairs, 2002) support and establish an action level of 50 mg/kg (50 ppm) for patulin in apple juice, apple juice concentrates, and apple juice products. With adherence to GMPs, these levels can readily be achieved. Patulin is only slightly reduced by thermal processing; therefore, it will be mostly unaffected by pasteurization of apple juice (McKinley and Carlton, 1991). The Codex Alimentarius is developing a draft *Code of Practice for the Reduction of Patulin Contamination in Apple Juice and Apple Juice Ingredients in Other Beverages*, which will be discussed at the 2003 meeting of the Codex Committee on Food Additives and Contaminants.

The Scientific Basis for Current Criteria

FDA asked the National Advisory Committee on Microbiological Criteria for Foods (NACMCF) to develop a juice performance standard based on the best available scientific data and information. This performance standard (FDA, 2001) was developed after consideration of public comments on the microbiological safety of juices. During subsequent discussions of NACMCF, it became clear that there were no data available on the levels of *E. coli* O157:H7—the microorganism of concern—in apple juice. Nevertheless, despite the lack of data on this pathogen, it was known that nonpathogenic (generic) *E. coli* can be isolated occasionally at low levels (i.e., < 10 cfu/mL) from apple juice. Based on these data, a level of 10 cfu/mL of the pathogenic strains was assumed to represent highly contaminated juice and, thus, the worst-case scenario. Using this level as the basis, a target concentration of *E. coli* O157:H7 in apple juice of less than one cell per 100-mL serving (considered a normal serving) plus an additional safety factor of 100 was adopted, resulting in a final target concentration of less than 1 cfu/10,000 mL of juice. Consequently, it was calculated that to reduce *E. coli* O157:H7 numbers from 10 cfu/mL to less than 1 cfu/10,000 mL, a process capable of achieving a minimum 5-D reduction would be required.

To validate that this performance standard was indeed the appropriate level of pathogen reduction, the working group explored a different scientific rationale. In particular, the estimate of 10 cfu/mL of juice for highly contaminated raw material was evaluated by calculating the theoretical level of *E. coli* O157:H7 that would be in the juice if 1 in 100 pieces of fruit were contaminated with 1 g of fecal material, assumed to be the primary source of contamination. Bovine feces have been shown to contain as many as 10,000 to 100,000 cfu/g of *E. coli* O157:H7. Even if as many as 1 fruit in 100 were contaminated, because 1 fruit produces approximately 100 mL of juice, the scenario above would result in 10,000 mL of juice contaminated at a level of 1 to 10 cfu/mL, as expected. The implemented 5-$\log_{10}$ reduction should then virtually eliminate the risk of disease from consumption of fruit juices.

Recognizing that citrus fruits with an intact skin may be processed so that pathogens on the surface are destroyed, and that pathogens are not reasonably likely to be present in the interior of the fruits, FDA allowed the use of surface treatment to achieve the 5-D pathogen reduction standard. If processors choose to use fruit surface treatments, FDA determined that an appropriate end-product sampling plan needed to be implemented as process control verification. FDA provided a detailed explanation of the derivation of the sampling plan for generic *E. coli* in citrus juices involving surface treatment of the whole fruit to achieve the 5-D pathogen reduction (Garthright et al., 2000). Briefly, two unpublished data sets, one from the University of Florida and the other from a survey by the Florida Department of Citrus, were used to establish estimated averages (and standard deviations) for *E. coli* Biotype I in orange juice. *E. coli* was selected because of its historical use as an indicator organism of fecal contamination and because with routine testing of juice, the probability of finding *E. coli* was significantly greater than the probability of finding *Salmonella*. Based on an assumed normal distribution of *E. coli* in the product and on assumed processing conditions, the calculated mean (1.2 $\log_{10}$ *E. coli*/mL) and standard deviations were used to estimate the probability of finding this organism in a 20-mL sample of untreated juice that had undergone a 1- to 5-D process. A 20-mL sample was chosen because it allowed detection of levels as low as 0.05 *E. coli*/mL (1.3 $\log_{10}$ *E. coli*/mL). A moving window approach was used to develop the sampling plan. With this approach, the probability of finding an occasional single positive sample even with a functioning 5-D process was acknowledged. A window was chosen such that finding two positives within the window when the 5-D process was functioning would be extremely rare and could be considered strong evidence of process failure. Monte Carlo simulations were used to select a window of seven tests that provided a high probability of identifying a process failure, while minimizing the probability that a false failure would occur. The assumptions made and the limitations were provided by FDA (Garthright et al., 2000).

The information on the scientific justification for the sampling plans for citrus juices that rely on surface treatments to achieve a 5-D pathogen reduction was published in a docket by FDA (Docket No. 97N-0511). This is an excellent example of using data and expert opinion to develop criteria or standards; the committee believes that this derivation could be used as a model when regulatory agencies develop other criteria or standards. In contrast, the justification for a 5-D pathogen reduction process is described only in a memorandum, with no reference to the scientific data from which the standard derives. As mentioned earlier, transparency of the criteria development process requires that the data and the assumptions made be clearly communicated.

The 50 μg/kg action level for patulin in apple juice, juice concentrates, and apple juice products was identified by FDA on the basis of a safety assessment (OPDFB, 2000) that agreed with the independent evaluation conducted at the international level by the FAO/WHO Joint Expert Committee on Food Additives (JECFA, 1996). The latter, in turn, was based on information derived from studies that indicated a no-observed-adverse-effect level for a cumulative patulin dose of 0.3 mg/kg body weight/wk (Becci et al., 1981). FDA defined this as the provisional tolerable weekly intake for patulin, from which a provisional tolerable daily intake of 0.043 mg/kg of body weight/d was derived. No reproductive or teratogenic effects were noted at dose levels up to 1.5 mg/kg of body weight in mice or rats. Genotoxicity assays using bacteria were generally negative, possibly due in part to the antibiotic properties of patulin, whereas many tests conducted using mammalian cells were positive, which prompted JECFA to conclude that patulin should be considered genotoxic. Early studies conducted in the 1940s had found patulin to be carcinogenic, but chronic oral studies in rats conducted later by FDA failed to confirm this (Becci et al., 1981).

LOW-ACID AND ACIDIFIED CANNED FOODS

Background

In the early 1900s, the technology to efficiently produce canned foods resulted in increased availability and popularity of these products. However, the science behind the thermal process was in its infancy, and thermal processes were often based on experience rather than experimental data. In addition, the primary focus was on limiting product spoilage, which was initially perceived as a greater problem than product safety. The facts that boiling temperatures were insufficient to eliminate *C. botulinum*, that this microorganism was widespread in the environment, that it was an anaerobe, and that most vegetables could serve as a vehicle for botulism were not known until the early 1900s (CDC, 1998; Geiger et al., 1922). Similarly, little was known about the illness and neither intensive care units nor antitoxin was available, which resulted in mortality rates of 60 to 70 percent. Outbreaks of botulism in 1919 and 1920, linked to commercially canned California ripe olives, contributed both to changes in regulation in that state and to research that greatly increased our knowledge of *C. botulinum* and of canning technology in general (Young, 1976). In the fall of 1919, botulism outbreaks involving commercially canned olives were reported in Ohio and Michigan, and similar outbreaks occurred in New York, Tennessee, Montana, and California in early 1920 (Young, 1976). In New York alone, six members of a family of eight died from eating seemingly "good" olives. These outbreaks led to widespread panic regarding the safety of olives and, to a lesser extent, of other canned foods. Some cities and states prohibited the sale of canned olives (Young, 1976).

These outbreaks and others exposed weaknesses in the 1906 Pure Food and Drug Act, for the law permitted seizure only when foods had been examined and found decomposed. Thus, the Bureau of Chemistry was limited to warning the public about the harm of eating "spoiled foods." Some industry members believed that the public was partly responsible because people had eaten spoiled olives; however, it was later confirmed that not all the toxic olives were spoiled (Young, 1976).

In December 1919, the National Canners Association (now the National Food Processors Association), the Canners League of California (now the California League of Food Processors), and the California Olive Association agreed to provide funds to support research on the epidemiology of botulism in the United States. This was one of the first comprehensive assessments of this topic, and Geiger and colleagues (1922) summarized the findings. Thus, research stimulated by the olive outbreaks and funded in large part by the canning industry resulted, in a relatively short period of time, in an improved understanding of the heat resistance of *C. botulinum*, the various factors that affected this resistance, and the bacterium's ability to grow in foods (Esty and Meyer, 1922).

At the time, it was common practice to preserve ripe, lye-treated olives ($pH > 7.0$) in glass jars and submerge them for 30 min in a boiling water bath, for the glass would not withstand high pressures (Young, 1976). Based on research conducted at the University of California, the processing of olives at 115.6°C (240° F) for 40 min was made mandatory in the state of California on August 7, 1920 (California State Board of Health, 1920). This regulation also gave the State Board of Health the authority to seize and quarantine all canned ripe olives not produced under these conditions. Current processing guidelines for ripe olives include heating at 115.6°C (240°F) for 60 min in No. 401 and 411 cans, with a minimum initial temperature of 21.1°C (70°F) (Downing, 1996).

Occasional outbreaks of botulism associated with commercially canned products continued to occur, but they were generally considered minor occurrences compared with the number of illnesses and deaths associated with home-canned products. In 1963, outbreaks of botulism associated with commercially smoked fish and with canned tuna (because of contamination through faulty seals) and canned liver paste (due to underprocessing because of an improperly calculated thermal process) resulted in a renewed interest in this microorganism (Gilbertson, 1964). In 1971, botulism was responsible for the death of one person and the prolonged illness of another after consumption of canned vichyssoise (potato) soup. A batch of underprocessed soup caused both cases of botulism; subsequently, the manufacturer went out of business (Gavin and Weddig, 1995; Paretti, 1972). Just months later, another U.S. processor discovered botulinal toxin in a few cans of chicken vegetable soup, but no cases of botulism were reported (Paretti, 1972). These incidents focused attention on the canning industry, leading to strengthening of GMP regulations for low-acid canned foods in 1973 and for acidified low-acid canned foods in 1979. These regulations were modeled after the California regulations, but also included a mandatory training component. This training component consists of required certification of retort operators and is currently offered by the Food Processors Institute (FPI, 2003), a nonprofit education provider for the National Food Processors Association.

Current Criteria and Standards

Regulations concerning canning of low-acid and acidified low-acid foods including produce, dairy products, and seafood are found in 21 C.F.R. parts 113 and 114. Equivalent regulations for meat products can be found in 9 C.F.R. parts 318G and 381X. These HACCP-based regulations provide considerable detail, from equipment design to allowable temperature-indicating devices.

The regulations require that hermetically sealed foods be "commercially sterile." (The term commercially sterile is defined as the application of heat sufficient to render the food free of microorganisms capable of reproducing in the food under normal nonrefrigerated conditions, and free of viable microorganisms—including spores—of public health significance.) Although not specifically stated, *C. botulinum* is recognized in the regulations as the most heat-resistant microorganism of public health significance, and the accepted minimum process to ensure safety is one that achieves a 12-D reduction in the number of spores of this microorganism in the food of interest (Stumbo, 1973). For acidified low-acid foods, defined as having a pH of 4.6 or below after equilibration, the key control parameter is the acidification step rather than the thermal process. Acidification of the food must be adequate so that the pH of the food will not permit the growth of microorganisms of public health significance (9 C.F.R. part 114). In addition to the reduction and control of potential growth of microorganisms, both 9 C.F.R. parts 113 and 114 mandate standardized training, registration of the processing facility at state and federal levels, filing of thermal processes, record keeping, and establishment of a recall program.

Botulism from commercially canned foods has been virtually eliminated since the implementation of these regulations, although occasional outbreaks do occur. For example, in 1978 and 1982, canned salmon caused single cases of botulism. The contamination occurred postprocess in both cases; one was from a damaged container and the other was from a malformation of the double seam on the bottom of the container (Gavin and Weddig, 1995). These sporadic cases led to increased regulatory focus on container manufacture and on the handling of containers by processors (Gavin and Weddig, 1995).

The Scientific Basis for Criteria

The initial published work used to establish thermal processes in canned foods is generally acknowledged to have been that of Esty and Meyer (1922). These researchers, using the limited bacteriological techniques available at the time, described the heat resistance of suspensions of 109 strains of *Bacillus botulinus* (now *Clostridium botulinum*) spores in phosphate buffer at temperatures above boiling. Of greatest significance was the development of a thermal destruction curve for a suspension of 60 billion spores of three of the most heat-resistant isolates. More than 1,800 small glass tubes were filled with 2 mL of the spore suspension and sealed. Multiple tubes were subjected to each of five temperatures for various lengths of time. After heating, the tubes were opened and the heated spore suspension was placed in nutrient medium, incubated for an appropriate period, and then analyzed for the presence of growth. The minimum time required to destroy this population of cells at each temperature was thus determined. Esty and Meyer made the significant observation that the data were logarithmic in the temperature range they evaluated. These data were later used to calculate that a thermal process at 250°F for 2.78 min (sometimes rounded up to 3.0 min and known as the F value) would eliminate a population of 6×10^{10} spores (theoretically, a 10.8-D process). This $F_{250°F}$ value and the calculated *z* value (the temperature difference required to change the F value by 1 $\log_{10}$) was generally used by the canning industry to establish equivalent processes at other temperatures. Esty and Meyer were attempting to achieve maximum levels of spore populations in their preparation that, in other experiments, ranged from 1×10^6 to 1×10^9. The level of 6.0×10^{10} used in their classic experiment appears to have been simply a level that they were able to achieve with this particular spore preparation. These data were later confirmed and, after introducing corrections for heating time, modified to an $F_{250°F}$ of 2.45 min and a *z* of 17.6°F (Townsend et al., 1938). These values were generally rounded up to 3 min and 18°F.

In 1950, Stumbo and coworkers published the first methods for determining and calculating D values for *C. botulinum*. The D value is the time required to destroy 90 percent of the cells in a suspension and, unlike the F value, it is not dependent upon the initial spore load. The D value for *C. botulinum* 62A in phosphate buffer at 250°F was reported to be 0.133 min by Stumbo and colleagues (1950) and 0.2 min by Schmidt (1964). By dividing Schmidt's D value of 0.2 into the $F_{250°F}$ value of 2.45 minutes of Townsend and colleagues (1938), a 12.25-D process was estimated. It is not clear whether this is the true origin of the accepted, but rather arbitrary, 12-D process; nevertheless, it appears to be an approximate account of how the scientific information evolved (Perkins, 1964; Stumbo, 1973). Stumbo (1973) noted that, with an estimated 1 spore per can of *C. botulinum,* this process results in a product for which the probability of this microorganism surviving is 1 in 1 trillion cans. Stumbo and coworkers (1975) later argued that a target of 1 viable spore in no more than 1 trillion cans should be determined using the following assumptions: that *C. botulinum* spores might be present at 1/g of food, and that the *z* value used to calculate the thermal processes should be 14°F and not 18°F. Their calculated thermal processes were, therefore, greater than those commercially applied at the time, particularly for larger can sizes where a 15-D process needed to be applied (due to an estimated thousands of cells per can) and at lower processing temperatures. Pflug and Odlaug (1978) challenged the assumptions of Stumbo and coworkers, arguing that a target of 1 viable spore in no more than 1 billion cans was adequate protection of public health. They also maintained that the epidemiological evidence supported the less conservative approach. They evaluated six outbreaks of botulism occurring from commercially processed canned foods between 1963 and 1974. All were attributed to the use of an incorrect process, a failure to deliver the scheduled thermal process, or postprocess contamination, and not to inadequate assumptions used to calculate the process (Pflug and Odlaug, 1978). Adequate training of personnel in the canning facility was emphasized as critical to the further reduction of botulism from commercially canned foods.

The D-value concept is still widely used to calculate thermal processes. However, the basic assumption that thermal inactivation of microbial spores or vegetative cells follows first-order kinetics (is linear) has recently been challenged (Peleg and Cole, 1998; van Boekel, 2002). This is particularly problematic when thermal death times are calculated by extrapolation. Although the use of the 12-D thermal process has a long history of safe use, its appropriateness should be scientifically reevaluated.

Technological innovations, through the use of alternative food-processing technologies (including microwave and radio frequency processing, ohmic and inductive heating, high pressure processing, pulsed electric fields, high voltage arc discharge, pulsed light technology, oscillating magnetic fields, ultraviolet light, ultrasound, and pulsed X-rays), are critical to the development of new fruit and vegetable products and the reduction and inactivation of pathogens of public health significance. As research and development continue to determine the efficacy of these processes for a variety of foods, it is important to recognize that any performance standards for these technologies require the following actions: (1) the use of pathogens most resistant to the technology, (2) a description of the mechanism of pathogen inactivation and its kinetics, (3) a determination of mechanisms to validate the effectiveness of microbial inactivation, (4) the identification of critical process factors, and (5) a description of the process deviations and corrective actions. Guidance must be provided by the agency on ways to validate the process. When assessing any nonthermal process for shelf-stable foods, the selection of an appropriate performance standard should be evaluated on scientific merit. Many thermal processes far exceed the 12-D process for *C. botulinum* in order to eliminate spoilage spores of microorganisms of greater heat resistance, a fact that is likely to hold true of nonthermal processes (Stumbo, 1973).

It is generally accepted that *C. botulinum* will not grow and produce toxin in foods having pH values of 4.6 or below (Kim and Foegeding, 1992). Dozier (1924) published the first comprehensive study on this topic, followed by Townsend and coworkers (1954). Both noted that a pH of 4.8 to 4.9 was the minimum for botulinal growth and toxin production in food. Since then, there have been a number of reports of *C. botulinum* growth and toxin production in laboratory media at pH values lower than 4.6 (Tanaka, 1982; Young-Perkins and Merson, 1987); however, media with high protein concentrations were necessary for growth and for toxin development to occur. The levels of protein in fruits and vegetables have not been shown to support the growth of *C. botulinum* at pH values lower than 4.6 (Kim and Foegeding, 1992). Outbreaks of botulism in acid foods are not entirely unknown (Odlaug and Pflug, 1978), but almost all have been associated with underprocessed, home-canned foods where it is suspected that surviving microorganisms may have altered the pH of the product, thus allowing *C. botulinum* to grow. Adequate acidification and thermal processes, as required by 9 C.F.R. part 114, should be sufficient to prevent botulism in these products.

SPROUTS

As a result of several disease outbreaks associated with the consumption of sprouts, FDA published a guidance document recommending that sprout producers proceed as follows: (1) grow source seed under GAPs, (2) store seeds under conditions that minimize contamination potential, (3) follow GMPs as per 21 C.F.R. part 110, (4) apply an appropriate seed treatment designed to reduce pathogens (such as 20,000 ppm calcium hypochlorite), (5) sample and test sprout irrigation water for *Salmonella* and *E. coli* O157:H7, and (6) develop and implement systems to facilitate trace-back and recall (CFSAN, 1999). Sprouts not produced using the guidance document can be considered adulterated under the Food, Drug, and Cosmetic Act. FDA issued a second document, also in 1999, expanding on some of the decontamination measures recommended in the first guidance document (NACMCF, 1999b).

PESTICIDE RESIDUES

Under the Food Quality Protection Act of 1996, the U.S. Environmental Protection Agency (EPA) must ensure that, before registering a new pesticide, it can be used with a reasonable certainty of no harm to human health and the environment. To determine its safety, more than 100 scientific studies and tests are required from the applicants, from which EPA sets tolerance levels (maximum pesticide residue levels) for residues in the food. The applicant provides information on the chemistry, safety, and tolerance of the new pesticide. In this way, in addition to environmental effects, long- and short-term potential human risks are evaluated. Pesticides are registered for use on specific crops.

Several factors must be addressed before a tolerance can be established, such as the aggregate exposure to the pesticide, the cumulative effects from pesticides with similar effects, increased susceptibilities of certain populations, and endocrine disruptor effects. These data are collected from industry as well as from state and federal monitoring programs. EPA then develops a comprehensive risk assessment (see Chapter 3 for a general description of the chemical risk assessment process) to determine the impact of the affected crops on the safety of the population and the environment. The risk assessment is then carefully reviewed by scientific experts and a decision is made to approve or reject the pesticide. For pesticides that are used in foods, EPA sets a tolerance, and FDA tests domestic and imported produce to verify compliance. Other FDA programs are designed to develop statistically valid information on pesticide residues that is used by EPA in its risk assessments for pesticides in foods.

The committee believes that the process to establish pesticide tolerances in produce is a good approach to ensure public health. The process of setting pesticide tolerances by EPA is in agreement with the committee's belief that food safety standards should be developed based on a combination of the best available science and expert opinion, and that this process should be a transparent one.

FOOD DEFECT ACTION LEVELS

The need to establish some type of defect levels for fruits and vegetables was recognized soon after passage of the 1906 Federal Food and Drug Act (Merrill and Hutt, 1980). Defect Action Levels were established by FDA as maximum levels of natural or unavoidable defects in foods for human use that present no health hazard (CFSAN, 1998). (See Appendix D for Defect Action Levels for selected fruits and vegetables.)

Some foods, even when produced under GMPs, contain natural or unavoidable defects that, at low levels, are not hazardous to health. Even with current technology, it is considered impractical or nearly impossible to produce foods entirely free of natural or unavoidable defects. FDA has established maximum levels for these defects in foods produced under current GMPs and uses these levels to decide whether to recommend regulatory action. The agency makes it clear in 21 C.F.R. part 110, subpart G, that "Defect action levels are established for foods whenever it is necessary and feasible to do so. These levels are subject to change upon the development of new technology or the availability of new information."

Compliance with defect action levels does not excuse violation of the statutory requirement (21 U.S.C. §402(a)(4)) that food not be prepared, packed, or held under unsanitary conditions or the regulatory requirements (21 C.F.R. part

110) that food manufacturers, distributors, and holders shall observe GMPs. Evidence indicating that such a violation exists causes the food to be adulterated, even though the amounts of natural or unavoidable defects are lower than the currently established defect action levels. FDA recommends that food manufacturers, distributors, and holders utilize quality control operations that reduce natural or unavoidable defects to the lowest level currently feasible.

INTERNATIONAL CRITERIA

There are various published international criteria that are applied to produce, as can be seen in Appendix E. However, there are a number of issues that make the value of these criteria difficult to interpret. First, they are applied at different stages, ranging from manufacturing, to retail, to the point of entry of imported produce into a country, or at unspecified points. For example, the point of application of standards for vegetables is either at the end of shelf-life, retail, or not specified, in France, Ireland, and Spain, respectively. Second, the legal status of these criteria—mandatory or guidance—is not specified. It is also unclear whether any of these criteria are being enforced and, if they are, whether they are effective or are being evaluated. In addition, there seem to be no organized efforts to harmonize these standards among nations or within international organizations.

The usefulness and scientific basis of some of these criteria with regard to public health can sometimes be questioned. For example, in Ireland there are criteria for *Vibrio parahaemolyticus* in dried fruits and vegetables and for *Campylobacter* in coleslaw, while Spain has criteria for *L. monocytogenes* in canned raw vegetables. Other examples of questionable produce safety criteria are a 200 cfu/g limit for nonpathogenic *Listeria* spp. in coleslaw, and a limit of 10^6 cfu/g of aerobic bacteria in mixed, prepared salads held at 30°C (see Appendix E).

DO PRODUCE AND JUICE PERFORMANCE STANDARDS IMPROVE PUBLIC HEALTH?

Tools for measuring the impact of food safety criteria on public health include public health surveillance of several types, special studies, and outbreak investigations (see Chapter 2). These activities can help define the burden of disease associated with specific pathogens and food groups, and can also serve to monitor the effectiveness of control programs. Because of the complexity of foodborne diseases, the effectiveness of these criteria is usually inferred, rather than directly demonstrated; nonetheless, basic public health surveillance offers a final check on the progress made in preventing foodborne diseases.

The committee recognizes that a clear example of the success of a performance standard is illustrated by the fact that after the establishment of the low-acid and acidified canned food rules and GMP regulations in the 1970s, only occasional cases of botulism attributable to these foods have occurred. The committee also believes that although the 12-D performance standard for low-acid canned foods might be too stringent in that it might compromise some quality attributes of certain canned foods, and therefore requires scientific reevaluation, the success of these criteria is nevertheless unquestionable.

Regarding the new juice regulations and sprouts guidance, the committee considers that it would be premature to try to evaluate their public health impact, for they were established just a few years ago. However, the fact that no disease outbreaks attributable to *Salmonella* or *E. coli* O157:H7 in juices have been reported to CDC since the juice regulation was implemented is noteworthy. In addition, all sprout outbreaks reported since the publication of the FDA guidelines have been associated with seed that was sanitized using methods other than those described in the guideline.

Likewise, industry guidance documents such as GAPs have recently been published and, therefore, although they are obviously valuable food safety tools, information on their use and possible impact is not yet available. For example, efforts to reduce the potential contamination of lettuce by water in hydrocoolers may have reduced the number of outbreaks. The committee believes that although the number and size of foodborne disease outbreaks associated with specific fresh produce or juice items will, in the future, offer a means of tracking progress in prevention, attributing changes in disease incidence to any specific factor continues to be a challenge because multiple confounding factors and safety measures are being implemented in parallel.

The committee reiterates its belief that, because of the multiple confounding factors, there is a need to develop a framework that allows for the timely sharing of data from surveillance programs on microbial contamination in specific food groups (in this case, fresh and fresh-cut produce and related products such as juices) and from human, animal, and environmental isolates, as well as eventual integration of such data. This framework, in addition to providing information for risk assessments and allocating the burden of disease among specific commodities, could also be used to monitor the progress, over time, of particular microbiological criteria in preventing the presence of hazardous levels of pathogens or toxins in produce (see Chapter 2).

The committee points to the need for a structured review process for guidance documents and regulations, with input from a wide variety of experts from industry, government, and academia, using the NACMCF model. This review process should be used to modify or rescind criteria as science evolves. For issues where the science is rapidly evolving (e.g., fresh produce, sprouts, juice) the review process should take place on a more frequent basis than in areas of relative scientific stability (e.g., thermally processed, low-acid canned foods). In all cases, and to facilitate the review process, the scientific justification for published guidance or regulations should be transparent and readily available, particularly when the data are limited.

The committee is aware that technological innovation based on nonthermal food-processing technologies is critical to the development of new fruit and vegetable products. However, the committee reiterates its recommendation that, prior to developing performance standards that accommodate process or other technical innovations, guidance must be provided to industry on process validation.

REFERENCES

AMS (Agricultural Marketing Service). 2001. *Microbiological Data Program. What is MDP*? Online. U.S. Department of Agriculture (USDA). Available at http://amsdev.ams.usda.gov/science/mpo/what.htm. Accessed September 19, 2002.

Becci PJ, Hess FG, Johnson WD, Gallo MA, Babish JG, Dailey RE, Parent RA. 1981. Long-term carcinogenicity study of patulin in the rat. *J Appl Toxicol* 1:256–261.

Besser RE, Lett SM, Weber JT, Doyle MP, Barrett TJ, Wells JG, Griffin PM. 1993. An outbreak of diarrhea and hemolytic uremic syndrome from *Escherichia coli* O157:H7 in fresh-pressed apple cider. *JAMA* 269:2217–2220.

Beuchat LR. 1998. *Surface Decontamination of Fruits and Vegetables Eaten Raw: A Review*. WHO/FSF/FOS/98.2. Geneva: World Health Organization.

Birkhead GS, Morse DL, Levine WC, Fudala JK, Kondracki SF, Chang HG, Shaydgani M, Novick L, Blake PA. 1993. Typhoid fever at a resort hotel in New York: A large outbreak with an unusual vehicle. *J Infect Dis* 167:1228–1232.

Buchanan RL, Edelson SG, Miller RL, Sapers GM. 1999. Contamination of intact apples after immersion in an aqueous environment containing *Escherichia coli* O157:H7. *J Food Prot* 62:444–450.

Butler ME. 2000. *Salmonella* outbreak leads to juice recall in Western states. *Food Chem News* 42:19.

CAC (Codex Alimentarius Commission). 2000. *Draft Code of Hygienic Practices for Primary Production, Harvesting, and Packaging for Fresh Fruits and Vegetables*. Rome: FAO. Pp.6–7.

California State Board of Health. 1920. Resolutions of the California State Board of Health on the packing of ripe olives in California. *Calif State Board Health Mon Bull* 16:35.

California Strawberry Commission. 1998. *Quality Assurance Program*. Watsonville, CA: California Strawberry Commission.

CAST (Council for Agricultural Science and Technology). 2003. *Mycotoxins: Risks in Plant, Animal and Human Systems*. Task Force Report No. 139. Ames, IA: CAST.

CDC (Centers for Disease Control and Prevention). 1975. *Salmonella typhimurium* outbreak traced to a commercial apple cider—New Jersey. *Morb Mortal Wkly Rep* 24:87–88.

CDC. 1995. *Outbreak of* Salmonella*—Hartford Infections among Travelers to Orlando, Florida*. EPI-AID Trip Rpt. 95–62. Atlanta, GA: CDC.

CDC. 1996. Outbreak of *Escherichia coli* O157:H7 infections associated with drinking unpasteurized commercial apple juice—British Columbia, California, Colorado, and Washington, October 1996. *Morb Mortal Wkly Rep* 45:975.

CDC. 1997. Outbreaks of *Escherichia coli* O157:H7 infection and cryptosporidiosis associated with drinking unpasteurized apple cider—Connecticut and New York, October 1996. *Morb Mortal Wkly Rep* 46:4–8.

CDC. 1998. *Botulism in the United States 1899—Handbook for Epidemiologists, Clinicians and Laboratory Workers*. Atlanta: CDC.

CDC. 1999. Oubreak of *Salmonella* serotype Muenchen infections associated with unpasteurized orange juice—United States and Canada, June 1999. *Morb Mortal Wkly Rep* 48:582–585.

CFSAN. 1998. *The Food Defect Action Levels.* Online. Food and Drug Administration (FDA). Available at http://www.cfsan.fda.gov/~dms/dalbook.html. Accessed August 10, 2002.

CFSAN. 1999. *Guidance to Industry. Reducing Microbial Food Safety Hazards for Sprouted Seeds.* Online. FDA. Available at http://www.cfsan.fda.gov/~dms/sprougd1.html. Accessed January 6, 2003.

CFSAN. 2001. *Survey of Domestic Fresh Produce: Interim Results (July 31, 2001).* Online. FDA. Available at http://www.cfsan.fda.gov/~dms/prodsur9.html. Accessed September 3, 2002.

Cody SH, Glynn K, Farrar JA, Cairns KL, Griffin PM, Kobayashi J, Fyfe M, Hoffman R, King AS, Lewis JH, Swaminathan B, Bryant RG, Vugia DJ. 1999. An outbreak of *Escherichia coli* O157:H7 infection from unpasteurized commercial apple juice. *Ann Intern Med* 130:202–209.

Cook KA, Dobbs TE, Hlady WG, Wells JG, Barrett TJ, Puhr ND, Lancette GA, Bodager DW, Toth WL, Genese CA, Highsmith AK, Pilot KE, Finelli L, Swerdlow DL. 1998. Outbreak of *Salmonella* serotype Hartford infections associated with unpasteurized orange juice. *JAMA* 280:1504–1509.

CSPI (Center for Science in the Public Interest). 2001. *Outbreak Alert: Closing the Gaps in Our Federal Food-Safety Net.* Washington DC: CSPI.

Creel RH. 1912. Vegetables as a possible factor in dissemination of typhoid fever. *Public Health Rep* 27:187–193.

Downing DL. 1996. *A Complete Course in Canning and Related Processes, 13th ed. Book III: Processing Procedures for Canned Food Products.* Baltimore: CTI Publications. P. 170.

Dozier CC. 1924. Optimum and limiting hydrogen-ion concentration for *B. botulinus* and quantitative estimation of its growth. IVI. *J Infect Dis* 35:105.

Duncan TG, Coull JA, Miller ER, Bancroft H. 1946. Outbreak of typhoid fever with orange juice as the vehicle illustrating the value of immunization. *Am J Public Health* 36:34–36.

Eisenstein AB, Aach RD, Jacobson W, Goldman A. 1963. An epidemic of infectious hepatitis in a general hospital. *JAMA* 185:171–174.

ERS (Economic Research Service). 2002. *Briefing Room. Vegetables and Melons: Trade.* Online. USDA. Available at http//www.ers.usda.gov/briefing/vegetables/trade.htm. Accessed September 19, 2002.

Esty JR, Meyer KF. 1922. The heat resistance of the spores of *B. botulinus* and allied anaerobes. XI. *J Infect Dis* 31:650–663.

FDA (Food and Drug Administration). 1998. Food labeling: Warning and notice statement: Labeling of juice products; final rule. *Fed Regist* 63:37029–37056.

FDA. 2001. Hazard analysis and critical control point (HACCP); Procedure for the safe and sanitary processing and importing of juice. Final rule. *Fed Regist* 66: 6137–6202.

FDA/USDA/CDC (U.S. Department of Agriculture/Centers for Disease Control and Prevention). 1998. *Guidance for Industry Guide to Minimize Microbial Food Safety Hazards for Fresh Fruits and Vegetables.* Online. Available at http://www.foodsafety.gov/~dms/prodguid.html. Accessed August 10, 2002.

FPI (Food Processors Institute). 2003. *Food Processors Institute Program Agenda.* Online. Available at http://www.fpi-food.org/courseschedule.cfm. Accessed January 6, 2003.

Garthright WE, Chirtel S, Graves Q. 2000. *Derivation of Sampling Plan to Meet the Testing Requirement in the Juice HACCP Final Rule for Citrus Juices that Rely Solely or in Part on Surface Treatments to Achieve the 5-Log Reduction Standard.* Washington, DC: Office of Plant and Dairy Food and Beverages, CFSAN, FDA.

Gavin EA, Weddig LM. 1995. *Canned Foods: Principles of Thermal Process Control, Acidification and Container Closure Evaluation*, 6th ed. Washington, DC: Food Processors Institute. Pp. 1–6.

Geiger JC, Dickson EC, Meyer KF. 1922. *The Epidemiology of Botulism.* Treasury Department, U.S. Public Health Service, Public Health Bulletin No. 127. Washington, DC: U.S. Government Printing Office.

Gilbertson WE. 1964. Opening remarks. In: Lewis KH, Cassell K, eds. *Botulism. Proceedings of a Symposium*. PHS Pub. No. 999-FP-1. Washington, DC: U.S. Government Printing Office.

IFPA (International Fresh-cut Produce Association). 1997. *Voluntary Food Safety Guidelines for Fresh Produce*. Alexandria, VA: IFPA.

IFPA. 2001. *Food Safety Guidelines for the Fresh-cut Produce Industry*, 4th ed. Alexandria, VA: IFPA.

IFT (Institute of Food Technologists). 2001. *Analysis and Evaluation of Preventive Control Measures for the Control and Reduction/Elimination of Microbial Hazards on Fresh and Fresh-cut Produce*. Chicago: IFT.

JECFA (Joint FAO/WHO Expert Committee on Food Additives). 1996. *Toxicological Evaluation of Certain Food Additives and Contaminants*. WHO Food Additives Series 35. Geneva: World Health Organization.

Jerardo A. 2002. *The Import Share of U.S.-Consumed Food Continues to Rise. Outlook Report.* Online. ERS, USDA. Available at http://www.ers.usda.gov/publications/fau/july02/fau6601/fau6601.pdf. Accessed September 19, 2002.

Kaufman PR, Handy CR, McLaughlin EW, Park K, Green GM. 2000. *Understanding the Dynamics of Produce Markets: Consumption and Consolidation Grow*. Online. ERS, USDA. Available at http://www.usda.gov/publications/ai6758/aib758.pdf. Accessed December 23, 2003.

Kim J, Foegeding PM. 1992. Principles of control. In: Hauschild AHW, Dodds KL, eds. Clostridium botulinum *Ecology and Control in Foods*. New York: Marcel Dekker. Pp. 121–176.

Litwak D. 1998. Is bigger better? *Supermarket Bus* 53:79–88.

Lovett J, Thompson RG, Boutin BK. 1975. Trimming as a means of removing patulin from fungus-rotted apples. *J Assoc Off Anal Chem* 58:909–911.

Lund BM. 1992. Ecosystems in vegetable foods. *J Appl Bacteriol Symp* 73:115S–126S.

McKinley ER, Carlton WW. 1991. Patulin. In: Sharma E, Salunkhe DK, eds. *Mycotoxins and Phytoalexins*. Atlanta: CRC Press.

Melnick CO. 1917. The possibility of typhoid infection through vegetables. *J Infect Dis* 21:28–38.

Merrill RA, Hutt PB. 1980. *Food and Drug Law*. Mineola, NY: The Foundation Press. P. 17.

Millard PS, Gensheimer KF, Addiss DG, Sosin DM, Beckett GA, Houck-Jankoski A, Hudson A. 1994. An outbreak of cryptosporidiosis from fresh-pressed apple cider. *JAMA* 272:1592–1596.

Morse FL. 1899. Health of towns. *Rep Bd Health Mass* 34:761.

NACMCF (National Advisory Committee on Microbiological Criteria for Foods). 1999a. Microbiological safety evaluations and recommendations on fresh produce. *Food Control* 10:117–143.

NACMCF. 1999b. *Microbiological Safety Evaluations and Recommendations on Sprouted Seeds*. Online. FDA. Available at http://www.cfsan.fda.gov/~mow/sprouts2.html. Accessed January 6, 2003.

NRC. 1985. *An Evaluation of the Role of Microbiological Criteria for Foods and Food Ingredients*. Washington, DC: National Academy Press.

Odlaug TE, Pflug IJ. 1978. *Clostridium botulinum* and acid foods. *J Food Prot* 41:566–573.

Office of Regulatory Affairs. 2002. *Compliance Policy Guidance for FDA Staff. Apple Juice, Apple Juice Concentrates, and Apple Juice Products—Adulteration with Patulin*. Online. FDA. Available at http://www.fda.gov/ora/compliance_ref/cpg/cpgfod/cpg510.150.htm. Accessed January 21, 2003.

OPDFB (Office of Plant and Dairy Foods and Beverages). 2000. *Patulin in Apple Juice, Apple Juice Concentrates and Apple Juice Products. (Draft) Guidance for FDA Components and Industry*. Online. CFSAN, FDA. Available at http://www.cfsan.fda.gov/~dms/patubckg2.html. Accessed December 22, 2002.

OPDFB. 2001. *FDA Survey of Imported Fresh Produce. FY 1999 Field Assignment.* Online. CFSAN, FDA. Available at http://www.cfsan.fda.gov/~dms/prodsur6.html. Accessed December 22, 2002.

OPDFB. 2002a. *Guidance for Industry. Juice HACCP Hazards and Controls Guidance. First Edition. Draft Guidance.* Online. CFSAN, FDA. Available at http://www.cfsan.fda.gov/~dms/juicgui3.html. Accessed February 13, 2003.

OPDFB. 2002b. *Guidance for Industry. Standardized Training Curriculum for Application of HACCP Principles to Juice Processing. Draft Guidance.* Online. CFSAN, FDA. Available at http://www.cfsan.fda.gov/~dms/juicgui5.html. Accessed February 13, 2003.

Paretti A. 1972. The Bon Vivant story. Statement by Andrew Paretti, President, Bon Vivant Soups, Inc. Filed with the Subcommittee on Public Health and Environment of the House Committee on Interstate and Foreign Commerce. *Food Prod Manage* 95:46–54, 56.

Parish ME. 1998. Coliforms, *Escherichia coli* and *Salmonella* serovars associated with a citrus-processing facility implicated in a salmonellosis outbreak. *J Food Prot* 61:280–284.

Peleg M, Cole MB. 1998. Reinterpretation of microbial survival curves. *Crit Rev Food Sci Nutr* 38:353–380.

Perkins WE. 1964. Prevention of botulism by thermal processing. In: Lewis KH, Cassel K, eds. *Botulism. Proceedings of a Symposium.* Cincinnatti, OH: U.S. Department of Health, Education, and Welfare.

Pflug IJ, Odlaug TE. 1978. A review of *z* and *F* values used to ensure the safety of low-acid canned food. *Food Technol* 32:63–70.

Pixley C. 1913. Typhoid fever from uncooked vegetables. *NY Med J* 98:328.

Rangarajan A, Bihn EA, Gravani RB, Scott DL, Pritts MP. 1999. *Food Safety Begins on the Farm: A Growers Guide. Good Agricultural Practices for Fresh Fruits and Vegetables.* Ithaca, NY: Cornell University.

Robbs PG, Bartz JA, Sargent SA, McFie G, Hodge NC. 1996. Potential inoculum sources for decay of fresh cut celery. *J Food Sci* 61:449–452, 455.

Rushing JW, Angulo FJ, Beuchat LR. 1996. Implementation of a HACCP program in a commercial fresh-market tomato packinghouse: A model for the industry. *Dairy Food Environ Sanit* 16:549–553.

Samish Z, Etinger-Tulczynska R. 1963. Distribution of bacteria within the tissue of healthy tomatoes. *Appl Microbiol* 11:7–10.

Schmidt CF. 1964. Spores of *C. botulinum*: Formation, resistance, germination. In: Lewis KH, Cassel K, eds. *Botulism. Proceedings of a Symposium.* Cincinnatti, OH: U.S. Department of Health, Education, and Welfare.

Solomon EB, Yaron S, Matthews KR. 2002. Transmission of *Escherichia coli* O157:H7 from contaminated manure and irrigation water to lettuce plant tissue and its subsequent internalization. *Appl Environ Microbiol* 68:397–400.

Stoloff L. 1975. Patulin, a contaminant of apple juice. *NY State Ag Exp Sta Spec Rep* 19:51–54.

Stumbo CR. 1973. *Thermobacteriology in Food Processing*, 2nd ed. San Diego: Academic Press. Pp. 131–132.

Stumbo CR, Murphy JR, Cochran J. 1950. Nature of thermal death time curves for P.A. 3679 and *Clostridium botulinum. Food Technol* 4: 321–326.

Stumbo CR, Purohit KS, Ramakrishnan TV. 1975. Thermal process lethality guide for low-acid foods in metal containers. *J Food Sci* 40:1316–1323.

Tabershaw IR, Schmelzer LL, Bruhn HB. 1967. Gastroenteritis from an orange juice preparation. *Arch Environ Health* 15:72–77.

Tanaka N. 1982. Toxin production by *Clostridium botulinum* in media at pH lower than 4.6. *J Food Prot* 45: 234–237.

Townsend CT, Esty JR, Baselt FC. 1938. Heat resistance studies on spores of putrefactive anaerobes in relation to determination of safe processes for canned foods. *Food Res* 3:323–346.

Townsend CT, Yee L, Mercer WA. 1954. Inhibition of the growth of *Clostridium botulinum* by acidification. *Food Res* 19:536.

van Boekel MAJS. 2002. On the use of the Weibull model to describe thermal inactivation of microbial vegetative cells. *Int J Food Microbiol* 74:139–159.

Warry JK. 1903. Enteric fever spread by watercress. *Lancet* 12:1671.

Young JH. 1976. Botulism and the ripe olive scare of 1919–1920. *Bull Hist Med* 50: 372–391.

Young-Perkins KE, Merson LR. 1987. *Clostridium botulinum* spore germination, outgrowth and toxin production below 4.6: Interactions between pH, total acidity and buffering capacity. *J Food Sci* 52:1084.

Zhuang R-Y, Beuchat LR, Angulo FJ. 1995. Fate of *Salmonella montevideo* on and in raw tomatoes as affected by temperature and treatment of chlorine. *Appl Environ Microbiol* 61:2127–2131.

7

Scientific Criteria and Performance Standards to Control Hazards in Dairy Products

High morbidity and mortality rates associated with diseases such as typhoid fever and infantile diarrhea, which may be contracted through consumption of microbiologically contaminated foods, led to initiation of food- and water-borne disease reporting in the United States more than 75 years ago (Olsen et al., 2000). Anecdotal observations that linked consumption of milk with the spread of disease spurred various scientists and physicians in the United States and around the world to undertake public health research to investigate the role of milk consumption in foodborne disease as early as the turn of the twentieth century. As a result of these investigations, consumption of unpasteurized milk was found to be associated with many serious diseases, including diphtheria, typhoid, tuberculosis, and brucellosis (Johnson et al., 1990).

The first reports of gastrointestinal disease outbreaks attributed to milk consumption were published by the Public Health Service (PHS) in 1925. These early reports provided evidence suggesting that to control milk-borne diseases, sanitation measures would need to be applied at all points in the food system, from the farm to the consumer (CFSAN, 2002). Further, these observations highlighted the need for technical research that would determine the bacterial destruction characteristics of food-processing treatments for pathogenic microbes likely to be present in raw milk (Enright et al., 1957; Gilman et al., 1946). The results of these studies led to the development of specific recommendations for pasteurization and other intervention strategies (described below) that were designed to protect the public from exposure to hazardous microorganisms that may be present in raw milk. In the case of cheese, however, investigations were initiated not because of the association between illness and cheeses made from unpasteurized

TABLE 7.1 Equivalent Temperature and Time Combinations for Milk Pasteurization According to U.S. Regulations

Temperature	Time	Temperature	Time
63°C (145°F)[a]	30 min	94°C (201°F)	0.1 sec
72°C (161°F)[a]	15 sec	96°C (204°F)	0.05 sec
89°C (191°F)	1.0 sec	100°C (212°F)	0.01 sec
90°C (194°F)	0.5 sec		

[a] If the fat content of the milk is 10% or more, or if it contains added sweeteners, the required minimum temperature must be increased by at least 3°C (5°F).
SOURCE: CFSAN (2002).

milk, but to assess the survival of *Brucella abortus* in the product (Gilman et al., 1946). In the past few decades, foodborne disease outbreaks have been linked to various cheeses and, therefore, the need to evaluate the survival of human pathogens during cheese manufacturing and aging has been revisited. In light of data indicating that certain pathogens (*Listeria monocytogenes* and *Escherichia coli* O157:H7) may survive the 60-day aging period in cheese, research is currently being conducted to determine if this process criterion is adequate to protect public health.

For the purpose of this report, "raw milk" is defined as milk, harvested from an animal, that may have been cooled to refrigeration temperatures or below, but that has not been subjected to processing with the objective of eliminating pathogenic bacteria that may be present. "Unpasteurized milk" is milk that may have been cooled or heated, but that has not been subjected to the minimal pasteurization processing conditions described in Table 7.1. While these terms are typically used interchangeably, unpasteurized milk is a broader term than raw milk as, for example, milk that can be processed into some types of cheeses may be subjected to heat treatments below minimum pasteurization conditions. Milk treated in this manner would be considered unpasteurized but not raw. (For a full discussion of the use of unpasteurized milk in dairy-product manufacturing, see later section, "Cheese and Other Dairy Food Products.")

MILK

Current Criteria and Standards

PHS implemented the Standard Milk Ordinance in 1924 to assist states and cities in the voluntary adoption of programs designed to control milk-borne disease. In 1950, the U.S. Surgeon General invited state milk-sanitation regulatory agencies to establish procedures for a voluntary Interstate Milk Shipper Certification Program, which resulted in the formation of the National Conference on Interstate Milk Shipments (NCIMS) and the Cooperative State-Public Health Service Program for the certification of interstate milk shippers (CFSAN, 2000). Responsibilities under this program were divided between state agencies and PHS. In 1969, the PHS responsibilities were transferred to the Food and Drug Administration (FDA). Currently, all states, the District of Columbia, and the United States trust territories participate in NCIMS.

PHS, and later FDA, recommended the application of the current Grade A Pasteurized Milk Ordinance, commonly referred to as the PMO (CFSAN, 2002), to provide national uniformity for milk sanitation standards. Milk products covered by the PMO include products such as creams, concentrated milks, yogurts, and low-fat and skim milks (CFSAN, 2002). FDA's Division of Dairy and Egg Safety, Office of Plant and Dairy Foods and Beverages, is responsible for the development of additional regulations to protect the safety of cheese and other dairy foods (infant formula, dried milk products, ice cream or other frozen desserts, butter, and cheese) that enter interstate commerce, but that are not specifically covered by the PMO.

The PMO covers production, transportation, processing, handling, sampling, examination, labeling, and sale of milk and milk products; the inspection of dairy farms and milk plants; the issuing and revocation of permits to milk producers, haulers, and distributors; and the fixing of penalties (CFSAN, 2002). The PMO is considered the reference for federal specifications for the procurement of milk and dairy products and as the sanitary regulation for dairy products served during interstate travel. It is also recognized by public health agencies and the dairy industry as the national standard for milk sanitation. As knowledge and experience is gained, modifications to the PMO are recommended during biennial NCIMS meetings, which then must be approved by FDA before incorporation into the PMO. Since 1924, the PMO has evolved with input from many sources, including federal, state, and local government health and agriculture departments, the dairy industry (from producers to associations), academic organizations, and individuals. Hence, the PMO is derived from broad-based consensus of current knowledge and experience with milk sanitation standards in the United States.

The implementation and enforcement of the PMO is another key element to protect the public from milk-borne illness. In this regard, FDA has no legal jurisdiction to enforce milk sanitation standards, except for interstate carriers and for products in interstate commerce.

In general, although state and local agencies bear the majority of enforcement responsibilities for dairy regulatory programs, they still commonly use the PMO as the basis for developing their programs. Since 1924, government, academia, and industry have worked together to address targeted research needs as new pathogens have been identified and to modify regulations when science-based research has revealed appropriate measures for destruction and control of microbiological hazards.

The development, implementation, and enforcement of the PMO provide a good model for an integrated "cow-to-cup" strategy for product safety assurance. In addition, this model also provides a specific structure and mechanism for biennial review of existing regulations directed toward the fluid milk industry.

Although FDA has the authority to enforce the implementation of the PMO standards in milk for interstate commerce, milk for local consumption is not subject to FDA oversight. Therefore, consumption of unpasteurized or raw milk continues to be an issue of concern, since it has been clearly established as a high-risk behavior for contracting foodborne illness.

The committee concludes that targeted educational programs that illustrate the hazards of raw milk and raw milk-product consumption for milk producers and for the general public are warranted.

The Public Health Objective of Fluid Milk Processing

The public health objective for milk pasteurization, as defined in the PMO, is to eliminate all nonspore-forming pathogens commonly associated with milk; nevertheless, the guidance document cautions that pasteurization may not destroy preformed toxins (CFSAN, 2002).

According to the PMO, an analysis of milk-borne outbreak data over the years indicates that the risk of contracting disease is about 50 times less when consuming pasteurized versus unpasteurized milk. Pasteurization, as first adopted in the United States, was defined in the 1939 Milk Ordinance and Code as "the process of heating every particle of milk to at least 143°F (61.7°C) and holding at such temperature for at least 30 minutes, or to at least 160°F (71.1°C) and holding at such temperature for at least 15 seconds, in approved and properly operated equipment" (PHS, 1940). These heat treatments were referred to as the "holding method" or vat/batch pasteurization, and the "flash method" or high-temperature, short-time pasteurization, respectively. Table 7.1 contains these and other equivalent temperature/time combinations allowed by U.S. regulations.

To address recognized scientific gaps regarding knowledge of the microbes associated with milk-borne disease, extensive research was conducted to determine the heat treatment required to kill *Mycobacterium tuberculosis* which, at the time, was considered to be the most heat-resistant pathogen associated with milk (Hammer, 1948). This work led to the widespread recognition of the public health significance of thermal milk processing and formed the basis for modern pasteurization processes (Hammer, 1948). In 1956, minimal pasteurization temperatures were slightly increased to those listed in Table 7.1 to assure destruction of *Coxiella burnetti*, the organism associated with Q fever, which was found to be more heat resistant than *M. tuberculosis* (Enright et al., 1957).

As described above, the PMO prescribes highly specific pasteurization conditions (i.e., time and temperature combinations), equivalent to process standards, to ensure the safety of dairy products.

The Scientific Basis for Current Pasteurization Requirements

The observation of a significant number of cases of Q fever attributed to the consumption of raw milk in the United States in the 1940s and 1950s inspired targeted research to precisely define conditions required for thermal destruction of *C. burnetii* (Enright et al., 1957). Q fever, which was first described in the mid-1930s, is a rickettsial disease characterized by chills, fever, weakness, and headache, with endocarditis as a possible complication in immunocompromised patients. *C. burnetti* is an obligate intracellular parasite that cannot multiply outside of living host cells; therefore, it cannot be cultured in laboratory media. While new detection strategies (e.g., polymerase chain reaction-based methods) are under development, current diagnostic strategies for Q fever are still based on the measurement of antibody titers for *C. burnetti* in blood samples taken from patients. High numbers of *C. burnetti*-specific antibodies in a patient's blood are considered to be indicative of exposure to this organism.

Experiments to ascertain the thermal destruction of *C. burnetti* are technically challenging because the presence of this organism in a heat-treated milk sample can only be measured indirectly by assessing the presence and concentration of antibodies in a host animal that has been inoculated with a sample of the milk. Current milk processing strategies, which are designed to destroy *C. burnetti* in raw milk, are the outcome of a collaborative project between PHS and the University of California in the mid-1950s. The objectives of this study were to determine the maximum number of *C. burnetti* that might be found in the milk of an infected cow, to develop a sensitive method for determining the presence of small numbers of *C. burnetti* in pasteurized milk, and to ascertain the thermal resistance of *C. burnetti* in whole raw milk to ensure the absence of viable organisms in processed milk products (Enright et al., 1957). The guinea pig was the host animal selected for monitoring residual levels of *C. burnetti* in heat-treated milk samples. Numbers of *C. burnetti* present in the milk were referred to as "infective guinea pig doses" because they were assessed through a determination of the highest tenfold milk dilution that caused an intraperitoneally inoculated guinea pig to have a significant rise (at least fourfold) in antibody titer to *C. burnetti* (Enright et al., 1957). The highest level of *C. burnetti* in milk of infected cows from samples collected around the state of California was determined to be 10,000 infective guinea pig doses. Therefore, to provide an additional margin of safety, the authors selected thermal destruction of 100,000 infective guinea pig doses as the goal for minimal pasteurization conditions (Enright et al., 1957). For the purpose of contrasting this thermal processing goal with other microbial destruction strategies described in this report, destruction of 100,000 infective guinea pig doses would be equivalent to a 5-D reduction in infective capacity for a given volume of milk. The pasteurization conditions described in Table 7.1 were found to result in destruction of 100,000 infective guinea pig doses of *C. burnetti*. Therefore, on July 16, 1956, the U.S. Assistant Surgeon

General released a recommendation for a minimum raw milk heat treatment of 145°F for 30 min or 161°F for 15 sec to ensure protection of the public from exposure to *C. burnetti* through consumption of milk. While the results reported by Enright and colleagues (1957) still serve as the scientific basis for current milk pasteurization practices, many processors apply time and temperature combinations that are above the minimum conditions (Douglas et al., 2000).

As discussed in Chapter 3 and mentioned in Chapters 4 and 5, the committee reiterates its belief that the implementation of performance standards that specify the reduction in numbers required for a targeted organism (e.g., a 5-D reduction for infective guinea pig doses for *C. burnetti*) in a food product (milk in this case), rather than specifying the precise conditions (i.e., process standards) for achieving that end, as currently practiced, could enable greater flexibility and innovation in the dairy industry, perhaps enabling the adoption of effective new processing technologies.

Emerging Food Safety Concerns That May Justify a Reexamination of Current Milk Pasteurization Conditions

As mentioned previously, currently applied thermal processing conditions for Grade A raw milk are designed to destroy the most heat-resistant of currently recognized nonspore-forming human pathogens, namely *C. burnetti*. However, some microbes that may be present in raw milk can survive pasteurization (Hammer et al., 1995). Spore-forming bacteria, including those of the *Bacillus* and *Clostridium* genera, are among the heat resistant organisms that can be isolated from pasteurized milk. While the public health risk associated with the presence of these organisms in processed milk products is considered insignificant under the current PMO, it is very important to recognize the fact that the pasteurization process is not intended to sterilize raw milk.

In addition to incomplete destruction of spore-forming bacteria, the efficacy of milk pasteurization in killing *M. avium* subspp. *paratuberculosis*, a bacterium that causes Johne's disease in cattle—but that has not been proven to cause human disease—is uncertain (Klijn et al., 2001; Mechor, 1997). Furthermore, although no evidence exists linking development of encephalopathy to consumption of milk from cows infected with bovine spongiform encephalopathy (commonly referred to as mad cow disease), current pasteurization conditions do not inactivate the causative prion. This prion, an infectious protein, shows little loss of infectivity even after prolonged exposure to temperatures up to 176°F (80°C) (Asher et al., 1986). Although mice injected with milk from bovine spongiform encephalopathy-infected cattle did not develop the disease nor have epidemiological analyses suggested transmission of the disease to calves via milk (Hillerton, 1997), the possibility of such a transmission route should not be totally ruled out.

A more recently emerging food pathogen is *Enterobacter sakazakii.* On April 12, 2002, FDA alerted health care professionals about this pathogen, which has been associated with consumption of milk-based infant formulas. *E. sakazakii* can cause sepsis, meningitis, or necrotizing enterocolitis in newborn infants, particularly in premature or immunodeficient infants. Investigations of multiple outbreaks of *E. sakazakii* infection occurring in neonatal intensive care units worldwide over the past several years have associated illnesses with milk-based powdered infant formulas. To date, FDA is not aware of *E. sakazakii* infections among healthy, full-term infants in home settings, nor have illnesses been associated with liquid infant formulas (FDA, 2002). The emergence of new or newly recognized human pathogens that may be transmitted through milk or through consumption of other animal products highlights the need for food safety regulations that can be changed in a timely and responsive fashion as new hazards are identified and characterized.

Other Fluid Milk Standards

Although adequate refrigeration, aseptic processing, and a specified sub-pasteurization heat treatment to separate cream prior to bulk shipment of milk are processes included in the PMO, only pasteurization and ultrapasteurization (defined in Table 7.2) are recognized by the PMO as acceptable processes for removing or deactivating microorganisms in milk (CFSAN, 2002).

In addition to specific recommendations for pasteurization conditions, chemical, bacteriological, and temperature standards have been established for grade A raw milk products intended for pasteurization, as well as for grade A pasteurized and bulk-shipped, heat-treated milk products (CFSAN, 2002). For these products, milk must be cooled to 7°C or less within two hours after milking. Further, the

TABLE 7.2 Minimum Temperature and Times for Fluid Milk Heat Treatments

Country	High-Temperature, Short-Time Pasteurization	Ultrapasteurization	Ultrahigh-Temperature Processing
United States[a]	72°C/15 sec	138°C/2 sec	Not defined[d]
European Economic Community[b]	71.7°C/15 sec	Not defined	135°C/1 sec
Australia/New Zealand[c]	72°C/15 sec	132°C/1 sec	132°C/1 sec

[a] CFSAN (2002).
[b] EEC (1994).
[c] ANZFA (2000).
[d] 21 C.F.R. part 113: "The thermal process and procedures for manufacturing UHT aseptically processed milk and milk products must comply with U.S. Food and Drug Administration requirements for sterilizing low acid foods."

blend temperature after the first and subsequent milkings cannot exceed 10°C. Pasteurized products must not exceed 7°C throughout distribution. Raw milk and pasteurized products cannot test positive for drug residues as specified in section 6 of the PMO (CFSAN, 2002), a chemical performance standard related to good on-farm practices. Residual phosphatase activity may be measured in pasteurized products to reflect pasteurization efficacy. Pasteurized products must have less than 350 munits/L phosphatase activity for fluid products and less than 500 munits/L for other milk products. Table 7.2 provides current standards from the United States, the European Economic Community (now the European Union), and Australia and New Zealand for minimum heat treatments for milk products. Table 7.3 provides microbial and somatic cells limits for raw milk intended for pasteurized products, and Table 7.4 provides microbial standards for pasteurized fluid milk products.

Somatic cell count limits for raw milk intended for pasteurized products are arguably a safety standard, as exceeding these limits may prevent effective application of a pasteurizing process. Similarly, the microbial standards for pasteurized fluid milk products (total bacteria and coliform bacteria) were not implemented on the basis of food safety per se; instead, the rationale behind these standards is that keeping total bacteria and coliform cell numbers within the specified limits reflects good management practices such as equipment cleanliness and sanitation or refrigeration control, which are essential elements of a food safety program.

TABLE 7.3 Microbial and Somatic Cell Count (SCC) Standards for Raw Milk Intended for Pasteurized Milk Products

Country	Producer Raw Milk[a]	Plant Raw Milk[b]
United States[c]	100,000 cfu/mL[d] 750,000 SCC[e]	300,000 cfu/mL
Canada[f]	50,000 cfu/mL 500,000 SCC	50,000 cfu/mL
European Economic Community[g]	100,000 cfu/mL 400,000 SCC	300,000 cfu/mL
Australia/New Zealand[h]	150,000 cfu/mL	150,000 cfu/mL

[a] Unpasteurized milk before it has left the holding tank on the farm.
[b] Unpasteurized milk after it has left the farm holding tank.
[c] CFSAN (2002).
[d] cfu/mL were measured by aerobic plate count.
[e] SCC must not exceed 1,000,000 in goat milk.
[f] CFIS (1997).
[g] EEC (1994).
[h] ANZFA (2000).

TABLE 7.4 Microbial Standards (per mL) for Pasteurized Milk Products

Country	Total Bacteria[a]	Coliform Bacteria[a]
United States[b]	20,000[c]	10, except in heat-treated, bulk milk transport tank shipments, which may not exceed 100
Canada[d]	m = 10,000	m = 1
	M = 25,000	M = 10
	n = 5	n = 5
	c = 2	c = 2
European Economic Community (EEC)[e]	After 5 d at 6°C	
	m = 50,000	m = 0
	M = 500,000	M = 5
	n = 5	n = 5
	c = 1	c = 1
Australia/New Zealand[f]	m = 50,000	m = 1
	M = 100,000	M = 10
	n = 5	n = 5
	c = 1	c = 1

[a] Total bacteria (as measured by aerobic plate count) and coliform bacteria counts given as the upper limit of cfu/mL for the United States. For Canada, EEC, and Australia/New Zealand, two-tiered limits are given, with allowable results based on n number of samples, where n = number of sample units (subsamples) to be examined per lot, m = maximum number of bacteria per g or mL of product that is of no concern (acceptable level of contamination), M = maximum number of bacteria per g or mL of product, that if exceeded by any one sample unit (subsamples) renders the lot in violation of the regulations, c = maximum number of sample units (subsamples) per lot that may have a bacterial concentration higher than the value for m but less than value for M without violation of the regulations.

[b] PHS (1999).

[c] Not applicable in cultured dairy products.

[d] CFIS (1997).

[e] EEC (1994).

[f] ANZFA (2000).

CHEESE AND OTHER DAIRY FOOD PRODUCTS

As with milk, FDA's Division of Dairy and Egg Safety, Office of Plant and Dairy Foods and Beverages is also responsible for the development and implementation of regulations to protect the safety of cheese and other dairy foods that enter interstate commerce. According to 21 C.F.R. §1240.61, no milk or milk products in final package form intended for direct human consumption shall enter interstate commerce unless they are manufactured from pasteurized milk or pasteurized milk ingredients, *except* where alternative procedures are provided for by regulation, such as in 21 C.F.R. part 133, which contains regulations for cheeses and related cheese products.

Standards of identity have been established for most natural cheeses, process cheeses, cheese foods, and cheese spreads (21 C.F.R. part 133). All cheeses belonging to a given variety must comply with the published standard and must be labeled with the name prescribed in the standard. In general, identity standards specify a maximum permissible moisture content and minimum milk fat content. A few natural cheeses are required to be made from pasteurized milk (e.g., Monterey Jack, cream cheese, mozzarella cheese); however, most, including many soft ripened cheeses (21 C.F.R. §133.182) and semi-soft cheeses (21 C.F.R. §133.187), may be made from either raw or pasteurized milk. The regulation states that "if cheese is labeled as 'heat treated,' 'unpasteurized,' 'raw milk,' or 'for manufacturing,' the milk may be raw or heated at temperatures below pasteurization. Cheese made from unpasteurized milk shall be cured for a period of 60 days at a temperature not less than 35°F. If the milk is held more than 2 hours between time of receipt or heat treatment and setting, it shall be cooled to 45°F or lower until time of setting" (7 C.F.R. §58.439). Standards of identity may stipulate a holding period longer than 60 days if further aging is required to develop the characteristics of the cheese variety.

The Scientific Basis for the 60-Day Aging Period for Cheeses Made with Unpasteurized Milk

Origins

Although not explicitly stated in the regulations, the 60-day holding period recommendation is intended to provide a measure of pathogen reduction in cheeses manufactured from milk that has not been pasteurized. This recommendation, which was first published in 1950 (15 C.F.R. §5653), was established by expert testimony provided during hearings that were conducted during the development of the current cheese standards of identity (Personal communication, J. Mowbray, FDA, September 25, 2002).

The scientific underpinnings of this recommendation are obscure, but appear to be derived at least partially from a study that investigated survival of *B. abortus* in Cheddar cheese (Gilman et al., 1946). This study reported that *B. abortus* survived for up to 6 months in cheeses that had been artificially inoculated at levels of approximately 1,000 cfu/mL and held at 4.4°C. Bacterial survival was monitored directly by culturing viable *B. abortus*, and indirectly by guinea pig infection. In these initial experiments, 6-month-old cheeses were reported as positive for *B. abortus*, but no numbers were given; guinea pig lesions were described as slight. When these cheeses had been held for 1 year, inoculated guinea pigs showed no sign of *B. abortus* infection (i.e., no blood agglutination reactions, no characteristic lesions, and no *B. abortus* recovery from the spleen). No *B. abortus* was recovered from commercial Limburger cheeses that had been held for 57 days (no temperature or other conditions were described), despite the fact that the milk used to manufacture two of the cheeses had tested positive for both viable *B. abortus* (no numbers given) and for guinea pig infection. Cheddar cheese made from milk that was naturally contaminated at levels of 700 to 800 cfu/mL was positive for culturable *B. abortus* (no numbers given) for 3 months. Viable *B. abortus* were recovered from some, but not all, of these test cheeses after 6 months; after 1 year, all guinea pigs were negative for signs of *B. abortus* infection. Cheeses made from milk collected from herds positive for *B. abortus* (no numbers given for initial levels of *B. abortus* in cheese milk) were negative (apparently for the presence of viable *B. abortus*, but the authors did not distinguish between this possibility or whether these negative results reflected guinea pig inoculation experiments) after storage for at least 41 days at temperatures ranging from 1.1°C to 2.7°C. Unfortunately, many of the cheeses that were intended for examination in this part of the study were not tested for the presence of *B. abortus*, as samples were lost. Further, initial cheese storage period lengths were not standardized, but rather ranged from 41 to 84 days, making it very difficult to compare results among the cheeses. As part of the manuscript discussion, the authors claimed that Cheddar cheese had not been proven as a vector for human brucellosis (undulant fever), and that typhoid fever epidemics had not been attributed to cheeses cured for more than 63 days. Therefore, despite their own laboratory results, they believed that the epidemiological evidence suggesting a lack of association between cheese consumption and disease provided strong support for an aging period of approximately 2 months for commercial cheeses. The final stated conclusion was that "an aging period of 60 days is reasonable assurance against the presence of viable *B. abortus* organisms in Cheddar cheese" (Gilman et al., 1946).

Emerging Food Safety Concerns

Recent evidence of the ability of bacterial pathogens to survive throughout a 60-day holding period has arisen from investigations of outbreaks of foodborne illnesses that have been traced back to aged cheeses, as well as from additional scientific research. Specifically, three outbreaks of salmonellosis following consumption of Cheddar cheese, two in Canada and one in the United States, suggest that various *Salmonella* strains can survive for extended periods in cheese products, as described below.

In the first outbreak, which was traced to Cheddar cheese manufactured in Kansas in 1976, raw milk had been held without refrigeration in the processing plant for 1 to 3 days prior to pasteurization and cheese manufacture. While it is not known for certain, total bacterial numbers in the prepasteurized, raw milk could have exceeded the thermal destruction capacity of the pasteurizing process. Microbiological analyses revealed the presence of *Salmonella* Heidelberg at very low levels (0.36–1.8 cfu/100 g of cheese) in the aged cheeses. The average pH of cheese batches bearing *Salmonella* was 5.6 vs. 5.4 for uncontaminated product;

thus, it is possible that slow acid production by starter cultures could have contributed to *Salmonella* survival. This outbreak resulted from numerous lapses in good manufacturing practices, and cannot be attributed solely to inadequacy of a 60-day holding period for pathogen reduction (Johnson et al., 1990). The second incident was comprised of a series of *Salmonella* outbreaks that occurred in Ontario, Canada, from 1980 to 1982. In these cases, *Salmonella* Muenster was isolated from raw-milk Cheddar cheese even after 125 days of curing at 41°F. In the third outbreak, which affected over 2,700 people in Canada in 1984, *S.* Typhimurium was isolated at very low levels from Cheddar cheese (0.39–9.3 cfu/100 g of cheese) that may have been prepared from a mix of raw and pasteurized milk. *S.* Typhimurium was found to persist in this cheese for 8 months at 41°F (Johnson et al., 1990).

In addition to the epidemiological evidence, research by Ryser and Marth (1987) and by Reitsma and Henning (1996) demonstrated the survival of *L. monocytogenes* and *E. coli* O157:H7 for more than 60 days in Cheddar cheese. Ryser and Marth (1987) showed that *L. monocytogenes* could persist for up to 434 days postprocessing in artificially contaminated Cheddar cheese. Together with the outbreak information, these laboratory findings suggest the possibility that various foodborne pathogens may be capable of surviving current raw-milk Cheddar cheese manufacturing practices. These data suggest the need for additional research on the persistence of pathogens during cheese manufacture and ripening, with a particular need to focus on survival of pathogens recognized as human hazards since 1946. As a consequence of the outbreaks described above, and due to reports in the scientific literature regarding pathogen persistence beyond 60 days, FDA is currently reviewing the 60-day aging policy. This policy review includes an examination of the literature to identify data gaps, research to confirm some findings and to fill identified data gaps, and input from stakeholders (Personal communication, J. Mowbray, FDA, September 25, 2002).

The committee recommends that for finished cheese products, a scientifically appropriate performance standard for the reduction of targeted pathogens that result from the processing strategies or aging periods be developed and implemented. The committee recommends that the cheese industry, FDA, and state authorities work together to conduct and/or sponsor research to assess pathogen reduction efficacies of cheese manufacturing conditions. The use of pasteurized milk in cheese manufacturing may provide an appropriate safe harbor for the manufacture of products for which adequate pathogen reduction may not occur during manufacture or during a holding period without an additional intervention.

In the meantime, to enable consumers to make informed decisions regarding consumption of unpasteurized milk products, the committee recommends that FDA and state authorities require cheeses manufactured from subpasteurized milk to be clearly and prominently labeled as such at the point of purchase.

Food Safety Policy for Imported Cheeses

FDA is charged with enforcing the Federal Food, Drug and Cosmetic Act, along with other laws that are designed to protect the health of consumers. These laws apply equally to domestic and imported products. Therefore, as with domestic products, imported foods must be pure, wholesome, safe to eat, and produced under sanitary conditions. All products must contain truthful and informative labeling in English. Under some circumstances, based on past history of a product or on other information indicating that a product may be violative, imported products may be detained upon arrival into the United States. FDA can identify and detain products from an entire country or geographic region if violative conditions appear to be widespread (this procedure is called "detention without physical examination"). Cheeses and other dairy foods have occasionally been subjected to detention. For example, due to widespread contamination with *L. monocytogenes*, French cheese was ordered to be detained in mid-1986. This action occurred despite a French program that already had been implemented in 1974, which allowed only plants that were certified by the French government to be following good manufacturing practices to export soft-ripened cheese to the United States. In January 1987, this certification program was expanded to include a requirement for the use of pasteurized milk in the manufacture of soft-ripened cheeses, as well as for *Listeria* testing of those products intended for export to the United States. Currently, only French processing plants that are certified by the French Ministry of Agriculture to export soft-ripened cheese manufactured from pasteurized milk can legally market their products in the United States. The FDA's Office of Regulatory Affairs maintains a listing of products that are currently subject to import action.

The Food and Drug Administration Food Compliance Program for Domestic and Imported Cheese and Cheese Products

In response to a stated increase in the association of cheese and cheese products with outbreaks of human illness, in 1998 FDA issued a Food Compliance Program document that detailed plans for inspecting domestic cheese firms; examining domestic and imported cheeses for microbiological contamination, phosphatase, and filth; and taking action on cheese lots when violations are detected (CFSAN, 1998). Sampling priorities were established in the following order: soft cheeses, hard cheeses, and cheese products. When cheese samples are taken as part of this program, mandated analyses include testing for *L. monocytogenes*, *Salmonella*, *E. coli*, enterotoxigenic *E. coli* (enterotoxigenic *E. coli* analyses are performed only when *E. coli* are present at levels of 10^4/g), *E. coli* O157:H7, *Staphylococcus aureus*, and phosphatase. The testing is performed as a result of a public health concern and with the objective of identifying contaminated product and keeping it off the market; therefore, the sampling is not designed for batch-to-batch or process verification purposes. Samples are collected during scheduled inspections when either of the following criteria are met: (1) the firm's products have a previous history of microbiological contamination (e.g., as a follow-up to a complaint or illness), or (2) sampling is conducted for some specific reason (e.g., observations during inspection indicate that sampling is warranted). This program is an example of a finished-product testing strategy initiated in response to illnesses associated with specific foods.

THE ROLE OF THE U.S. DEPARTMENT OF AGRICULTURE IN DAIRY PRODUCT QUALITY AND WHOLESOMENESS

Dairy Products Grading and Inspection Program

In addition to FDA oversight of dairy product safety, many U.S. dairy plants participate in a voluntary grading and inspection program offered by the U.S. Department of Agriculture (USDA) through its Agricultural Marketing Service (AMS). USDA inspection and grading services are performed under the regulations in 7 C.F.R. part 58. The overarching goal of the AMS inspection and grading program is "to aid in the marketing of milk and dairy products by providing a common language of trade through the development, improvement, and interpretation of standards, specifications, and quality improvement programs" (AMS, 2002). The specific objectives of the program are to develop, maintain, and disseminate (1) sanitary requirements and model regulations to enhance the availability of safe, wholesome, high-quality dairy products, (2) definitions for product quality and wholesomeness, (3) requirements for participation in the USDA-Approved Dairy Plant Program, and (4) model state requirements for sanitary production and processing of manufacturing grade milk and milk products.

The USDA grading program was initiated in the early 1900s as a consequence of a recognized need for a common language for dairy product characteristics. The Office of Markets, which predates the AMS, was established in 1913 to lay the groundwork for dairy market news and product standardization and grading. The Dairy Grading Branch of AMS currently administers this program. Plants participating in this program are inspected at least twice yearly. Plant inspections are unannounced and cover more than 100 items, including milk supply, plant facilities, equipment condition, sanitary practices, and processing procedures. AMS publishes specifications to guide dairy plants toward meeting approval requirements (Dairy Division, 2002). In some cases, buyers may require that products meet specifications or grade standards. Therefore, despite a fee required to participate, this voluntary program is widely used by the dairy industry (AMS, 2002) because it provides guidance regarding how to achieve these quality standards.

Although almost all dairy products can be inspected or graded, the products most commonly inspected and graded are butter, Cheddar cheese, and instant and regular nonfat dry milk (AMS, 2002). Official USDA grades (e.g., U.S. Grade AA for butter and Cheddar cheese and U.S. Extra Grade for nonfat dry milk) are derived from uniform standards of quality developed by the Standardization Branch of USDA. An official USDA grade indicates the product's quality by use of designated letters such as "AA" or words such as "extra" (AMS, 2002). Product specifications reflect minimum acceptable requirements for dairy products for which official grade standards have not been determined. The official USDA quality approved shield can be applied to products that meet the requirements of a specification. USDA standards and specifications are designed to ensure that products are free from defects that affect usability, which include, but are not limited to, the state of preservation of the product, cleanliness, wholesomeness, and fitness for human food (7 C.F.R. part 58).

Development of USDA product standards and specifications is usually initiated by requests from outside USDA, often as a consequence of the development of a new product or a change in processing technology (AMS, 2002). Many requests are industry-driven, but other groups may initiate the process as well. Standard and specification development includes four elements: (1) research to determine quality factors and the range of quality encountered for the product, (2) investigation of production practices, including types of processing operations, packing, and equipment used, and consumer buying practices, (3) a statistical plan for product sampling, and (4) interviews with producers, packers, processors, shippers, receivers, consumers, and scientists. The standards and specifications are field-tested after the research is completed. At the end of this process, the standard or specification is published in the *Federal Register*. Standards and specifications increasingly rely upon scientific measurements, microscopic examinations, and written descriptions of quality aspects, but the process is still largely subjective (AMS, 2002). Conformance to standards and grades is largely based on the grader's perception of product taste, smell, appearance, and feel. Standards and specifications are reviewed and updated periodically to reflect changes in technology and milk quality (AMS, 2002).

Milk for Manufacturing Purposes

Milk for manufacturing purposes includes "milk produced for processing and manufacturing into products for human consumption but not subject to Grade A or comparable requirements" (AMS, 2002). USDA has established bacterial standards for milk to be used for manufacturing purposes. The goal of these requirements is to promote uniformity in state dairy regulations and laws, which should promote national uniformity in the sanitary processing of milk for manufacturing purposes. Enforcement of manufacturing milk regulations lies solely with the states. Lists of recommended microbiological standards for raw milk intended for manufacturing purposes and of AMS dairy product grade standards are presented in the tables in Appendixes F and G.

THE USE OF CURRENT STANDARDS AND CRITERIA UNDER HACCP

As described earlier, through evolution of the PMO and other dairy standards, the dairy industry has a long history of application of regulations to ensure the safety of its products intended for interstate commerce. Nevertheless, NCIMS has proposed testing the Hazard Analysis and Critical Control Point (HACCP) system under NCIMS as an alternative to the traditional dairy inspection/rating/check system. In 1997, NCIMS conference delegates voted to evaluate the possibility of implementing HACCP systems in the dairy industry, and in 1999 they voted to implement a voluntary HACCP pilot program. The NCIMS HACCP committee has had oversight responsibilities for implementation of this pilot program since 1999. One of the greatest challenges facing the dairy industry has been the incorporation of HACCP into the regulatory format already in place. The NCIMS proposal has been developed in ways that harmonize HACCP with traditional NCIMS requirements, in terms of regulatory reciprocity and oversight. For example, NCIMS proposes that the role of FDA in dairy HACCP could be similar to its current oversight and technical assistance role in the NCIMS system. The current regulatory authority is envisioned to perform the HACCP auditing function to verify that HACCP plans are effective.

Implementation of HACCP requires establishing prerequisite programs such as Good Manufacturing Practices and Standard Sanitary Operating Procedures. Various aspects of these programs (e.g., safety of process water, condition and cleanliness of food contact surfaces, prevention of cross-contamination, control of employee health conditions and personal hygiene facilities, proper labeling and storage of toxic compounds, and pest exclusion) are already addressed in various sections of the existing PMO. Hence, the dairy industry already has in place the background Good Manufacturing Practices and Standard Sanitary Operating Procedures to reduce the potential occurrence of food safety hazards. The most likely critical control points for dairy processing operations will be pasteurization time and temperature conditions and control of raw and processed product storage temperatures. Microbial specifications and standards have been and will continue to be used for regulatory purposes in the dairy industry; however, microbiological CCPs are unlikely to be adopted in the dairy industry.

In July 1999, applications to participate in the dairy HACCP pilot program were sent to all 50 states by the NCIMS HACCP committee. Of 16 dairy industry applicants, 6 plants representing 6 states were chosen to participate. To provide essential ongoing technical support for the participating plants and state regulators, NCIMS and FDA's State Training Branch have held HACCP training workshops for program participants. Further, the NCIMS HACCP established a Technical Resource Team comprised of FDA, state, and industry representatives. Questions are generally submitted by e-mail, and responses are posted on the NCIMS HACCP website (CFSAN, 2003). In May 2001, the NCIMS Conference extended the pilot program to 2003 and expanded the program to invite all Grade A plants to participate. The pilot program now includes 15 plants in 10 states. The dairy processing industry's continued participation in this program will help to promote the continued availability of the NCIMS HACCP program as a voluntary alternative to the more prescriptive PMO program.

The committee commends the dairy industry for voluntarily implementing a HACCP pilot program and strongly encourages timely adoption of HACCP systems throughout various sectors of the dairy processing industry. Adoption of performance standards for pathogen reduction, such as that proposed for cheese manufacturing, would more appropriately fit into a HACCP framework than in the dairy industry's current regulatory system.

ARE THE STANDARDS AND SCIENTIFIC CRITERIA FOR MILK AND DAIRY PRODUCTS ACHIEVING THEIR GOAL?

The committee recognizes that the application of regulations within the evolving PMO has been directly credited with reducing the incidence of milk-borne disease (Olsen et al., 2000). To illustrate this point, the 1999 revision of the PMO stated that 25 percent of all disease outbreaks due to contaminated food and water were a consequence of consumption of milk products in 1938, but that, more recently, the prevalence of milk-borne disease has dropped to less than 1 percent of reported outbreaks.

While dairy foods appear to be responsible for a relatively small proportion of U.S. foodborne-illness outbreaks that currently are successfully tracked to their source, occasional outbreaks of illness from consumption of contaminated dairy products do occur. The outbreaks listed in Table 7.5 do not provide a comprehensive listing of dairy food-associated illnesses since 1985, but rather provide a description of a selection of outbreaks associated with an international variety of dairy products, a variety of foodborne pathogens, and a variety of routes of product contamination. The goal of the table is to illustrate routes of entry for foodborne pathogens in dairy products. Determination of patterns among outbreak incidents may assist in identifying the most effective interventions and allocation of resources to further reduce dairy food-associated illnesses.

Of the 20 outbreaks listed in Table 7.5, 11 are associated with consumption of raw milk products or of products contaminated by raw milk or by close contact with farm animals. These outbreaks further illustrate the possibility of the presence of microbiological hazards in unpasteurized milk, as well as the need to develop effective interventions to control pathogens on the farm. Nine outbreaks (including some of those associated with raw milk product consumption) were associated with postpasteurization contamination of processed products. Post-pasteurization contamination usually results from lapses in cleaning and sanitizing procedures or from human food handling or processing errors that compromise product safety. The outbreak in 1988 brings into question the adequacy of current

TABLE 7.5 Outbreaks of Foodborne Disease Associated with Dairy Products

Year	Product and/or Source
1985	Mexican-style soft cheese, illegally imported, raw milk suspected
1985	Mexican-style white cheese, environment and equipment grossly contaminated, even after clean-up; raw-milk delivery allegedly exceeded pasteurization capacity
1985	Pasteurized 2% milk; postpasteurization contamination; pipe cross-connection appears to have allowed raw milk to commingle with pasteurized
1988	Pasteurized milk; spores of *Bacillus* survived pasteurization and grew during subsequent storage at refrigeration temperatures
1989	Mozzarella manufactured at a single plant, or cross-contaminated by a batch from that plant; low-level contamination of nationally distributed food product caused geographically dispersed foodborne outbreak that was difficult to detect
1992	Imported Irish soft unpasteurized cows' milk cheese (import into UK temporarily stopped, resumed after manufacturer decided to pasteurize milk used in production of cheese for export)
1994	Chocolate milk, leaking equipment, *L. monocytogenes* in plant environment, poor sanitation, postpasteurization contamination, insufficient cooling
1994	Unpasteurized soft cheese cross-contaminated by chicken carcass (chickens dressed by cheese makers)
1994	Ice cream, contaminated through transport of pasteurized ice cream premix in tanker trailers that had previously carried nonpasteurized liquid eggs containing *S.* Enteritidis
1996	Formula dried milk for infants, international outbreak
1997	Raw milk, contaminated by cows at dairy of origin
1997	Mexican-style soft cheese made with raw milk
1998	Fresh cheese curds, unpasteurized, mislabeled as pasteurized
2000	Bottled pasteurized milk, possibly postpasteurization contamination from pigs via rinsing with untreated well water
2000	Fluid milk products; milk products formulated with skim milk powder bearing staphylococcal enterotoxin A
2000	Morbier cheese, one batch from a single processing plant incriminated (unpasteurized)
2001	Mexican-style soft cheese
2002	Raw milk obtained through cow-lease program, strategy used to circumvent legislation that prohibits sale of unpasteurized milk in this state
2002	Visit to dairy farm with *E. coli*-infected cows and calves
2003	Farmstead Gouda cheese; source under investigation

Organism	Number of Cases	Location	Reference
Brucella melitensis	9	TX	Altekruse et al., 1998
Listeria monocytogenes	145	CA	Boor, 1997
Salmonella Typhimurium	16,000 culture confirmed; 168,791 to 197,581 cases estimated	IL	Ryan et al., 1987
B. cereus	280	The Netherlands	Van Netten et al., 1990
S. Javiana, *S.* Oranienberg	164	WI, MN, MI, NY	Hedberg et al., 1992
S. Dublin	42	UK (South-east England)	Maguire et al., 1992
L. monocytogenes	45	IL	Dalton et al., 1997
S. Berta	82	Ontario	Ellis et al., 1998
S. Enteritidis	224,000 (estimate)	MN	Hennessy et al., 1996
S. Anatum	19	France, UK	Threlfall et al., 1998
E. coli O157:H7	6	OR	Keene et al., 1997
S. Typhimurium DT104	54	WA	Villar et al., 1999
E. coli O157:H7	55	WI	Durch et al., 2000
Yersinia enterocolitica	10	VT, NH	Ackers et al., 2000
Staphylococcal enterotoxin A, produced by *S. aureus*	14,700	Japan	Asao et al., 2002
S. Typhimurium	113	France	De Valk et al., 2000
L. monocytogenes	3 NC	Boggs et al., 2001	
Campylobacter jejuni	5 WI	CDC, 2002	
E. coli O157:H7	51	PA	Crump et al., 2002
E. coli O157:H7	11	Alberta	CFIA, 2003

pasteurization practices for destruction of spore-forming organisms (e.g., *Bacillus cereus*) that can reproduce in fluid milk, particularly in those products that may be stored at refrigeration temperatures for extended times. In general, the presence of spore-forming organisms in raw milk that might not be destroyed by pasteurization has not been considered a significant public health risk (CFSAN, 2002). Additional research, targeted at exploring the survival and outgrowth of spore-forming pathogens in conventionally pasteurized milk that is at refrigeration temperatures for more than 7 days, may be warranted. Finally, one large-scale outbreak in 2000 resulted from poor manufacturing practices in combination with reprocessing of past-code-date fluid milk products. Out-of-date cartons of fluid milk that had been delivered to a powdered milk processing plant were reportedly opened by hand and poured into vats that were not properly refrigerated. A subsequent power outage prevented the milk from being pasteurized for many hours. As a consequence, the milk was held for an extended period at temperatures permissive for bacterial growth. *S. aureus* was probably introduced into the milk during handling. This organism is predicted to have multiplied to levels necessary for enterotoxin production (> 100,000/mL) in the warm milk. After the electricity was restored, the milk was pasteurized, but conventional pasteurization conditions do not inactivate staphylococcal enterotoxin A. The milk was then dried into powdered milk ingredients. The resulting powdered milk ingredients were used to formulate fluid milk products, which also were pasteurized. The presence and persistence of the enterotoxin from the powdered milk ingredients in the pasteurized fluid milk products illustrates the toxin's ability to withstand conventional heat processing treatments and highlights the importance of preventing bacterial contamination of, and maintaining temperature control over, perishable food products.

The committee concludes that the reduction in foodborne illnesses associated with milk consumption in the United States is primarily a consequence of the near universal implementation of milk pasteurization for commercial fluid milk products, and also reflects the implementation of sanitation programs in processing plants that are designed to protect pasteurized milk from recontamination with pathogenic microbes. The committee further recognizes that despite the clear link that has been established between raw milk consumption and foodborne illnesses, some consumers continue to drink raw milk. The committee recommends that state and local authorities ban the sale of unpasteurized milk because of its inherent risks. Because most unpasteurized milk is sold or consumed at the farm, targeted educational programs that illustrate the hazards of raw milk consumption are warranted. FDA and state authorities should consider requiring clear and concise labeling to identify cheeses manufactured from unpasteurized milk to assist members of the public in making informed choices regarding food purchase and consumption.

ECONOMIC AND ADMINISTRATIVE FEASIBILITY OF MILK PASTEURIZATION

Virtually all fluid milk processors that ship milk products via interstate commerce have invested in equipment for pasteurizing their product. Manufacturers of cheese from milk that has not been pasteurized must hold the product for a minimum of 60 days at a temperature not less than 35°F. The expense of holding this inventory for the required time is part of the input cost of cheese manufacturing. As a measure for controlling numbers of bacterial pathogens, pasteurization of fluid milk and other products and holding times for cheeses are economically feasible and commonly applied.

REFERENCES

Ackers ML, Schoenfeld S, Markman J, Smith MG, Nicholson MA, DeWitt W, Cameron DN, Griffin PM, Slutsker L. 2000. An outbreak of *Yersinia enterocolitica* O:8 infections associated with pasteurized milk. *J Infect Dis* 181:1834–1837.

Altekruse SF, Timbo BB, Mowbray JC, Bean NH, Potter ME. 1998. Cheese-associated outbreaks of human illness in the United States, 1973 to 1992: Sanitary manufacturing practices protect consumers. *J Food Prot* 61:1405–1407.

AMS (Agricultural Marketing Service). 2002. *Standardization Program Objectives*. Online. U.S. Department of Agriculture (USDA). Available at http://www.ams.usda.gov/dairy/stand.htm. Accessed December 31, 2002.

ANZFA (Australia/New Zealand Food Authority). 2000. *Food Standards Code. Standard H1—Milk and Liquid Milk Products*. Online. Available at http://anzfa.gov.au/FoodStandardCode/code/parth/H1.htm. Accessed October 9, 2000.

Asao T, Kumeda Y, Kawai T, Shibata T, Oda H, Haruki K, Nakazawa H, Kozaki S. 2002. An extensive outbreak of staphylococcal food poisoning due to low-fat milk in Japan: Estimation of enterotoxin A in the incriminated milk and powdered skim milk. *Epidemiol Infect* 130:33–40.

Asher DM, Gibbs CJ Jr, Gajdusek DC. 1986. Slow viral infections: Safe handling of the agents of subacute spongiform encephalopathies. In: Miller BM, ed. *Laboratory Safety: Principles and Practices*. Washington, DC: American Society of Microbiology. Pp. 59–71.

Boggs JD, Whitwam RE, Hale LM, Briscoe RP, Kahn SE, MacCormack JN, Maillard J-M, Grayson SC, Sigmon KS, Rardon JW, Saah JR. 2001. Outbreak of listeriosis associated with homemade Mexican-style cheese—North Carolina, October 2000–January 2001. *Morb Mortal Wkly Rep* 50:560–562.

Boor KJ. 1997. Pathogenic microorganisms of concern to the dairy industry. *Dairy Food Environ Sanit* 17:714–717.

CDC. 2002. Outbreak of *Campylobacter jejuni* infections associated with drinking unpasteurized milk procured through a cow-leasing program—Wisconsin, 2001. *Morb Mortal Wkly Rep* 51:548–549.

CFIA (Canadian Food Inspection Agency). 2003. *Health Hazard Alert. Eyot Creek Farm Natural Farmstead Gouda Cheese May Contain Dangerous Bacteria*. Online. Available at http://www.inspection.gc.ca/english/corpaffr/recarapp/2003/20030128ee.shtml. Accessed March 12, 2003.

CFIS (Canadian Food Inspection System). 1997. *National Dairy Regulation and Code, Production and Processing Regulation October 1, 1997. Part 2. Processing*. Online. Available at http://www.cfis.agr.ca/english/regcode/prod_2ehtm#PartII. Accessed March 12, 2003.

CFSAN (Center for Food Safety and Applied Nutrition). 1998. *Food Compliance Program. Domestic and Imported Cheese and Cheese Products.* Online. Food and Drug Administration (FDA). Available at http://www.cfsan.fda.gov/~comm/cp03037.html. Accessed September 30, 2002.

CFSAN. 2000. *Food Compliance Program. Milk Safety Program.* Online. FDA. Available at http://www.cfsan.fda.gov/~comm/cp18003.html. Accessed September 30, 2002.

CFSAN. 2002. *Grade "A" Pasteurized Milk Ordinance. 2001 Revision.* Online. FDA. Available at http://www.cfsan.fda.gov/~ear/pmo01toc.html. Accessed September 30, 2002.

CFSAN. 2003. *Hazard Analysis and Critical Control Point.* Online. FDA. Available at http://www.cfsan.fda.gov/~lrd/haccp.html. Accessed March 17, 2003.

Crump JA, Sulka AC, Langer AJ, Schaben C, Crielly AS, Gage R, Baysinger M, Moll M, Withers G, Toney DM, Hunter SB, Hoekstra RM, Wong SK, Griffin PM, van Gilder TJ. 2002. An outbreak of *Escherichia coli* O157:H7 infections among visitors to a dairy farm. *N Engl J Med* 347:555–560.

Dairy Division. 2002. *General Specifications for Dairy Plants Approved for USDA Inspection and Grading Service. Effective August 28, 2002.* Online. AMS, FDA. Available at http://www.ams.usda.gov/dairy/genpecs.pdf. Accessed December 31, 2002.

Dalton CB, Austin CC, Sobel J, Hayes PS, Bibb WF, Graves LM, Swaminathan B, Proctor ME, Griffin PM. 1997. An outbreak of gastroenteritis and fever due to *Listeria monocytogenes* in milk. *N Engl J Med* 336:100–105.

De Valk H, Delarocque-Astagneau E, Colomb G, Ple S, Godard E, Vaillant V, Haeghbaert S, Bouvet PH, Grimont F, Grimont P, Desenclos JC. 2000. A community-wide outbreak of *Salmonella enterica* serotype Typhimurium infection associated with eating a raw milk soft cheese in France. *Epidemiol Infect* 124:1–7.

Douglas SA, Gray MJ, Crandall AD, Boor KJ. 2000. Characterization of chocolate milk spoilage patterns. *J Food Prot* 63:516–521.

Durch J, Ringhand T, Manner K, Barnett M, Proctor M, Ahrabi-Fard S, Davis J, Boxrud D. 2000. Outbreak of *Escherichia coli* O157:H7 infection associated with eating fresh cheese curds—Wisconsin, June 1998. *Morb Mortal Wkly Rep* 49:911–913.

EEC (European Economic Community). 1994. *Council Directive 92/46/EEC of June 16, 1992. Laying Down the Health Rules for the Production and Placing on the Market of Raw Milk, Heat-Treated Milk and Milk Based Products.* Online. Available at http://europa.eu.int/comm/food/fs/sfp/mr/mr03_en.pdf. Accessed March 12, 2003.

Ellis A, Preston M, Borczyk A, Miller B, Stone P, Hatton B, Chagla A, Hockin J. 1998. A community outbreak of *Salmonella berta* associated with a soft cheese product. *Epidemiol Infect* 120:29–35.

Enright JB, Sadler WW, Thomas RC. 1957. *Thermal Inactivation of* Coxiella burnetii *and its Relation to Pasteurization of Milk.* Public Health Monograph No. 47. Washington, DC: U.S. Government Printing Office.

FDA. 2002. *FDA Warns About Possible* Enterobacter sakazakii *Infections in Hospitalized Newborns Fed Powdered Infant Formulas.* Online. Available at http://www.fda.gov/bbs/topics/ANSWERS/2002/ANS01146.html. Accessed September 30, 2002.

Gilman HL, Dahlberg AC, Marquardt JC. 1946. The occurrence and survival of *Brucella abortus* in Cheddar and Limburger cheese. *J Dairy Sci* 29:71–85.

Hammer BW. 1948. *Dairy Bacteriology*, 3rd ed. New York: John Wiley and Sons. Pp. 275–280.

Hammer P, Lembke F, Suhren G, Heeschen W. 1995. Characterization of a heat resistant mesophilic *Bacillus* species affecting the quality of UHT milk. In: *Heat Treatments and Alternative Methods.* Proceedings of the IDF Symposium. Brussels: International Dairy Federation. Pp. 9–16.

Hedberg CW, Korlath JA, D'Aoust JY, White KE, Schell WL, Miller MR, Cameron DN, MacDonald KL, Osterholm MT. 1992. A multistate outbreak of *Salmonella* Javiana and *Salmonella* Oranienburg infections due to consumption of contaminated cheese. *JAMA* 268:3203–3207.

Hennessy TW, Hedberg CW, Slutsker L, White KE, Besser-Wiek JM, Moen ME, Feldman J, Coleman WW, Edmonson LM, MacDonald KL, Osterholm MT. 1996. A national outbreak of *Salmonella enteritidis* infections from ice cream. The Investigation Team. *N Engl J Med* 334:1281–1286.

Hillerton JE. 1997. Milk as a risk factor for BSE. In: *Proceedings of the 36th Annual Meeting of the National Mastitis Council.* Madison, WI: National Mastitis Council. Pp. 33–41.

Johnson EA, Nelson JH, Johnson M. 1990. Microbiological safety of cheese made from heat-treated milk, Part II. Microbiology. *J Food Prot* 53:519–540.

Keene WE, Hedberg K, Herriott DE, Hancock DD, McKay RW, Barrett TJ, Fleming DW. 1997. A prolonged outbreak of *Escherichia coli* O157:H7 infections caused by commercially distributed raw milk. *J Infect Dis* 176:815–818.

Klijn N, Herrwegh AAPM, DeJong P. 2001. Heat inactivation data for *Mycobacterium avium* subsp. *paratuberculosis*: Implications for interpretation. *J Appl Microbiol* 91:697–704.

Maguire H, Cowden J, Jacob M, Rowe B, Roberts D, Bruce J, Mitchell E. 1992. An outbreak of *Salmonella* Dublin infection in England and Wales associated with a soft unpasteurized cows' milk cheese. *Epidemiol Infect* 109:389–396.

Mechor GD. 1997. Milk as a risk factor for Crohn's disease. In: *Proceedings of the 36th Annual Meeting of the National Mastitis Council.* Madison, WI: National Mastitis Council. Pp. 50–55.

Olsen SJ, MacKinon LC, Goulding JS, Bean NH, Slutsker L. 2000. Surveillance for foodborne disease outbreaks—United States, 1993–1997. *Morb Mortal Wkly Rep* 49:1–51.

PHS (Public Health Service). 1940. *Ordinance and Code.* Public Health Bulletin #220, 1939 ed. Washington, DC: PHS.

Reitsma CJ, Henning DR. 1996. Survival of enterohemorrhagic *Escherichia coli* O157:H7 during the manufacture and curing of Cheddar cheese. *J Food Prot* 59:460–464.

Ryan CA, Nickels MK, Hargrett-Bean NT, Potter ME, Endo T, Mayer L, Langkop CW, Gibson C, McDonald RC, Kenney RT, Puhr ND, McDonnell PJ, Martin RJ, Cohen ML, Blake PA. 1987. Massive outbreak of antimicrobial-resistant salmonellosis traced to pasteurized milk. *JAMA* 258:3269–3274.

Ryser ET, Marth EH. 1987. Behavior of *Listeria monocytogenes* during the manufacture and ripening of Cheddar cheese. *J Food Prot* 50:7–13.

Threlfall EJ, Ward LR, Hampton MD, Ridley AM, Rowe B, Roberts D, Gilbert RJ, van Sommeren P, Wall PG, Grimon P. 1998. Molecular fingerprinting defines a strain of *Salmonella enterica* serotype Anatum responsible for an international outbreak associated with formula-dried milk. *Epidemiol Infect* 121:289–293.

Van Netten P, van de Moosdijk A, van Hoensel P, Mossel DAA, Perales I. 1990. Psychrotrophic strains of *Bacillus cereus* producing enterotoxin. *J Appl Bacteriol* 69:73–79.

Villar RG, Macek MD, Simons S, Hayes PS, Goldoft MJ, Lewis JH, Rowan LL, Hursh D, Patnode M, Mead PS. 1999. Investigation of multidrug-resistant *Salmonella* serotype Typhimurium DT104 infections linked to raw-milk cheese in Washington State. *JAMA* 281:1811–1816.

8

Overall Findings and Recommendations

The U.S. food safety regulatory system has developed over a period spanning more than a century. The regulatory focus has shifted from an overriding concern about filth and fraud to issues regarding food safety as it relates to wholesomeness and control of contaminants, particularly those of chemical and microbiological origin. Because the regulatory authority for food is divided among several agencies and is based on legislation enacted under the technical, societal, and political circumstances of the times of their enactment, there are vast differences in the regulations being applied to various food groups and in the way the agencies interpret and enforce such regulations. These differences in the regulatory framework, together with the differences in origin, processing, and characteristics of the food groups selected for the study, explain the committee's decision to discuss and evaluate the current safety criteria individually for each food group.

However, the committee also recognizes that there are issues regarding the establishment of food safety criteria that are common to all food groups being studied that should be addressed separately from those specific to each selected food group. Although most issues regarding policy were intentionally excluded from the individual commodity discussions, the committee considered some policy issues closely related to the success of scientific criteria. Thus, the committee concluded that the authority of regulatory agencies to enact and enforce food safety criteria within the current regulatory system, and the effectiveness and consistency of such enforcement, were inextricably linked to its charge and needed consideration. In addition, discussions regarding the need to regulate food safety based on science and to link food safety criteria to overall public health objectives were so central to the committee's charge that these issues constituted the core of the discussions.

THE NEED FOR REGULATORY AGENCIES TO HAVE THE AUTHORITY AND FLEXIBILITY TO ENACT, ENFORCE, AND UPDATE FOOD SAFETY CRITERIA

During its deliberations, the committee concluded that legal challenges to actions taken by regulatory agencies in response to violations of established food safety criteria have cast doubt on the authority of the agencies to enforce some current criteria (e.g., performance standards). While the committee did not undertake an analysis of the merits of these challenges, it concluded that the doubts created by these challenges should be promptly addressed through Congressional action.

- **Congress should give regulatory agencies the clear authority to establish, and enforce compliance with, science-based food safety criteria, including performance standards.**

Furthermore, the committee concluded that the current process to modify existing food safety criteria is too rigid to allow appropriate and timely updating of these regulations to keep up with the fast pace of scientific and technological progress.

- **Congress should give the regulatory agencies the flexibility needed within the administrative process to update food safety criteria, including performance standards, so that new scientific knowledge and technological innovation can be timely incorporated in an efficient manner into these regulations.** This flexibility is needed to incorporate new processing or assessment techniques and to allow the agencies the ability to change performance standards to align them with the best contemporary scientific knowledge.

LINKING FOOD SAFETY CRITERIA TO PUBLIC HEALTH OBJECTIVES

The committee concluded that defining the means to measure the effectiveness of a new regulation is an essential factor for consideration during its development.

- **Any food safety criterion should be coupled with some sort of verification measure so that the effectiveness of the criterion can be assessed.**

Food safety criteria have the common objective of protecting or improving public health. Therefore, the committee concludes that **science-based food safety criteria must be clearly linked to the public health problem they are designed to address.** To accomplish this, a cause/effect relationship needs to be established between contaminants in foods and human disease, that is, to allocate the burden of foodborne disease among foods and food groups. Knowing the contribution of each food or food group to this burden would allow the selection (or promote the development) of appropriate interventions and set the basis for establishing criteria such as performance standards. This knowledge would also allow regulators to (1) focus on those foods that present the highest risk, and (2) target effective interventions at Critical Control Points (CCPs) in the production, processing, and distribution continuum of such foods. Moreover, **such a link would allow the regulatory agencies and industry to measure the effectiveness of the selected interventions**, and corresponding criteria, such as performance standards, in controlling the particular hazard and thus improving public health.

- **Congress should require the development of a comprehensive national plan to harmonize the foodborne disease surveillance that is conducted by public health agencies with the monitoring of pathogens across the food production, processing, and distribution continuum that is conducted by food safety regulatory agencies, and allocate the funds to develop and implement this plan.**

This plan would aim to establish the burden of foodborne disease and would be a concerted effort between public health and food safety regulatory authorities.

- **To implement such a plan, Congress should allocate funds to expand the current foodborne disease surveillance programs such as FoodNet, PulseNet, foodborne outbreak reporting and data sharing, and other national foodborne disease surveillance systems conducted by public health authorities.**
- **In addition, Congress should allocate funds for the food safety regulatory agencies to establish and maintain databases on pathogen contamination at various stages in the production/consumption continuum of domestic and imported foods and food groups frequently associated with foodborne disease. This effort should include studies to characterize the points in the production/consumption continuum of such foods where contamination is most likely to occur, so that the limited current knowledge of the microbial ecology of pathogens and cross-contamination pathways may be advanced. This knowledge will be the basis to identify CCPs that would serve to achieve a particular public health objective.**

DEVELOPING AND MONITORING SCIENCE-BASED FOOD SAFETY CRITERIA

An executive order exists that requires regulatory agencies to develop food safety criteria based on science. The committee recognizes that a first major step in this direction has been the introduction of the Hazard Analysis and Critical Control Points (HACCP) system in various areas of the food industry.

- **The committee strongly recommends that the regulatory agencies continue to introduce and audit the implementation of HACCP in all sectors of the food industry, as appropriate.**

HACCP

The committee concluded that the positive balance of progress in food safety after implementation of HACCP, as measured by overall reductions in several major foodborne diseases, is a tribute to the efforts of industry and the regulatory agencies to improve food safety. This progress confirms the committee's belief that **industry and food safety regulatory agencies alike must continue to focus on prevention, reduction, or elimination of foodborne hazards along the food continuum through a science-based food safety assurance system**. However, the committee also recognizes that there is still much to be done concerning the way HACCP is being implemented by industry and the way compliance with established criteria is being enforced by the agencies. Among the problems being encountered in HACCP implementation, the committee concluded that inadequate HACCP plan specificity for a given operation, in some cases, may be the root of certain miscommunications and problems in complying with HACCP regulations. There is also inconsistency in the approach taken by the U.S. Department of Agriculture (USDA) and the Food and Drug Administration (FDA) regarding HACCP implementation. This should be addressed.

- **Continued training in HACCP principles to assure proper implementation by industry personnel and consistent interpretation and monitoring of compliance by inspectors from the regulatory agencies is necessary.**

In addition, the committee recognizes that one of the longstanding limitations of HACCP is that the actual level of hazard control may not be clearly stated in the HACCP plan. That is, there is little or no guidance on the level of hazard control expected in an adequately designed and implemented HACCP plan because the "acceptable level" to which a hazard must be reduced at a CCP is undefined by HACCP. The committee concludes that, as currently done with certain performance standards, use of the evolving Food Safety Objective (FSO) concept could, in some cases, help remedy this problem by clearly defining the level of control needed for adequate Good Manufacturing Practices (GMP), Prerequisite Programs, and HACCP systems.

Strategies for Developing Science-Based Food Safety Criteria

Regarding the strategies available to the regulatory agencies to develop science-based food safety criteria, the committee concludes that it is seldom possible for regulators to base new regulations strictly on laboratory data or using only expert opinion.

- **Recognizing that it is impossible to fill all data gaps, the committee recommends that regulatory agencies use a strategy that combines the use of the best available data and the best expert judgment as an appropriate, science-based means to establish food safety regulations.**

The committee recommends that the following process be used to develop food safety regulations:

1. **Clearly document the public health objective and the appropriate level of protection.**
2. **Obtain or generate the best scientific knowledge through the use of laboratory or field studies, risk assessments, and similar food safety tools.**
3. **Minimize knowledge gaps by conducting pilot programs of the proposed performance standard, by maintaining databases of critical information, or by conducting risk assessments that can be used to develop performance standards, and by including science-based expertise if needed.**
4. **Explicitly state the nature, limits, and extent of the scientific uncertainties.**
5. **Explicitly identify the assumptions, criteria, and expertise used to address the uncertainties in formulating the performance standard.**

The process described above would have a high degree of transparency and provide an appropriate strategy to establish regulations in a timely manner.

- **The committee emphasizes that transparency—that is, effective communication of the underlying reasons for establishing food safety**

control measures, as well as the expected outcome of these measures, to all stakeholders—greatly contributes to acceptance of the measures. In addition, to maximize transparency in developing new food safety regulations when limitations in data occur, transparency should include documenting the limitations of the data, describing the assumptions used to fill in the data gaps, and making this information available to the public. This process should actively involve the best scientists in the field.

- **Similarly, for flexibility, the committee recommends that the regulatory agencies periodically evaluate and update food safety criteria. To this end, Congress should enable regulatory agencies to incorporate flexibility into the administrative process, so that these criteria can be adjusted efficiently to meet future public health goals.** The Pasteurized Milk Ordinance and the Conference for Food Protection provide models of a specific structure and mechanism for biennial review of existing regulations.

The committee also discussed what constitutes appropriate data to support the development of science-based food safety criteria. There are several ways through which regulatory agencies may obtain appropriate data:

- **Regulatory agencies can conduct or fund pilot studies or risk assessments, or collect appropriate data if these data are not available.**
- **Regulatory agencies should develop and maintain databases on the prevalence of specific contaminants for critical commodities.**
- **Congress should provide adequate resources to develop and maintain these databases.**

Chapters 2, 4, and 6 describe the particular need and justification to maintain current databases on major food groups, or to develop new ones. In addition to maintaining these databases, regulatory agencies must continually analyze these data using basic time series analyses, techniques that are standard in Statistical Process Control (SPC) methods.

The committee also discussed a number of critical issues that must be addressed and controlled to ensure good analytical results whether the data are collected for monitoring purposes for baseline development or for verification purposes. **Ensuring that validated testing and monitoring methods are used is essential when developing standards or for verifying processes.**

The committee recognizes that consideration of unique methodology issues is necessary when "zero tolerance" is used as a performance standard. The concept of a zero-tolerance performance standard is inextricably linked to the sensitivity of the method employed to detect the offending hazard, as well as to the sampling strategy employed. Sampling protocols must take into account that a large sample is needed to ensure the absence of the hazard, and that the sample must be representative of the material being tested.

There are various tools that would facilitate the development of science-based food safety criteria or their implementation and monitoring within a HACCP system; these tools are described below.

Risk Assessment

Among the food safety tools discussed by the committee, microbial risk assessment was deemed to offer a systematic approach to estimating the impact of pathogenic microorganisms in the food chain. **Microbial risk assessment may help find the most effective solutions for lowering consumer exposure to foodborne microbiological hazards**. Microbial Risk Assessment is rapidly evolving into a major scientific methodology on which to base food safety criteria. However, the committee emphasizes that **defining microbial dose–response relationships for foodborne pathogens is essential if more accurate microbial risk assessment results are desired**. Allocation of resources to fund basic research studies defining these microbial dose–response relationships would help to remedy this deficiency.

Data on microbial cross-contamination rates suitable for quantitative risk assessment are only now starting to become available. Precise localization of where such cross-contamination occurs would require multiple sampling points in the food production system.

- **The committee calls on USDA and FDA to undertake or fund studies to characterize the points in the food continuum where control may be most effective and could have the greatest impact on reducing foodborne disease for food–pathogen combinations where insufficient knowledge has prevented intervention.**

The committee recognizes that no data from a system analogous to the National Residue Program exist for use in microbial risk assessments, and concludes that **a national residue system may represent a useful working model on which a national pathogen system could be based.** Just as the national residue system can be used to validate chemical risk assessments, such a national pathogen system would be invaluable in validating microbial risk assessments. Various other **data gaps have been identified that must be addressed before microbial risk characterization will be seen to be as effective as chemical risk characterization**. However, the committee recognizes that when data are not available for part of the food production chain, there are strategies such as the use of predictive models, the use of surrogate data, stochastic simulation using probabilistic distributions, and the use of expert opinions and consults (sometimes referred to as qualitative risk assessment), to fill such data gaps.

- **Data gaps should not prevent a risk assessment from being initiated, completed, and serving a useful purpose. However, these data gaps must be communicated to those requesting the microbial risk assessment, so that they will be aware of its limitations.**

The inherently iterative nature of risk assessments allows continual updating as more and better quality data become available, thereby increasing their effectiveness as tools for policy making.

Food Safety Objectives

The committee examined another evolving food safety tool, the Food Safety Objective (FSO) concept. Regulatory agencies may find that FSOs represent a useful concept for establishing a theoretical framework to relate performance standards to public health objectives. Conceptually, an FSO could be established on the basis of a quantitative risk assessment of the hazard of interest and would be consistent with the level of consumer protection that the regulatory agency deems appropriate to fulfill the public health objective. This concept may be useful to regulators in developing performance standards for application at the processing plant level (processing safety objective) such that an appropriate level of protection against a hazard is achieved in a food product at the time it is consumed. FSOs may also be useful to industry in selecting interventions that would ensure that the FSO is achieved, and to the regulators in monitoring compliance with criteria such as performance standards. **FSOs are important because they enable translation of public health goals into measurements that food processors are directly able to effect. This is a novel approach that may allow regulators to close the gap left by HACCP when it defined a CCP as any point, stage, or step along the food production/processing/distribution continuum where a hazard can be prevented, eliminated, or reduced to an acceptable level, but left the acceptable level undefined.** An FSO provides the basis for defining this level.

- **The committee recommends that regulatory agencies examine the potential application of the FSO concept when appropriate.**

FSOs can play an important role in modern food safety management by linking information from the risk assessment processes with measures to control the identified risk. As more information becomes available, risk assessments should be updated and FSOs adjusted accordingly. Thus, the committee concludes that the FSO concept may be a useful tool for developing policies that are consistent with current science and could offer an alternative approach to food safety management focusing on the protection of human health, while offering flexibility in achieving that goal.

Statistical Process Control

Because manufacturing processes tend to vary over time, processors and regulators determine compliance with a performance standard either through end-product testing or process control. Because most food product testing is destructive, food processors and regulators use acceptance sampling when testing rather than 100 percent inspection. Acceptance sampling assumes that the product characteristic that is being measured exhibits relatively stable variation; thus, it is not designed to identify "hot spots" (i.e., when microorganisms or toxins are concentrated in a very small portion of the lot), sporadic food safety hazards, or food hazards that occur at very low levels in a production lot—scenarios that are likely to occur with many foodborne microbial hazards. Although end-product testing by itself does very little to improve the safety of individual batches of food, microbiological testing has an absolutely critical role to play in HACCP plan verification and verification of scientific criteria.

The committee recognizes the value of SPC as a scientific method that can help the processor to improve the process and the regulator to ensure compliance with food safety criteria. Processors may use it to verify control of a food-processing system and to provide information that can be used to critically examine the system so that appropriate actions can be taken to reduce the likelihood of manufacturing unsafe food products. The committee also recognizes the potential benefit that could be derived from the use of SPC principles linked to continuous improvement by food processors, to continually reduce the risk of producing unsafe food products, and possibly also to reduce production costs. In addition, the committee believes that for regulators, the most effective procedure to determine whether a food processor is complying with a performance standard is to analyze process and product data using control charts, histograms, and process capability indices. SPC, linked to continuous improvement, provides a very robust methodology that is easy to monitor from a regulatory perspective.

Therefore, the committee concludes that food safety regulations should incorporate the concepts of SPC linked to continuous improvement, and they should require that food processors analyze and maintain records to ensure that their processes (1) exhibit stable and predictable variation, and (2) are capable of meeting performance standards. The regulatory agencies, in turn, must ensure that their professional staff assigned to inspecting or auditing food-processing plants are trained to enable them to determine whether a processing plant is properly using SPC techniques to monitor performance standards and is capable of meeting the performance standards.

- **The committee recommends the adoption of SPC principles linked to continuous improvement by food processors, as well as incorporation of such principles by the regulatory agencies into food safety regulations and into the agencies' compliance monitoring procedures of food processors.**

Food Safety Economics

The committee recognizes that the bulk of current food safety economics research has not focused on the impact of individual performance standards isolated from overall food safety policy or program (mostly HACCP-based regulations). Therefore, **the committee concludes that, at present, it is difficult to quantify the unique costs and benefits of particular performance standards implemented as part of a broader regulatory change**. In order to complete such evaluations it would be necessary to have representative, detailed cost data linked to actual improvements solely due to the particular performance standard under review. Research in this area is needed.

New Diagnostic Tools

Modern regulatory systems depend on technology to detect deviations from regulatory criteria. Rapid advances in the field of diagnostic technology underscore the committee's belief that there is a need for flexibility in any food safety regulatory approach and development of performance standards. Currently, there is a perception on the part of regulatory agencies that identification of a pathogen for regulatory purposes is not "real" unless a microorganism is isolated.

- **Regulations need to be changed to recognize that molecular analytical methods and other rapid methods can produce results of comparable or greater accuracy than those obtained with traditional culture techniques, and there must be provision for the use of data obtained with such methods in regulatory actions. Any regulatory approaches, including the establishment of performance standards, must have built into them sufficient flexibility to take advantage of the improvements in diagnostics that will almost certainly occur.**

The committee points out that there are limits to what science can deliver. While science will continue to search for and discover answers to problems involving foodborne illness, inexpensive answers are often unavailable or impractical. Where to draw the line between reasonably cost-effective requirements that should be implemented and those that would be beneficial but would have too great an impact on food prices is a question for politics rather than science.

SCIENTIFIC CRITERIA IN MEAT AND POULTRY, SEAFOOD, PRODUCE, AND DAIRY PRODUCTS

The committee, through its two subcommittees on meat and poultry and on seafood, produce and related products, and dairy products, examined the main safety criteria, including performance standards, currently applicable to each one of the sectors of food processing selected for consideration in this report. In so doing, the committee answered specific questions posed by USDA and FDA in their respective charges to the committee, as described in the following sections.

Safety Criteria for Meat and Poultry

The Approach to Meat and Poultry Safety

Under the Federal Meat Inspection Act and the Poultry Products Inspection Act, the USDA, through its Food Safety and Inspection Service (FSIS), inspects all domestic meat and poultry to be sold in interstate commerce in the United States. It also inspects plants that export meat or poultry to the United States. In addition, there are 27 states that operate state meat and poultry inspection programs. All of these plants operate under a HACCP system.

Microbiological testing of product samples obtained by the federal and state programs is conducted at USDA-approved laboratories. The committee notes that these are lagging indicators of process performance by meat or poultry plants because samples are taken after the product is prepared and packaged and, even with rapid methods, there is a significant lag time between the collection of the sample and the analysis of the laboratory data. **Although microbiological samples provide both the plant and regulatory agency with a "score card" for plant performance, if further significant gains in the safety of the U.S. meat and poultry supply are to be realized, meat and poultry establishments need to implement more effective process control measures**. As mentioned earlier, these process control measures should be linked to a systematic continuous improvement process to achieve the necessary level of safety demanded by the U.S. consumer. In addition, the committee concludes that the regulatory enforcement of HACCP and associated microbiological performance standards must be conducted adequately and in a timely manner if it is to achieve its goal of reducing microbial contamination of raw meat and poultry products and, hence, of improving public health.

Raw Meat and Poultry Process Control Criteria

The committee concurs that there is general agreement within the scientific community that generic *Escherichia coli* is likely the best indicator of fecal contamination of carcasses. In addition, the committee deems that the FSIS rationale used in developing the generic *E coli* process control criteria for raw meat and poultry made reasonable assumptions and proceeded in a logical fashion. However, in some instances, the committee notes that if the populations of generic *E. coli* are extremely low, the testing may no longer be providing the valuable information that would allow the processor to continue making improvements in the process.

- **The committee recommends that a reevaluation of the criteria be conducted to identify either an alternate system of testing or another indicator of carcass hygiene when the populations of generic *E. coli* are extremely low and the testing may no longer be providing the valuable information that the processor needs to continue making improvements in the process. In addition, the committee recommends the implementation of similar criteria for generic *E. coli* in ground product; these criteria should be developed using the generic *E. coli* criteria for carcasses as the model.**

Furthermore, the committee recognizes that the data from generic *E. coli* testing of carcasses collected by industry are not within the public domain, and therefore are not available for review and for use by processors in comparing their performance with that of their peers.

- **The committee recommends that an anonymous national database be created to collect the available generic *E. coli* data on carcasses so that industry and regulatory and public health agencies have benchmarks available for comparative purposes. The committee further recommends that this database be operated by a nonregulatory government agency or under contract to a university or nonprofit organization. The new data on generic *E. coli* in ground product recommended above should be handled in the same manner as those for carcasses.**

Pathogen Reduction Criteria

The stated purpose of the *Salmonella* performance standards is to promote a reduction in the levels of *Salmonella* on raw meat. On this basis, **the committee concludes that the *Salmonella* performance standards are valid**. As for generic *E. coli*, **however, the committee recognizes that when the populations or incidence of salmonellae are extremely low, the testing may no longer provide the information needed by the processor to continue making improvements in the process.**

- **Because of the importance of the baseline data, the committee recommends that a new baseline survey be conducted on a periodic basis to evaluate the microbiological status of carcass, trim, ground product, and ready-to-eat products, both at the site of production and at retail. It is important that data for this new baseline be collected in such a way as to address two concerns. First, it should be possible to compare the results of the new baseline to the old baseline to determine if the situation is improving, worsening, or remains unchanged. Second,**

the new baseline should be as representative and statistically valid as possible and should correct sampling deficiencies that were present in the first baseline study.

The committee concludes that recent data on the prevalence of *Salmonella* in raw meat and poultry, assessed on the basis of the proportion of inspected meat production facilities passing the *Salmonella* performance standard from 1998 to 2000 and compared with the defining pre-HACCP baseline prevalence data, are encouraging. Despite some significant limitations in the data sets collected, the committee recognizes that the vast number of data sets collected clearly indicate a decrease in *Salmonella*-positive samples since the implementation of the *Salmonella* performance standards.

- **Given the lack of a clear cause and effect relationship between *Salmonella* standards and the observed public health gains, and considering the importance of measuring the public health impact of pathogen reduction performance standards, the committee reiterates its recommendation to expand and harmonize foodborne disease surveillance and monitoring of microbial contamination of foods. The resulting data should allow a comparison of microbial serotypes in isolates from animals, humans, and foods as a means to enable regulatory and public health agencies to allocate the burden of foodborne disease to specific foods or classes of foods and thus provide a measure of the effectiveness of specific food safety criteria.**

The committee concludes that the *Salmonella* performance standard for ground products may not reflect the overall quality of the grinding operation, but rather the quality of the incoming raw materials. *Salmonella* testing of ground beef provides verification of the total system—live animal production through grinding—but not the grinding operation alone.

- **The committee recommends that a *Salmonella* performance standard or other appropriate criterion be developed for beef trim intended for grinding. In addition, the committee recommends that the current *Salmonella* performance standard for ground beef be reevaluated after appropriate interventions and the trim performance standard are in place. Further research should be conducted to determine an appropriate performance standard for ground beef at the grind operation.**
- **Furthermore, the committee recommends that all meat intended for trim for ground products, especially ground beef, be exposed to some form of verified intervention. This also applies to meat derived from heads, which currently may not be subject to any intervention.**

Adulteration of Ground Beef: Escherichia coli *O157:H7*

The committee recognizes that the low infectious dose attributed to *E. coli* O157:H7 and the potential severity of the disease it causes make the presence of this pathogen in foods a serious human health hazard. The committee also recognizes that the grinding process does not necessarily introduce this pathogen into the product but does redistribute it if present; however, the USDA interpretation of the code regarding this pathogen as an adulterant is to place the zero tolerance enforcement after meat grinding. Furthermore, the committee notes that recent FoodNet data suggest that occurrence of illness due to *E. coli* O157:H7 has not declined during the past five years, raising questions as to whether the current testing of ground beef for *E. coli* O157:H7 is achieving its desired goal. Under these circumstances, the committee feels that it is important to emphasize the need for testing and interventions prior to the grinding operation. If the contamination of the raw material used for ground beef (trim) could be reduced, or if contaminated trim could be diverted to other processes, then the potential contamination in fresh ground beef reaching the consumer would be reduced. The current survey testing at the retail level serves a purpose as a means of monitoring progress on this issue with ground beef. However, there is also a need for more effective monitoring of the process itself.

- The committee points to the urgent need for research on the ecology of *E. coli* O157:H7 and other close serotypes in beef, from the farm through transportation, lairage, slaughter, decontamination treatments, and into the trim, and recommends that USDA promptly undertake or fund such research. Parallel research to develop better interventions for trim destined for ground product, especially ground beef, should be urgently conducted as well. **Until such information on the ecology and mode of transmission of this pathogen is available, and other effective preventive or corrective controls can be applied, only cooking to a high enough temperature or irradiation to a high enough dose can ensure the safety of ground beef. Considerably more education of the public and particularly of commercial and noncommercial food service managers and workers is needed. The irradiation process does not replace the need for proper cooking. The committee urges regulatory and health authorities to (1) advise those members of the public who would prefer to minimize the risk of this product to cook irradiated and nonirradiated ground beef products to the appropriate temperature, (2) require that these products be clearly labeled with a warning of the potential for harm if not properly cooked, and (3) expand educational efforts to the public and to target commercial and noncommercial food service managers and workers.**

Lethality: Standards for the Production of Certain Meat and Poultry Products

The committee deemed that the FSIS approach in developing this standard was not scientifically justified and has resulted in an excessively conservative performance standard. Also, in examining the safe harbor treatments allowed for use by processors who cannot or do not wish to validate their own treatments, the committee expressed concern about the need to ensure proper adaptation of such treatments to the particular processor's HACCP plan.

Stabilization: Performance Standards for the Production of Certain Meat and Poultry Products

The committee considers the method used by FSIS to achieve the specified reductions in *Salmonella* in ready-to-eat poultry and beef products confusing and hard to use in determining the validity of either the data or the assumptions made in setting this standard. Therefore, the committee did not critically review this performance standard or assess the validity of the assumptions made during its development. The committee points out that this case illustrates the need for greater transparency in the development of food safety criteria, as mentioned earlier. This directive does not cover cured meat products but is being universally applied to them by inspection personnel.

Animal Drug Residues

The committee recognizes that regulatory review of the use of drugs in food animals is continuing. **The committee concurs that the approved tolerance level constitutes the performance standard for those chemicals that are used in animals and have such a tolerance level.**

Sanitation Standards

The committee concludes that, although described as "standards," the actual language in the sanitation regulations includes numerous references to "adequate," "preventing sources of adulteration," and "sufficient." Therefore, these regulations provide little in the way of a descriptive and objective "standard" and are better characterized as "guides."

Economic Cost–Benefit of the Pathogen Reduction/HACCP Rule

As mentioned earlier, **the committee concludes that more research is needed before a proper cost–benefit analysis of specific food safety criteria can be isolated from the general effects of a wider regulation such as the Pathogen Reduction (PR)/HACCP rule.** However, the committee points out that future economic impact assessments of such regulations, when considering the effectiveness of novel interventions, should rely on data gathered at the processing plant level and not only from laboratory or theoretical assessments.

Additional Approaches to Reduce Microbial Hazards in Meat and Poultry

The committee considered the need to move toward an integrated approach to meat and poultry safety. It concluded that efforts to reduce preslaughter contamination are likely to be an important part of a comprehensive, farm-to-table food safety strategy, not only to reduce pathogen load at the slaughter plant, but also to prevent the hazard from direct contact with infected animals, from runoff from feedlots and farms, and from contaminated water supplies.

- **The committee recommends that USDA conduct or fund research on the role of nonfecal carriage and commingling prior to and after slaughter to elucidate the factors that contribute to the microbial contamination of live animals, carcasses, and products.**
- **The committee also recommends a research focus on intervention trials at all stages of the production process of meat and poultry products.**

This is consistent with the committee's view that industry and the regulatory agencies should continue to place greater emphasis on contamination prevention rather than relying on inspection and end-product testing to ensure the safety of meat and poultry.

Safety Criteria for Seafood

There are currently over 350 species of fish that are commonly consumed. This diversity is expressed as a broad spectrum of sensory attributes, product forms, and preparations that are particular to seafood. Seafood presents unique safety concerns that arise from both the intrinsic characteristics of the animals and the environmental conditions from which they are harvested. In addition, conditions and handling at harvest and processing, as well as during distribution and preparation, may enhance or reduce the risk of seafood-borne disease.

The Approach to Seafood Safety

Unlike meat and poultry, the inspection system for seafood safety is under the jurisdiction of FDA. This system also differs from that in the meat and poultry industry in that regulatory inspections are not performed on a continuous, on-site basis.

Anticipating that the seafood industry would need assistance in HACCP plan development and implementation, FDA issued the *Fish and Fisheries Products Hazards and Control Guide*, commonly referred to as "the Guide." The committee recognizes that the Guide is an innovative and useful document that effectively assists seafood processors with the development of their HACCP plans.

To improve the utility of the *Fish and Fisheries Products Hazards and Control Guide*, the committee recommends that FDA consider the following measures:

- **Introduce a more collaborative process in further developing the Guide. To this effect, the committee recommends that FDA appoint a Hazards and Control Guide Advisory Committee.**
- **Further address the issues of expert capability and process.**
- **Develop a protocol to guide process validation. This protocol must address criteria for distinguishing the creditability of processing authorities, sampling plans, experimental designs, and appropriate methodologies. Validation and verification guidelines, including recommendations for adequate analytical methods and sampling plans, should also accompany the recommended controls in the Guide.**
- **Develop a protocol to recognize the application of analytical methodologies, such as new, rapid test procedures that can be utilized in process validation and in routine verification.**
- **Enhance communications to ensure awareness, understanding, and consistent application of the Guide.**

In addition, the committee believes that **screening limited quantities of seafood products at points of entry is not consistent with the preventive concept of HACCP; hence, prevention of seafood safety hazards in imported seafood must place greater emphasis on intervention prior to shipment.**

- **The committee recommends that FDA give immediate attention to the application of the Guide to ensure food safety equivalence in international seafood commerce. The committee believes that the intent of the Guide and its contents need to be clarified to U.S. trading partners.**

Aware that international collaboration is essential to enhance seafood safety, the committee recommends that FDA initiate an International Seafood Safety Exchange Program to foster international collaboration in seafood safety research and training. A common topic for initial consideration could be the development of Best Aquaculture Practices. The existing FDA Guide, as well as relevant documents already published by other organizations, could be used as models.

Criteria for Control of Chemical Contaminants and Toxins in Seafood

The committee examined current safety criteria applicable to seafood including tolerances, action levels, and guidelines, and concluded that the specific scientific basis for each of them differs, depending mainly on the availability of data about a hazard. The tolerance for methyl mercury content in fish (1.0 ppm) for example, is appropriately based on the level necessary for consumer safety, whereas the labeling requirement for sulfite residues (10 ppm) is also appropriately based on the lower limit of analytical capability.

All seafood safety criteria established prior to the seafood HACCP rule remain in place within the current regulatory system. Therefore, processors must produce seafood that comply with all relevant food safety criteria. The committee recognizes that, in most cases, these criteria cannot be used as critical limits for CCPs in HACCP plans, but can be used as verification criteria when end-product testing is warranted. Thus, direct monitoring of chemical contaminants using analytical tests would often be impractical as a CCP because of the significant variability in concentration for some of these contaminants among geographic areas. However, this geographical variability makes it possible to reduce consumer exposure to such contaminants through restrictions of harvesting sites. Therefore, **the committee concludes that harvest location restrictions are meaningful and effective controls for chemical contaminants in seafood.**

The committee also recognizes that chemical hazards that are not of environmental origin, such as scombrotoxin, require a different control strategy. Because monitoring of histamine levels in each fish received at a processing plant would not be viable, **the committee concludes that an alternate procedure based on review of the harvest records, both time and temperature, associated with each lot of fish is an acceptable procedure for monitoring histamine levels in seafood within a HACCP system.**

Criteria for Control of Vibrio vulnificus *and* V. parahaemolyticus *in Raw Oysters*

As with chemical contaminants, control of pathogenic microorganisms in shellfish is based on restrictions of harvesting sites. The fecal coliform standard for shellfish harvesting waters, in turn, is based on the potential presence of microbial pathogens.

The important role that innovation may play in enhancing seafood safety in the future is illustrated by the strategy adopted for control of *V. vulnificus* and the related species, *V. parahaemolyticus*, in raw oysters. **The committee concludes that the mandate for postharvest treatment in the model ordinance to reduce illnesses from consumption of raw oysters is a unique and novel approach to enhancing seafood safety.**

Safety Criteria for Produce and Related Products

Fruits and vegetables provide many health benefits and are an important component of the American diet. Consumption of these products in the United States has increased considerably in the past two decades, with corresponding increases in the volume of imports. Producers have responded to this increased demand not only by growing new varieties of fruits and vegetables, but they have also introduced novelty produce items in the marketplace and developed a large niche for fresh-cut produce.

Although fresh produce and juices were not traditionally thought to be important vehicles of foodborne disease, this notion has changed in recent years. Fresh produce safety is of special concern to the public health community because fruits and vegetables often do not receive any treatment specifically designed to kill all microbial pathogens prior to consumption.

The Approach to Produce Safety

There are virtually no criteria or standards for microbiological safety currently being applied to fresh produce or fresh-cut produce in the United States other than those pertaining to sprouts and fruit juices. The committee recognizes that to minimize foodborne disease from being transmitted through fresh produce, it is necessary to prevent initial contamination of these products and to control the potential amplification of pathogens in them throughout the production and distribution chain. Intervention strategies currently being applied in the fresh produce industry are Good Agricultural Practices in the field and packing houses and GMPs in fresh-cut operations. **The committee recognizes that the principles that make up the current Good Agricultural Practices recommendations are necessarily general given the broad range of fruits and vegetables and their growing conditions,** and, like GMPs, they focus on minimizing the potential for microbial contamination. The committee also recognizes that data gaps on risks associated with many specific practices in the fresh produce sector make it difficult to assess which intervention strategies could provide the greatest reduction in risk. Among these, the committee discussed the issue of potential internalization of pathogenic bacteria during growth or processing of produce and concluded that research is urgently needed in this area.

- **The committee recommends that FDA conduct or support additional studies to determine whether the internalization of bacteria represents a significant safety hazard in fruits and vegetables.**

There have been few attempts to integrate the various steps associated with production and processing of fresh produce into a farm-to-table HACCP system. Several HACCP plans have been developed for sprouted seeds, shredded lettuce, and tomatoes, but complete validation of these plans has not yet been accomplished. **The committee concludes that currently available data are insufficient to develop validated HACCP plans for most fresh produce items. Also, prerequisite programs, such as Good Agricultural Practices and GMPs, which provide the foundation for HACCP systems, are still being defined and evaluated for their effectiveness on farms and in orchards.** It is expected that data from ongoing research in this area will provide valuable information to supplement the basic guidelines.

In view of the trend toward greater importation of fruits and vegetables into the United States, the committee expressed concern about harmonization of food safety standards for imported produce. Several international efforts in this direction are underway, and some efforts are being made by FDA to survey pathogen contamination in imported produce. Domestic surveys are also being conducted by FDA and USDA to establish a microbiological baseline to assess the risk of contamination in the domestic supply; however such efforts need integration.

- **The committee reiterates that there is a need to develop a framework that allows timely sharing of data from surveillance programs on microbial contamination in specific high-risk fresh and fresh-cut produce and related products and from human, animal, and environmental isolates, and eventual integration of such data.**
- **The committee further points to the need for a structured review process for guidance documents and regulations, with input from a wide variety of experts from industry, government, and academia, using the National Advisory Committee on Microbiological Criteria for Foods model. This review process should be used to modify or rescind criteria as science evolves.**

Pathogen Reduction Criteria in Fruit and Vegetable Juices

As a consequence of foodborne disease outbreaks associated with raw juices processed at commercial facilities, FDA introduced regulations for all juices produced for inter- or intrastate sale. This regulation mandates that juice be produced under a HACCP plan having supporting GMPs and Sanitation Standard Operating Procedures. In addition, it requires that juice processors achieve at least a 5-$\log_{10}$ reduction (referred to as a 5-D process) in numbers of the pertinent microorganism, defined as "the most resistant microorganism of public health significance that is likely to occur in the juice." Although thermal treatments are most commonly used to ensure the required 5-D reduction, other processes will be accepted if appropriately validated. FDA issued a *Juice Hazards and Control Guidance Document* that provides some background on validating these alternate treatments, which was complemented with an educational program developed by the Juice HACCP Alliance.

Processors of raw citrus juices are allowed to use surface decontamination methods to achieve part of the 5-D pathogen reduction requirement under circumstances specified in the rule. **The publication by FDA of information explaining the scientific justification of the sampling plans for citrus juices that rely on surface treatments to achieve a 5-D pathogen reduction is an excellent example of using data and expert opinion to develop criteria or standards; the committee believes that this derivation could be used as a model when regulatory agencies develop other criteria or standards.** In contrast, the justification for a 5-D pathogen reduction process for citrus juices is described in a memorandum, with no reference to the scientific data from which the standard derives. As mentioned earlier, transparency of the criteria development process requires that the data and the assumptions made be clearly communicated.

The committee concludes that it would be premature to try to evaluate the public health impact of the new juice regulations. However, the fact that no disease outbreaks attributable to *Salmonella* or *E. coli* O157:H7 in juices have been reported to the Centers for Disease Control and Prevention since the juice regulation was implemented is noteworthy.

Control of Patulin in Fruit Juices

The committee concludes that the action level established by FDA for patulin in apple juice, apple juice concentrates, and apple juice products, 50 μg/kg (50 ppm), is appropriate. This level can readily be achieved with proper adherence to GMPs.

Criteria for Low-Acid and Acidified Canned Foods

For low-acid canned foods, a 12-D pathogen reduction thermal process must be applied. This regulation includes other foods besides vegetables. For acidified low-acid foods, defined as having a pH of 4.6 or below after equilibration, the key control parameter is the acidification step rather than the thermal process. Acidification of the food must be adequate so that the pH will not permit the growth of microorganisms of public health significance. Other requirements for these foods include standardized training of retort operators, registration of the canning facility at state and federal levels, filing of thermal processes, record keeping, and establishment of a recall program.

The committee recognizes that a clear example of the success of a performance standard is illustrated by the fact that after the establishment of the low-acid and acidified canned food rules and GMP regulations in the 1970s, only occasional cases of botulism attributable to these foods have occurred. The committee also believes that the 12-D performance standard for low-acid canned food might be too stringent and thus might compromise some quality attributes of certain canned foods; therefore, it should be

reevaluated. The committee is aware that technological innovation based on nonthermal food-processing technologies is critical to the development of new fruit and vegetable products. However, **the committee reiterates its recommendation that, prior to developing performance standards that accommodate process or other technical innovations, guidance must be provided to industry on process validation.**

Criteria for Sprouts

As a result of several disease outbreaks associated with the consumption of sprouts, FDA published the document *Guidance to Industry—Reducing Microbial Food Safety Hazards for Sprouted Seeds*, which recommends specific measures that sprout producers should apply to minimize pathogen contamination and growth during sprout production. **The committee recognizes that proper application of this guidance enhances the safety of sprouts, but that it would be premature to assess the effectiveness of the guidance. Nevertheless, the committee notes that all sprout outbreaks reported since the publication of the FDA guidelines have been associated with seed that was sanitized using methods other than those described in the guideline.**

Pesticide Residues

The committee believes that the process used to establish pesticide tolerances in produce is a good approach to ensure public health. **The process of setting pesticide tolerances by the U.S. Environmental Protection Agency is in agreement with the committee's belief that food safety standards should be developed based on a combination of the best available science and expert opinion, and that this process should be a transparent one.**

Safety Criteria for Dairy Products

Anecdotal observations that linked consumption of milk with the spread of disease spurred various scientists and physicians in the United States and around the world to undertake research to investigate the role of milk consumption in foodborne disease as early as the turn of the twentieth century. Consumption of unpasteurized milk was found to be associated with many serious diseases, including diphtheria, typhoid, tuberculosis, and brucellosis. Early reports provided evidence suggesting that control of milk-borne diseases required application of sanitation measures at all points in the food system, from the farm to the consumer. These observations also highlighted the need for technical research to determine the bacterial destruction characteristics of food-processing treatments for pathogenic microbes likely to be present in raw milk. The results of these studies led to pasteurization and other intervention strategies designed to protect the public from exposure to hazardous microorganisms that may be present in raw milk.

The Approach to Milk and Other Dairy Products Safety

Criteria for the safety of milk and other dairy products are defined in the "Grade A Pasteurized Milk Ordinance," commonly referred to as the PMO. The PMO is considered the reference for federal specifications for the procurement of milk and dairy products and as the sanitary regulation for dairy products served by carriers during interstate travel. It is also recognized by public health agencies and the dairy industry as the national standard for milk sanitation. This ordinance is administered by the National Conference on Interstate Milk Shipments and the Cooperative State Public Health Service Program for certification of interstate milk shippers, with FDA having oversight responsibility. Currently, all states, the District of Columbia, and the United States trust territories participate in the National Conference.

The committee recognizes that development, implementation, and enforcement of the PMO has been directly credited with reducing the incidence of milk-borne disease, and that the PMO is a good model for an integrated strategy for product safety assurance. In addition, this model also provides a specific structure and mechanism for biennial review of existing regulations directed toward the fluid milk industry. Nevertheless, the committee notes that milk for local consumption is not subject to FDA oversight. Therefore, consumption of unpasteurized (raw) milk continues to be an issue of concern. The committee concludes that targeted educational programs that illustrate the hazards of raw milk and raw milk-product consumption for milk producers and for the general public are warranted.

Through evolution of the PMO and other dairy standards, the dairy industry has a long history of application of regulations to ensure the safety of its products intended for interstate commerce. Nevertheless, the National Conference has proposed its own testing of HACCP as an alternative to the traditional dairy inspection/rating/check system. The committee concludes that one of the greatest challenges facing the dairy industry is the incorporation of HACCP into the regulatory format already in place, and commends the dairy industry for voluntarily implementing a HACCP pilot program. In addition, the committee strongly encourages the timely adoption of HACCP systems throughout various sectors of the dairy processing industry. Adoption of performance standards for pathogen reduction, such as that proposed for cheese manufacturing, would more appropriately fit into a HACCP framework than in the dairy industry's current regulatory system.

Criteria for Control of Hazards in Milk and Milk Products

In addition to specific recommendations for pasteurization conditions specified in the PMO, chemical, bacteriological, and temperature standards have been established for grade A raw milk products intended for pasteurization, as well as for grade A pasteurized and bulk-shipped, heat-treated milk products. Concerning the strict process requirements for milk pasteurization, the committee reiterates its belief that implementation of performance standards that specify the reduction in numbers required for a targeted organism in a food product, rather than specifying the precise conditions for achieving that end (as currently practiced), could allow greater flexibility and innovation in the dairy industry, perhaps enabling the adoption of effective new processing technologies.

Despite the success of pasteurization in ensuring milk safety, **the committee notes that, in addition to incomplete destruction of spore-forming bacteria, the efficacy of pasteurization in destroying other highly heat-resistant microbes that may be present in raw milk, such as *Mycobacterium avium* subspp. *Paratuberculosis,* requires FDA attention**. Recent illness outbreaks linked to dairy foods that had been successfully pasteurized, but then subjected to postpasteurization contamination with bacteria such as *Listeria monocytogenes* or *Salmonella*, highlight the critical need for application of effective processing-plant sanitation programs to prevent postprocessing contamination of these products. Somatic cell count limits for raw milk intended for pasteurized products are arguably a safety standard, as exceeding these limits may prevent effective application of a pasteurizing process. Similarly, the microbial standards for pasteurized fluid milk products—total bacteria and coliform bacteria—are considered a reflection of good management. The committee notes that despite the clear link that has been established between raw milk consumption and foodborne illnesses, some consumers continue to drink raw milk.

- **To further decrease the association between dairy products and foodborne illnesses, the committee recommends that FDA and public health agencies target educational programs to communicate to consumers that drinking raw milk represents a form of risky food-consumption behavior.**
- **In addition, state and local health authorities should ban the sale of unpasteurized milk.**

Criteria for Control of Hazards in Cheese

Current regulations state that no milk or milk products in final package form intended for direct human consumption shall enter interstate commerce unless they are manufactured from pasteurized milk or pasteurized milk ingredients, except where alternative procedures are provided for by regulation. Moreover, standards of identity have been established for most natural cheeses, process cheeses, cheese foods, and cheese spreads.

The committee examined the requirement that cheese made from unpasteurized milk be cured for a period of 60 days at a temperature not less than 35°F, and concludes that the scientific basis for this requirement is unclear.

- **The committee recommends the development and implementation of a scientifically appropriate performance standard for the reduction of targeted pathogens in finished cheese products that result from the processing strategies or aging periods employed in the manufacture of the products.**

The cheese industry and FDA should work together to conduct or sponsor research to assess pathogen reduction efficacies of cheese manufacturing conditions.

The use of pasteurized milk in cheese manufacturing may provide an appropriate safe harbor for the manufacture of products for which adequate pathogen reduction may not occur during manufacture or a holding period without an additional intervention.

- **In the meantime, to enable consumers to make informed decisions regarding consumption of unpasteurized milk products, the committee recommends that FDA and state authorities require cheeses manufactured from subpasteurized milk to be clearly and prominently labeled as such at the point of purchase.**

Appendix A

Current and Proposed Definitions of Key Food Safety Terms

One of the important tasks of the committee was to establish the definitions of food safety terms to be used throughout this report. Definitions of key food safety terms from a variety of agencies and organizations were thoroughly reviewed and are listed in Table A.1. To assure uniformity and consistency, the committee decided to adopt most of the definitions published by the International Commission on Microbiological Criteria for Foods (ICMSF, 2002), which are widely accepted throughout the global food safety community. There are a few terms that were specifically defined by the committee, one that was modified from the ICMSF definition, one that was adopted from the Codex Alimentarius Commission, and one that was used in a presentation to the committee (Personal communication, R. Buchanan, Food and Drug Administration, February 5, 2002). These definitions are explained below.

A microbiological criterion defines the acceptability of a product or a food lot, based on the absence or presence or number of microorganisms, including parasites, and/or the quantity of their toxins/metabolites, per unit of mass, volume, area, or lot (CAC, 1997). Microbiological criteria usually fall into three categories and include microbiological standards, guidelines, and specifications.

Microbiological standards are used to determine the acceptability of a food with regard to a regulation or policy. These standards are established by regulatory authorities and define the microbiological content that foods must meet to be in compliance with a regulation or policy. Foods not meeting the standard are in violation of the regulation or policy and are subject to removal from the market (ICMSF, 2002).

TABLE A-1 Definition of Terms

Term	Committee Consensus	ICMSF[a]	NRC[b]	FDA[c]
Appropriate level of protection	The level of protection deemed appropriate by the country establishing a sanitary or phytosanitary measure to protect human, animal, or plant life or health within its territory			
Control point	Any step at which biological, chemical, or physical factors can be controlled			
Criterion	A requirement on which a judgment or decision can be made			
Critical control point (CCP)	A step at which control can be applied and is essential to prevent or eliminate a food safety hazard or reduce it to an acceptable level			A point, step, or procedure in a food process at which a control measure can be applied and at which control is essential to reduce an identified food hazard to an acceptable level

FSIS[d]	NACMCF[e]	Codex[f]	WTO[g]	EC[h]
			The level of protection deemed appropriate by the country establishing a sanitary or phytosanitary measure to protect human, animal, or plant life or health within its territory	
	Any step at which biological, chemical, or physical factors can be controlled			
	A requirement on which a judgment or decision can be made			
A point, step, or procedure in a food process at which control can be applied and, as a result, a food safety hazard can be prevented, eliminated, or reduced to acceptable levels	A step at which control can be applied and is essential to prevent or eliminate a food safety hazard or reduce it to an acceptable level	A step at which control can be applied and is essential to prevent or eliminate a food safety hazard or reduce it to an acceptable level		

continued

TABLE A-1 Continued

Term	Committee Consensus	ICMSF[a]	NRC[b]	FDA[c]
Defect action level	Maximum level of natural or unavoidable defect in foods for human use that presents no health hazard			Maximum levels of natural or unavoidable defects in foods for human use that present no health hazard
Food safety objective (FSO)	A statement of the maximum frequency and/or concentration of a hazard in a food at the time of consumption that is considered tolerable for consumers	A statement of the maximum frequency and/or concentration of a microbiological hazard in a food at the time of consumption that provides the appropriate level of protection		

FSIS[d]	NACMCF[e]	Codex[f]	WTO[g]	EC[h]
				A statement of the frequency or concentration of a microbiological hazard in a food appropriate for consumer protection

continued

TABLE A-1 Continued

Term	Committee Consensus	ICMSF[a]	NRC[b]	FDA[c]
Microbiological criterion	A criterion that defines the acceptability of a product or food lot, based on the absence or presence or number of microorganisms, including parasites, and/or the quantity of their toxins/ metabolites, per unit of mass volume, area, or lot	A microbiological criterion defines the acceptability of a product or food lot, based on the absence or presence or number of microorganisms, including parasites, and/or quantity of their toxins/ metabolites, per unit(s) of mass, volume, area or lot	A yardstick on which a judgment or decision can be made: a microbiological criterion will stipulate that a type of microorganism, group of microorganisms or toxin produced by a microorganism must either not be present at all, be present in only a limited number of samples, or be present as less than specified number or amount in a given quantity of a food or food ingredient	

FSIS[d]	NACMCF[e]	Codex[f]	WTO[g]	EC[h]
Microbiological criteria are not regulatory standards, but are benchmarks for evaluating test results				A microbiological criterion for food-stuffs defines the acceptability of a process, product or food lot based on the absence or presence, or number of microorganisms and/or quantity of their toxins/ metabolites, per unit(s) of mass, volume or area

continued

TABLE A-1 Continued

Term	Committee Consensus	ICMSF[a]	NRC[b]	FDA[c]
Microbiological guideline	An advisory microbiological criterion used to inform food operators of the microbiological content that can be expected in food when best practices are applied	An advisory criterion used to inform food operators of the microbiological content that can be expected in a food when best practices are applied	A criterion that often is used by the food industry or a regulatory agency to monitor a manufacturing process. Guidelines function as alert mechanisms to signal whether microbiological conditions prevailing at critical control points or in the finished product are within the normal range	
Microbiological specification	Part of a purchasing agreement between a buyer and a supplier of a food; such criteria may be mandatory or advisory according to use	Part of a purchasing agreement between a buyer and a supplier of a food; such criteria may be mandatory or advisory according to use	A microbiological criterion that is used as a purchase requirement whereby conformance with it becomes a condition of purchase between a buyer and vendor of a food or ingredient; such criteria may be either mandatory or advisory	

FSIS[d]	NACMCF[e]	Codex[f]	WTO[g]	EC[h]
				Criteria included in legislation or regulations which are intended to guide the manufacturer and help to ensure good hygienic practice

continued

TABLE A-1 Continued

Term	Committee Consensus	ICMSF[a]	NRC[b]	FDA[c]
Microbiological standard	A mandatory microbiological criterion that is incorporated into a law, regulation, or ordinance	A mandatory criterion that is incorporated into a law or ordinance	A microbiological criterion that is a part of a law, ordinance or administrative regulation. A standard is a mandatory criterion. Failure to comply with it constitutes a violation of the law, ordinance, or regulation and will be subject to the enforcement policy of the regulatory agency having jurisdiction	
Monitor	The act of conducting a planned sequence of observations or measurements of control parameters to assess whether a CCP is under control	The act of conducting a planned sequence of observations or measurements of control parameters to assess whether a CCP is under control		To conduct a planned sequence of observations or measurement to assess whether a process, point, or procedure is under control and to produce an accurate record for use in verification

FSIS[d]	NACMCF[e]	Codex[f]	WTO[g]	EC[h]
A criterion that is part of a regulation; is a legal requirement				Criteria included in legislation or regulations where failure to comply with them can result in rejection of the food
Monitoring consists of observations or measurements taken to assess whether a CCP is within the established critical limit	To conduct a planned sequence of observations or measurements to assess whether a CCP is under control and to produce an accurate record for future use in verification	The act of conducting a planned sequence of observations or measurements of control parameters to assess whether a CCP is under control		

continued

TABLE A-1 Continued

Term	Committee Consensus	ICMSF[a]	NRC[b]	FDA[c]
Performance criterion	The required outcome of a step, or combination of steps, that contributes to assuring a food safety objective is met	The required outcome of a step, or combination of steps, that contribute to assuring a food safety objective is met		A public health goal that is based on relating the level of stringency with achieving some level of control over the public health impact of the hazard; it requires being able to qualitatively or quantitatively relate the level of hazard in a food with its public health impact
Performance standard	The degree to which a step or combination of steps in the production, processing, distribution, and/or preparation of a food must operate to achieve the required level of control over a hazard			The degree to which a step or combination of steps in the production, processing, distribution, and/or preparation of a food MUST operate to achieve the desired level of control over a hazard

FSIS[d]	NACMCF[e]	Codex[f]	WTO[g]	EC[h]
Performance standards prescribe the objectives or levels of performance (such as pathogen reduction standards for raw product) establishments must achieve	Defines the expected level of control at one or more steps in a process; establishing and meeting performance standards can be a means of reaching public health goals to reduce foodborne illness; the stringency of a performance standard should be proportional to the risk and stated public health goals			

continued

TABLE A-1 Continued

Term	Committee Consensus	ICMSF[a]	NRC[b]	FDA[c]
Process criteria	The control parameters of a step, or combination of steps, that can be applied to achieve a performance criterion	The control parameters of a step, or combination of steps, that can be applied to achieve a performance criterion		
Processing safety objective	The FSO minus projected pathogen growth	The FSO minus projected pathogen growth		
Product criterion	A parameter of a food that can be used to assess the acceptability of a lot or consignment	A parameter of a food that can be used to assess the acceptability of a lot or consignment		
Public health goal	The desired outcome associated with reducing the burden of disease in society			
Public health objective	A measurable population-based target for maintaining or improving health			

FSIS[d]	NACMCF[e]	Codex[f]	WTO[g]	EC[h]

continued

TABLE A-1 Continued

Term	Committee Consensus	ICMSF[a]	NRC[b]	FDA[c]
Tolerable level of risk	The level of risk proposed following consideration of the public health impact, technological feasibility, economic implications, and that which society regards as reasonable in the context of, and in comparison with, other risks in everyday life	The level of risk proposed following consideration of public health impact, technological feasibility, economic implications, and that which society regards as reasonable in the context of, and in comparison with, other risks in everyday life		
Validation	Obtaining evidence that the elements of the Hazard Analysis and Critical Control Point (HACCP) plan are effective	Obtaining evidence that the elements of the HACCP plan are effective		Element of verification focused on collecting and evaluating scientific and technical information to determine whether the HACCP plan, when properly implemented, will effectively control the identified food hazards

FSIS[d]	NACMCF[e]	Codex[f]	WTO[g]	EC[h]
The scientific and technical process for determining that the CCPs and associated critical limits are adequate and sufficient to control likely hazards	The element of verification focused on collecting and evaluating scientific and technical information to determine if the HACCP plan, when properly implemented, will effectively control the hazards	Obtaining evidence that the elements of the HACCP plan are effective		

continued

TABLE A-1 Continued

Term	Committee Consensus	ICMSF[a]	NRC[b]	FDA[c]
Verification	The application of methods, procedures, tests, and other evaluations, in addition to monitoring, to determine compliance with the HACCP plan	The application of methods, procedures, tests, and other evaluations, in addition to monitoring, to determine compliance with the HACCP plan		Those activities, other than monitoring, that establish the validity of the HACCP plan and that the system is operating according to the plan
Zero tolerance	Lay audience perception of the absence of a hazard that cannot be scientifically assured, but is operationally defined as the absence of a hazard in a specified amount of food as determined by a specific method			

[a] ICMSF = International Commission on Microbiological Criteria for Foods (ICMSF, 1997, 1998, 2002).
[b] NRC = National Research Council (NRC, 1985).
[c] FDA = Food and Drug Administration (FDA, 1995, 2001).
[d] USDA = U.S. Department of Agriculture (USDA, 1996).
[e] NACMCF = National Advisory Committee on Microbiological Criteria for Foods (NACMCF, 1997, 2002).
[f] Codex = Codex Alimentarius Commission (CAC, 1997).
[g] WTO = World Trade Organization (WTO, 1995).
[h] EC = European Commission (EC, 1999).

FSIS[d]	NACMCF[e]	Codex[f]	WTO[g]	EC[h]
	Those activities, other than monitoring, that determine the validity of the HACCP plan and that the system is operating according to the plan	The application of methods, procedures, tests, and other evaluations, in addition to monitoring, to determine compliance with the HACCP plan		

Microbiological guidelines are usually established by a regulatory authority, industry trade association, or a company to indicate the expected microbial content of a food when best practices are applied. Food companies use microbiological guidelines as a basis to design their control systems. These guidelines are advisory in nature and may not lead to rejection of a food (ICMSF, 2002).

Microbiological specifications are used by buyers of a food or ingredient to reduce the likelihood of purchasing a product that may be of unacceptable safety or quality. Microbiological specifications can define the microbiological limits for an ingredient so that when it is used, the final product will meet all the requirements for safety and quality. Buyers throughout the food system establish microbiological specifications for materials they purchase. In most cases, specifications are advisory and the materials are sampled periodically. When microbiologically sensitive ingredients are purchased, each incoming lot may be sampled and tested (ICMSF, 2002).

A performance standard is the degree to which a step or combination of steps in the production, processing, distribution, and/or preparation of a food must operate to achieve the desired level of control over a hazard (Personal communication, R. Buchanan, Food and Drug Administration, February 5, 2002). The term performance standard does not appear anywhere in the U.S. Department of Agriculture Pathogen Reduction/Hazard Analysis and Critical Control Point Final Rule (USDA, 1996), but was incorporated from regulations used in other industries.

It should be noted that the committee defined a food safety objective as a statement of the maximum frequency and/or hazard in a food at the time of consumption that is considered tolerable for consumer protection. This is broader and less restrictive than the ICMSF definition of the term because it includes microbiological, chemical, and physical hazards. It should also be noted that the committee changed the word "acceptable" to "tolerable" because contamination of food is seldom acceptable; it cannot be deemed "appropriate" either.

A public health objective is a measurable population-based target for maintaining or improving health, while a public health goal is the desired outcome associated with reducing the burden of disease in society.

The committee defined the term zero tolerance as the lay audience perception of the absence of a hazard that cannot be scientifically assured but is operationally defined as the absence of a hazard in a specified amount of food as determined by a specific method.

REFERENCES

CAC (Codex Alimentarius Commission). 1997. *Hazard Analysis and Critical Control Point System and Guidelines for its Application.* Annex to CAC/RCP 1-1969, Rev. 3-1997. Rome: CAC.

EC (European Commission). 1999. *The Evaluation of Microbiological Criteria for Food Products of Animal Origin for Human Consumption.* Online. Available at http://europa.eu.int/comm/food/fs/sc/scv/out26_en.pdf. Accessed March 14, 2003.

FDA (Food and Drug Administration). 1995. Procedures for the safe and sanitary processing and importing of fish and fishery products; Final rule. *Fed Regist* 60:65095–65202.

FDA. 2001. HACCP procedures for the safe and sanitary processing and importing of juice: Final rule. *Fed Regist* 66:6137–6202.

FSIS (Food Safety and Inspection Service). 1996. Pathogen reduction; Hazard analysis and critical control point (HACCP) systems; Final rule. *Fed Regist* 61:38805–38855.

ICMSF (International Commission on Microbiological Specification for Foods). 1997. Establishment of microbiological safety criteria for foods in international trade. *World Health Stat Q* 50:119–123 .

ICMSF. 1998. Potential Application of Risk Assessment Techniques to Microbiological Issues Related to International Trade in Food and Food Products. *J Food Prot* 61:1075–1086.

ICMSF. 2002. *Microorganisms in Foods 7. Microbiological Testing in Food Safety Management.* New York: Klewer Academic/Plenum Publishers.

NACMCF (National Advisory Committee on Microbiological Criteria for Foods). 1997. Hazard analysis and critical control point principles and application guidelines. *J Food Prot* 61:1246-1259.

NACMCF. 2002. Final. Response to the Questions Posed by FSIS Regarding Performance Standards with Particular Reference to Ground Beef Products. Online. FSIS, U.S. Department of Agriculture. Available at http://www.fsis.usda.gov/OPHS/nacmcf/2002/rep_stand2.pdf. Accessed March 12, 2003.

NRC (National Research Council). 1985. *An Evaluation of the Role of Microbiological Criteria for Foods and Food Ingredients.* Washington, DC: National Academy Press.

USDA (U.S. Department of Agriculture). 1996. Pathogen reduction; Hazard analysis and critical control point (HACC) systems; Final rule. *Fed Regist* 61:38805–38989.

WTO (World Trade Organization). 1995. *Agreement on the Application of Sanitary and Phytosanitary Measures (SPS).* Geneva: WTO.

Appendix B

Sanitation Performance Standards

The following are excerpts from FSIS Directive 11000.1 (FSIS, 2000).

A. Grounds and Pest Control

1. What are the regulatory performance standards for grounds and pest control?

Section 416.2 (a) states that "The grounds about an establishment must be maintained to prevent conditions that could lead to insanitary conditions, adulteration of product, or interfere with inspection by FSIS [Food Safety Inspection Service] program employees. Establishments must have in place a pest management program to prevent harborage and breeding of pests on the grounds and within establishment facilities. Pest control substances used must be safe and effective under the conditions of use and not be applied or stored in a manner that will result in the adulteration of product or the creation of insanitary conditions."

2. What do the performance standards mean?

Proper maintenance of the grounds about an establishment is essential for ensuring good sanitation. However, establishments are responsible for preventing sources of adulteration of product even if the cause of the adulteration originates from conditions outside the designated boundaries of the establishment.

The pest management program does not have to be written.

B. Construction

1. What are the regulatory performance standards for construction?

Section 416.2 (b) states: "(1) Establishment buildings, including their structures, rooms, and compartments must be of sound construction, be kept in good repair, and be of sufficient size to allow for processing, handling, and storage of product in a manner that does not result in product adulteration or the creation of insanitary conditions.

(2) Walls, floors, and ceilings within establishments must be built of durable materials impervious to moisture and be cleaned and sanitized as necessary to prevent adulteration of product or the creation of insanitary conditions.

(3) Walls, floors, ceilings, doors, windows, and other outside openings must be constructed and maintained to prevent the entrance of vermin, such as flies, rats, and mice.

(4) Rooms or compartments in which edible product is processed, handled, or stored must be separate and distinct from rooms or compartments in which inedible product is processed, handled or stored, to the extent necessary to prevent product adulteration and the creation of insanitary conditions."

2. What do these performance standards mean?

The establishment buildings must be sound and kept in good repair to prevent insanitary conditions or the adulteration of product. Establishments currently maintaining sanitary conditions will not be required to make changes to their construction or layout because of this performance standard. Establishments can process, handle, or store edible and inedible product in the same room as long as they are separated by time or space, in a manner sufficient to prevent the adulteration of the edible product or the creation of insanitary conditions.

C. Light

1. What are the regulatory performance standards for lighting?

Section 416.2 (c) states that "Lighting of good quality and sufficient intensity to ensure that sanitary conditions are maintained and that product is not adulterated must be provided in areas where food is processed, handled, stored, or examined; where equipment and utensils are cleaned; and in hand-washing areas, dressing and locker rooms, and toilets."

2. What do the performance standards mean?

We have abolished the specific lighting requirements in the poultry regulations and have combined the separate meat and poultry lighting requirements into one performance standard. While we are giving establishments flexibility in determining lighting requirements, lighting must be adequate in quality and well distributed to allow for the monitoring of sanitary conditions and processing conditions, and to examine product for evidence of adulteration.

D. Ventilation

1. What are the regulatory performance standards for ventilation?

Section 416.2 (d) states that "Ventilation adequate to control odors, vapors, and condensation to the extent necessary to prevent adulteration of product and the creation of insanitary conditions must be provided."

2. What does the performance standard mean?

We do not expect that an establishment's ventilation will be able to completely eliminate all odors, vapors, and condensation but it must control them as far as necessary to prevent adulteration of product or the creation of insanitary conditions.

E. Plumbing and Sewage

1. What are the regulatory performance standards?

a. Section 416.2 (e) states: "Plumbing systems must be installed and maintained to:

(1) Carry sufficient quantities of water to required locations throughout the establishment;
(2) Properly convey sewage and liquid disposable waste from the establishment;
(3) Prevent adulteration of product, water supplies, equipment, and utensils and prevent the creation of insanitary conditions throughout the establishment;
(4) Provide adequate floor drainage in all areas where floors are subject to flooding type cleaning or where normal operations release or discharge water or other liquid waste on the floor;
(5) Prevent back-flow conditions in and cross-connection between piping systems that discharge waste water or sewage and piping systems that carry water for product manufacturing; and
(6) Prevent the backup of sewer gases."

b. Section 416.2 (f) states that "Sewage must be disposed into a sewage system separate from all other drainage lines or disposed of through other means sufficient to prevent backup of sewage into areas where product is processed, handled, or stored. When the sewage disposal system is a private system requiring approval by a State or local health authority, the establishment must furnish FSIS with the letter of approval from that authority upon request."

2. What do the performance standards mean?

It is the responsibility of the establishment to ensure that plumbing and sewage systems provide an adequate supply of potable water and remove waste and sewage from the establishment without adulterating product or creating insanitary conditions.

F. Water Supply and Water, Ice, and Solution Reuse

1. What are the regulatory performance standards for water supply and water, ice, and solution reuse?

Section 416.2 (g) states: "(1) A supply of running water that complies with the National Primary Drinking Water regulations (40 CFR part 141), at a suitable temperature and under pressure as needed, must be provided in all areas where required (for processing product, for cleaning rooms and equipment, utensils, and packaging materials, for employee sanitary facilities, etc.). If an establishment uses a municipal water supply, it must make available to FSIS, upon request, a water report, issued under the authority of the State or local health agency, certifying or attesting to the potability of the water supply. If an establishment uses a private well for its water supply, it must make available to FSIS, upon request, documentation certifying the potability of the water supply that has been renewed at least semi-annually.

(2) Water, ice, and solutions (such as brine, liquid smoke, or propylene glycol) used to chill or cook ready-to-eat product may be reused for the same purpose, provided that they are maintained free of pathogenic organisms and fecal coliform organisms and that other physical, chemical, and microbiological contamination have been reduced to prevent adulteration of product.

(3) Water, ice, and solutions to chill or wash raw product may be reused for the same purpose provided that measures are taken to reduce physical, chemical, or microbiological contamination so as to prevent contamination or adulteration of product.

Reuse that has come into contact with raw product may not be used on ready-to-eat product.

(4) Reconditioned water that has never contained human waste and that has been treated by an onsite advanced waste water treatment facility may be used on

raw product, except in product formulation, and throughout the facility in edible and inedible production areas, provided that measures are taken to ensure that this water meets the criteria prescribed in paragraph (g)(1) of this section. Product, facilities, equipment, and utensils coming in contact with this water must undergo a separate final rinse with nonreconditioned water that meets the criteria prescribed in paragraph (g)(1) of this section.

(5) Any water that has never contained human waste and that is free of pathogenic organisms may be used in edible and inedible product areas, provided it does not contact edible product. For example, such reuse water may be used to move heavy solids, to flush the bottom of open evisceration troughs, or to wash antemortem areas, livestock pens, trucks, poultry cages, picker aprons, picking room floors, and similar areas within the establishment.

(6) Water that does not meet the use conditions of paragraphs (g)(1) through (g)(5) of this section may not be used in areas where edible product is handled or prepared or in any manner that would allow it to adulterate edible product or create insanitary conditions."

2. What do the performance standards mean?

The water performance standard makes transparent the current requirement that potable water comply with EPA's [Environmental Protection Agency] National Primary Drinking Water regulations. Certifications of water potability provided by the state or local governments or other responsible entities will show whether water meets the EPA requirements.

Some meat and poultry establishments use private wells for their water supply. EPA does not require testing for these water sources. Usually the state or local governments do not test the wells for potability. Most establishments can obtain the needed documentation from private laboratories. The regulations require that documentation certifying the potability of water from private systems be renewed at least semi-annually. Establishments can reuse water in a manner that will neither adulterate product nor create insanitary conditions. FSIS permitted under the old regulations certain uses of nonpotable water. For example, an establishment recirculating water in a chill tank for raw poultry might add chlorine to the water to reduce the number of pathogens. An establishment reusing ice to chill raw poultry might bag the ice to prevent it from contacting product. FSIS is making final performance standards that will provide for the reuse of water in numerous processing contexts, provided that the establishment takes actions necessary to ensure that product is not adulterated by the water and that sanitation is not compromised.

In many cases establishments will document and monitor water reuse activities as part of their HACCP [Hazard Analysis and Critical Control Point] plans (See 417.2), because the water treatments or conditioning will eliminate or reduce hazards they have determined would be otherwise reasonably likely to occur. The requirements that water be reused only "for the same purpose" refers to whether water is reused for processing ready-to-eat or not ready-to-eat products; it does not prohibit the reuse of water for different processes. For example, an establishment could reuse poultry chiller water in a scalding tank. An establishment could not, however, reuse poultry chiller water for cooking or cooling packaged ready-to-eat product.

G. Dressing Room/Lavatory

1. What are the regulatory performance standards for dressing rooms and lavatories?

a. Section 416.2 (h) states: "(1) Dressing rooms, toilet rooms and urinals must be sufficient in number, ample in size, conveniently located, and maintained in a sanitary condition and in good repair at all times to ensure cleanliness of all persons handling any product. They must be separate from the rooms and compartments in which products are processed, stored, or handled.

(2) Lavatories with running hot and cold water, soap, and towels, must be placed in or near toilet and urinal rooms and at such other places in the establishment as necessary to ensure cleanliness of all persons handling any product.

(3) Refuse receptacles must be constructed and maintained in a manner that protects against the creation of insanitary conditions and the adulteration of product."

2. What do the performance standards mean?

OSHA [Occupational Safety and Health Administration] has always had standards for lavatories in their regulations (29 CFR 1910.141). These standards should be followed when establishments are constructed. FSIS will no longer dictate the number of lavatories required. Lavatory facilities need to be maintained by the establishment in good repair and in a sanitary manner.

H. Equipment/Utensils

1. What are the regulatory performance standards for equipment and utensils?

a. Section 416.3 states: "(a) Equipment and utensils used for processing or otherwise handling edible product or ingredients must be of such material and construction to facilitate thorough cleaning and to ensure that their use will not cause the adulteration of product during processing, handling, or storage. Equipment and utensils must be maintained in sanitary condition so as not to adulterate product.

(b) Equipment or utensils must not be constructed, located, or operated in a manner that prevents FSIS inspection program employees from inspecting the equipment or utensils to determine whether they are in sanitary condition.

(c) Receptacles used for storing inedible material must be of such material and construction that their use will not result in the adulteration of any edible product or in the creation of insanitary conditions. Such receptacles must not be used for storing any edible product and must bear conspicuous and distinctive marking to identify permitted uses."

2. What do the performance standards mean?

Establishments have the flexibility to choose whatever method they want to clean utensils and equipment to ensure that they are maintained in sanitary condition so as not to adulterate product. We have eliminated the requirement that utensils and equipment used to dress diseased meat carcasses be cleaned with either 180 degree F water or an approved disinfectant. FSIS no longer requires a specific method for the cleaning of utensils and equipment used to dress diseased meat carcasses, although they must still be maintained in a sanitary condition.

I. Sanitary Operations

1. What are the regulatory performance standards for sanitary operations?

Section 416.4 states: "(a) All food-contact surfaces, including food-contact surfaces of utensils and equipment, must be cleaned and sanitized as frequently as necessary to prevent the creation of insanitary conditions and the adulteration of product.

(b) Non-food-contact surfaces of facilities, equipment, and utensils used in the operation of the establishment must be cleaned and sanitized as frequently as necessary to prevent the creation of insanitary conditions and the adulteration of product.

(c) Cleaning compounds, sanitizing agents, processing aids, and other chemicals used by an establishment must be safe and effective under the conditions of use. Such chemicals must be used, handled, and stored in a manner that will not adulterate product or create insanitary conditions. Documentation substantiating the safety of a chemical's use in a food processing environment must be available to FSIS inspection program employees for review." (In most cases the documentation will be "Material Safety Data Sheet." You do not keep these documents in your office files.)

(d) "Product must be protected from adulteration during processing, handling, storage, loading, and unloading at and during transportation from official establishments."

2. What do the performance standards mean?

Usually, an establishment cleans up its operations once a day; however, some establishments have for some time conducted chemical cleanup procedures less than once a day. Currently, establishments may use extended cleanup procedures without prior approval of FSIS. FSIS expects an establishment to incorporate extended cleanup procedures into its Sanitation SOPs [Standard Operating Procedures] (See 416.12). To ensure that extended cleanup procedures prevent insanitation and the adulteration of product, most establishments will probably conduct microbiological and chemical sampling that evaluates the effectiveness of the extended cleanup. The establishment's Sanitation SOPs records would include the microbiological and chemical data that distinguish acceptable sanitary conditions from marginal or unacceptable sanitary conditions. (See 416.14). During the normal course of an establishment's operations meat and poultry products should not come in contact with non-food contact surfaces. Still if non-food contact surfaces are not properly cleaned and sanitized, insanitary conditions could result, leading to the potential adulteration of product. We have discontinued approving all nonfood compounds and proprietary substances before use in official meat and poultry establishments. We are continuing to require that meat and poultry products be neither adulterated nor misbranded through the misuse of proprietary substances and nonfood compounds.

Documentation substantiating the safety of a chemical's use in a food-processing environment must be available for your review. The documentation will vary with the nature and intended use of that chemical. For example, for a pesticide, an establishment should have documentation showing that the compound is registered with EPA and the label information for the pesticide. For a chemical sanitizer used on food contact surfaces, an establishment should have documentation showing that the compound complies with the relevant Food and Drug Administration regulations in 21 CFR 178.1010. (Sanitizers meeting this requirement are usually identified as "Food Grade.")

Meat and poultry establishments are responsible for ensuring that all proprietary substances and nonfood compounds are safe for their intended use and used appropriately.

Establishments are free to choose whatever scientifically supportable method they find effective in limiting microbial growth in their operations.

J. Employee Hygiene

1. What are the regulatory performance standards for employee hygiene?

Section 416.5 states: "(a) Cleanliness. All persons working in contact with product, food-contact surfaces and product-packaging materials must adhere to hygienic practices while on duty to prevent adulteration of product and the creation of insanitary conditions.

(b) Clothing. Aprons, frocks, and other outer clothing worn by persons who handle product must be of material that is disposable or readily cleaned. Clean garments must be worn at the start of each working day and garments must be changed during the day as often as necessary to prevent adulteration of product and the creation of insanitary conditions.

(c) Disease control. Any person who has or appears to have an infectious disease, open lesion, including boils, sores, or infected wounds, or any other abnormal source of microbial contamination, must be excluded from any operations which could result in product adulteration and the creation of insanitary conditions until the condition is corrected."

2. What do the performance standards mean?

Specific types of unhygienic practices have been removed from the regulations. You continue to have the authority to take action against any unhygienic practice that could result in insanitary conditions or adulterated product.

K. Custom Exempt Facilities

1. What are the regulatory performance standards for custom exempt facilities?

Section 303.1 (2) (i) states: "Establishments that conduct custom operations must be maintained and operated in accordance with the provisions of §§ 416.1 through 416.6, except for § 416.2 (g) (2) through (6) of this chapter, regarding water reuse and any provisions of part 416 of this chapter relating to inspection or supervision of specified activities or other action by a Program employee. If custom operations are conducted in an official establishment, however, all of the provisions of Part 416 of this chapter shall apply to those operations."

2. What does the performance standard mean?

Custom exempt facilities must comply with the sanitation performance standards except for sections 416.2 (g) paragraphs (1) through (6) about water reuse. The establishment conducting custom exempt/retail exempt activities should also operate in accordance with time/space separation and adequate procedures to ensure that product does not bear the mark of inspection.

REFERENCE

FSIS (Food Safety and Inspection Service). 2000. *FSIS Directive 11000.1 Sanitation Performance Standards*. Online. U.S. Department of Agriculture. Available at http://www.fsis.usda.gov/OPPDE/rdad/FSISDirectives/FSISDir11000.1.pdf. Accessed May 15, 2002.

Appendix C

Food and Drug Administration and Environmental Protection Agency Guidance Levels for Seafood

TABLE C-1 Microbiological and Chemical Guidelines/Tolerances in Seafood

Product	Guideline/Tolerance	Reference
Ready to eat fishery products (minimal cooking by consumer)	Enterotoxigenic *Escherichia coli* (ETEC): 1×10^3 ETEC/g, LT or ST positive	Compliance Program 7303.842
	Listeria monocytogenes: presence of organism	Compliance Program 7303.842
	Vibrio cholerae: presence of toxigenic 01 or non-01	Compliance Program 7303.842
	V. parahaemolyticus: level $\geq 1 \times 10^4$/g (Kanagawa positive or negative)	Compliance Program 7303.842
	V. vulnificus: presence of pathogenic organism	Compliance Program 7303.842
All fish	*Salmonella* species: presence of organism	Compliance Policy Guide Section 555.300
	1. *Staphylococcus aureus:* positive for staphylococcal enterotoxin, or 2. *S. aureus* level $\geq 10^4$/g (most probable number [MPN])	Compliance Program 7303.842

continued

TABLE C-1 Continued

Product	Guideline/Tolerance	Reference
All fish (continued)	*Clostridium botulinum:* 1. Presence of viable spores or vegetative cells in products that will support their growth; or, 2. Presence of toxin	Compliance Program 7303.842
	Polychlorinated biphenyls: 2.0 ppm (edible portion)[a]	21 CFR 109.30
	Chlordane: 0.3 ppm (edible portion)	Compliance Policy Guide Section 575.100
	Chlordecone: 0.4 ppm crabmeat and 0.3 ppm in other fish (edible portion)	Compliance Policy Guide Section 575.100
	DDT, TDE and DDE: 5.0 ppm (edible portion)	Compliance Policy Guide Section 575.100
	Heptachlor and heptachlor epoxide: 0.3 ppm (edible portion)	Compliance Policy Guide Section 575.100
	Mirex: 0.1 ppm (edible portion)	Compliance Policy Guide Section 575.100
	Diquat: 0.1 ppm[a]	40 CFR 180.226
	2,4-D: 1.0 ppm[a]	40 CFR 180.142
	Sulfamerazine: no residue permitted	21 CFR 556.660
	Unsanctioned drugs[b]: no residue permitted	Compliance Policy Guide Section 615.200
	Methyl mercury: 1.0 ppm	Compliance Policy Guide Section 540.600
	Paralytic shellfish poison: 0.8 ppm (80 μg/100 g) saxitoxin equivalent	Compliance Policy Guide Section 540.250 and Compliance Program 7303.842
	Amnesic shellfish poison: 20 ppm domoic acid, except in the viscera of dungeness crab, where 30 ppm is permitted	Compliance Program 7303.842
Salt-cured, air-dried uneviscerated fish	Not permitted in commerce (small fish exemption)	Compliance Policy Guide Section 540.650
Tuna, mahi mahi, and related fish	Histamine: 500 ppm set based on toxicity; 50 ppm set as defect action level, because histamine is generally not uniformly distributed in a decomposed fish; therefore, if 50 ppm is found in one section, there is the possibility that other units may exceed 500 ppm	Compliance Policy Guide Section 540.525

TABLE C-1 Continued

Product	Guideline/Tolerance	Reference
Fin fish	Glyphosate: 0.25 ppm[a] Simazine: 12 ppm[a]	40 CFR 180.364 40 CFR 180.213a
Fin fish and shellfish	Aldrin and dieldrin: 0.3 ppm (edible portion)	Compliance Policy Guide Section 575.100
Fin fish and crayfish	Fluridone: 0.5 ppm[a]	40 CFR 180.420
Frog legs	Benzene hexachloride: 0.3 ppm (edible portion)	Compliance Policy Guide Section 575.100
Shellfish	Glyphosate: 3.0 ppm[a]	40 CFR 180.364
Salmonids, catfish and lobster	Oxytetracycline: 2.0 ppm	21 CFR 556.500
Salmonids and catfish	Sulfadimethoxine/ormetoprim combination: 0.1 ppm	21 CFR 556.640
Crustacea	Toxic elements: 76 ppm arsenic, 3 ppm cadmium, 12 ppm chromium, 1.5 ppm lead, 70 ppm nickel	Food and Drug Administration Guidance Documents
Clams and oysters, fresh or frozen, imports	Microbiological: 1. *E. coli:* MPN of 230/100 g (average of subs or 3 or more of 5 subs) 2. Aerobic plate count (APC): 500,000/g (average of subs or 3 or more of 5 subs)	Compliance Policy Guide Section 560.600
Clams, oysters, and mussels, fresh or frozen, domestic	Microbiological: 1. *E. coli* or fecal coliform: 1 or more of 5 subs exceeding MPN of 330/100 g or 2 or more exceeding 230/100 g 2. APC: 1 or more of 5 subs exceeding 1,500,000/g or 2 or more exceeding 500,000/g	Compliance Program 7303.842
Clams, oysters, and mussels	Toxic elements: 86 ppm arsenic, 4 ppm cadmium, 13 ppm chromium, 1.7 ppm lead, 80 ppm nickel	FDA Guidance Documents

continued

TABLE C-1 Continued

Product	Guideline/Tolerance	Reference
Clams, mussels and oysters, fresh, frozen, or canned	Neurotoxic shellfish poison: 0.8 ppm (20 mouse units/100 g) brevetoxin-2 equivalent	National Shellfish Sanitation Program Manual of Operations

NOTE: The term "fish" refers to fresh or saltwater fin fish, crustaceans, other forms of aquatic animal life other than birds or mammals, and all mollusks, as defined in 21 C.F.R. §123.3(d).
[a] These values are tolerances.
[b] Sanctioned drugs are approved drugs, low regulatory priority drugs, and drugs used under an investigational new drug application.
SOURCE: CFSAN (2001).

TABLE C-2 Limiting Conditions for Pathogen Growth in Seafood

Pathogen	Min a_w	Min pH	Max pH	Max % Salt	Min Temp	Max Temp	Oxygen Requirement
Bacillus cereus	0.92	4.3	9.3	18	39.2°F 4°C	131°F 55°C	Aerobe
Campylobacter jejuni	0.987	4.9	9.5	1.5	86°F 30°C	113°F 45°C	Microaerophilic[a]
Clostridium botulinum, type A, and proteolytic B and F	0.935	4.6	9	10	50°F 10°C	118.4°F 48°C	Anaerobe[b]
C. botulinum, type E, and nonproteolytic B and F	0.97	5	9	5	37.9°F 3.3°C	113°F 45°C	Anaerobe[b]
C. perfringens	0.93	5	9	7	50°F 10°C	125.6°F 52°C	Anaerobe[b]
Pathogenic strains of *Escherichia coli*	0.95	4	9	6.5	44.6°F 7.0°C	120.9°F 49.4°C	Facultative anaerobe[c]
Listeria monocytogenes	0.92	4.4	9.4	10	31.3°F –0.4°C	113°F 45°C	Facultative anaerobe[c]
Salmonella spp.	0.94	3.7	9.5	8	41.4°F 5.2°C	115.2°F 46.2°C	Facultative anaerobe[c]
Shigella spp.	0.96	4.8	9.3	5.2	43°F 6.1°C	116.8°F 47.1°C	Facultative anaerobe[c]
Staphylococcus aureus growth	0.83	4	10	25	44.6°F 7°C	122°F 50°C	Facultative anaerobe[c]
S. aureus toxin	0.85	4	9.8	10	50°F 10°C	118°F 48°C	
Vibrio cholerae	0.97	5	10	6	50°F 10°C	109.4°F 43°C	Facultative anaerobe[c]
V. parahaemolyticus	0.94	4.8	11	10	41°F 5°C	111°F 44°C	Facultative anaerobe[c]
V. vulnificus	0.96	5	10	5	46.4°F 8°C	109.4°F 43°C	Facultative anaerobe[c]
Yersinia enterocolitica	0.945	4.2	10	7	29.7°F –1.3°C	107.6°F 42°C	Facultative anaerobe[c]

[a] Requires limited levels of oxygen.
[b] Requires the absence of oxygen.
[c] Grows either with or without oxygen.
SOURCE: CFSAN (2001).

TABLE C-3 Time and Temperature Guidance for Controlling Pathogen Growth and Toxin Formation in Seafood

Potentially Hazardous Condition	Product Temperature	Maximum Cumulative Exposure Time
Growth of *Campylobacter jejuni*	86–93°F (30–34°C)	48 hours
	Above 93°F (above 34°C)	12 hours
Germination, growth, and toxin formation by *Clostridium botulinum* type A, and proteolytic B and F	50–70°F (10–21°C)	12 hours[a]
	Above 70°F (above 21°C)	4 hours[a]
Germination, growth, and toxin formation by *C. botulinum* type E, and nonproteolytic B and F	37.9–50°F (3.3–10°C)	24 hours
	51–70°F (11–21°C)	12 hours
	Above 70°F (above 21°C)	4 hours[a]
Growth of pathogenic strains of *Escherichia coli*	44.6–50°F (7–10°C)	14 days
	51–70°F (11–21°C)	6 hours
	Above 70°F (above 21°C)	3 hours
Growth of *Listeria monocytogenes*	31.3–50°F (–0.4–10°C)	2 days
	51–70°F (11–21°C)	12 hours[a]
	Above 70°F (above 21°C)	3 hours[a]
Growth of *Salmonella* spp.	41.4–50°F (5.2–10°C)	14 days
	51–70°F (11–21°C)	6 hours
	Above 70°F (above 21°C)	3 hours
Growth of *Shigella* spp.	43–50°F (6.1–10°C)	14 days[a]
	51–70°F (11–21°C)	6 hours[a]
	Above 70°F (above 21°C)	3 hours[a]
Growth and toxin formation by *Staphylococcus aureus*	44.6–50°F (7–10°C)	14 days
	51–70°F (11–21°C)	12 hours[a]
	Above 70°F (above 21°C)	3 hours
Growth of *Vibrio cholerae*	50°F (10°C)	21 days
	51–70°F (11–21°C)	6 hours[a]
	Above 70°F (above 21°C)	2 hours[a]
Growth of *V. parahaemolyticus*	41–50°F (5–10°C)	21 days
	51–70°F (11–21°C)	6 hours[a]
	Above 70°F (above 21°C)	2 hours[a]
Growth of *V. vulnificus*	46.4–50°F (8–10°C)	21 days
	51–70°F (11–21°C)	6 hours
	Above 70°F (above 21°C)	2 hours
Growth of *Yersinia enterocolitica*	29.7–50°F (–1.3–10°C)	1 day
	51–70°F (11–21°C)	6 hours
	Above 70°F (above 21°C)	2.5 hours

[a] Additional data needed.
SOURCE: CFSAN (2001).

REFERENCE

CFSAN (Center for Food Safety and Applied Nutrition). 2001. *Fish and Fishery Products Hazards and Controls Guidance, 3rd ed.* Online. Food and Drug Administration. Available at http://www.cfsan.fda.gov/~comm/haccp4.html. Accessed December 27, 2002.

Appendix D

Food Defect Action Levels in Produce

TABLE D-1 Food and Drug Administration Levels of Natural or Unavoidable Defects in Fruit and Vegetable Products that Present No Health Hazards for Humans

Product	Defect	Defect Action Level	Defect Source (Significance)
Apple butter	Mold	Average of mold count is 12% or more	Postharvest infection
	Rodent filth	Average of 4 or more rodent hairs/100 g	Postharvest and/or processing contamination
	Insects	Average of 5 or more whole or equivalent insects (not counting mites, aphids, thrips, or scale insects)/100 g	Whole or equivalent insects: pre-/postharvest and processing insect infestation
Apricots, canned	Insect filth	Average of 2% or more by count has been damaged or infected by insects	Preharvest insect infestation
Asparagus, canned or frozen	Insect filth	10% by count of spears or pieces are infested with 6 or more asparagus beetle eggs and/or sacs	Preharvest insect infestation
	Insects	Asparagus contains an average of 40 or more thrips/100 g, insects (whole or equivalent) 3 mm or longer have an average aggregate length of 7 mm or longer/100 g	Preharvest insect infestation
Beets, canned	Rot	Average of 5% or more pieces by weight with dry rot	Preharvest mold infection
Berries, drupelet, canned and frozen (blackberries, raspberries, etc.)	Mold	Average mold count is 60% or more	Postharvest infection
	Insects and larvae	Average of 4 or more larvae/500 g Average of 10 or more whole insects or equivalent/500 g excluding thrips, aphids, and mites	Preharvest insect infestation
Berries, lingon, canned (European cranberry)	Insect larvae	Average of 3 or more larvae/lb in a minimum of 12 subsamples	Preharvest insect infestation
Berries, multer, canned	Insects	Average of 40 or more thrips/#2 can in all subsamples and 20% of subsamples are materially infested	Preharvest infestation
Broccoli, frozen	Insects and mites	Average of 60 or more aphids and/or thrips and/or mites/100 g	Preharvest insect infestation
Brussels sprouts, frozen	Insects	Average of 30 or more aphids and/or thrips/100 g	Preharvest infestation

Cherries, brined and maraschino, fresh, canned, or frozen	Insect filth	Average of 5% or more pieces are rejects due to maggots; average of 7% or more pieces are rejects due to insects other than maggots	Preharvest insect infestation Insect reject: pre- and/or postharvest insect infestation
	Rot	Average of 7% or more pieces are rejects due to rot	Rot reject: preharvest mold infection
Citrus fruit juices, canned	Mold	Average mold count is 10% or more	Processing contamination
	Insects and insect eggs	Five or more Drosophila and other fly eggs/250 ml or 1 or more maggots/250 ml	Postharvest insect infestation
Corn, sweet corn, canned	Insect larvae	Insect larvae (corn ear worm or corn borer) 2 or more 3 mm or longer larvae, cast skins, larval or cast skin fragments of corn ear worms or corn borer and the aggregate length of such larvae, cast skins, larval or cast skin fragments exceeds 12 mm in 24 lb (24 #303 cans or equivalent)	Preharvest insect infestation
Currants	Insect filth	5% or more, by count, wormy in the average of the subsamples	Preharvest insect infestation
Date material, chopped, sliced, or macerated	Insects	10 or more dead insects (whole or equivalent) in 1 or more subsamples; 5 or more dead insects (whole or equivalent)/100 g	Pre- and/or postharvest and/or processing insect infestation
	Pits	2 or more pits and/or pit fragments 2 mm or longer measured in the longest dimension/900 g	Processing
Dates, pitted	Multiple	Average of 5% or more dates by count are rejects (moldy, dead insects, insect excreta, sour, dirty, and/or worthless) as determined by macroscopic sequential examination	Insects, insect excreta, and mold: pre- and/or postharvest and/or processing Sour and worthless: preharvest Dirt: harvest contamination
	Pits	Average of 2 or more pits and/or pit fragments 2 mm or longer in the longest dimension/100 dates	Processing
Dates, whole	Multiple	Average of 5% or more dates by count are rejects (moldy, dead insects, insect excreta, sour, dirty, and/or worthless) as determined by microscopic sequential examination	Insect excreta and mold: pre- and/or postharvest and/or processing Sour and worthless: preharvest Dirt: harvest contamination

continued

TABLE D-1 Continued

Product	Defect	Defect Action Level	Defect Source (Significance)
Figs	Insect filth, mold, dirty fruit, or pieces of fruit	Average of 10% or more by count are insect-infested and/or moldy and/or dirty fruit or pieces of fruit	Insect infestation: pre- and/or postharvest infestation Mold: preharvest infection Dirt: harvest contamination Mold: potential health hazard, may contain mycotoxin-producing fungi
Greens, canned	Mildew	Average of 10% or more of leaves, by count or weight, showing mildew over $^1/_2$ in in diameter	Preharvest infection
Nectars, apricot, peach and pear	Mold	Average mold count is 12% or more	Preharvest infection
Olives, pitted	Pits	Average of 1.3% or more by count of olives with whole pits and/or pit fragments 2 mm or longer measured in the longest dimension	Processing
Olives, imported green	Insect damage	7% or more olives by count showing damage by olive fruit fly	Preharvest insect infestation
Olives, salad	Pits	Average of 1.3% or more olives by count of olives with whole pits and/or pit fragments 2 mm or longer measured in the longest dimension	Processing
Olives, salt-cured	Insects	Average of 10% or more olives by count with 10 or more scale insects each Average of 25% or more olives by count are moldy	Preharvest infestation, postharvest and/or processing infection
Olives, black, imported	Insect damage	10% or more olives by count showing damage by olive fruit fly	Preharvest insect infestation
Peaches, canned and frozen	Mold Insect damage; insects	Average of 3% or more fruit by count are wormy or moldy In 12 1-pound cans or equivalent, 1 or more larvae and/or larval fragments whose aggregate length exceeds 5 mm	Pre- and/or postharvest infection Insect damage: preharvest insect infestation Larvae: preharvest insect infestation

Peas, black-eyed, cowpeas, field peas, dried	Insect damage	Average of 10% or more by count of class 6 damage or higher in minimum of 12 subsamples	Pre- and/or postharvest insect infestation
Peas, cowpeas, black-eyed peas (succulent), canned	Insect larvae	Average of 5 or more cowpea curculio larvae or the equivalent/#2 can	Pre- and/or postharvest and/or processing insect infestation
Peas and beans, dried	Insect filth	Average of 5% or more by count insect-infested and/or insect-damaged by storage insects in minimum of 12 subsamples	Pre- and/or postharvest and/or processing infestation
Pineapple, canned	Mold	Average mold count is 20% or more; the mold count of any 1 subsample is 60% or more	Processing mold contamination
Pineapple, juice	Mold	Average mold count is 15% or more; the mold count of any 1 subsample is 40% or more	Processing mold contamination
Plums, canned	Rot	Average of 5% or more plums by count with rot spots larger than the area of a circle 12 mm in diameter	Pre- and/or postharvest infection
Prunes, dried and dehydrated, low moisture	Multiple defects	Average of 10 subsamples is 5% or more prunes by count are rejects (insect-infested, moldy or decomposed, dirty, and/or otherwise unfit)	Insect infestation: preharvest infestation Moldy and decomposed: preharvest infection Dirty: harvest contamination Otherwise unfit preharvest condition
Prunes, pitted	Pits	Average of 2% or more by count with whole pits and/or pit fragments 2 mm or longer and 4 or more of 10 subsamples of pitted prunes have 2% or more by count with whole pits and/or pit fragments 2 mm or longer	Processing
Puree, apricot, peach, and pear	Mold	Average mold count is 12% or more	Pre- and/or postharvest and/or processing infection
Raisins, natural and golden	Mold	Average of 10 subsamples is 5% or more, by count, moldy raisins	Postharvest and/or processing infection
	Sand and grit	Average of 40 mg or more of sand and grit/100 g of natural or golden bleached raisins	Postharvest contamination

continued

TABLE D-1 Continued

Product	Defect	Defect Action Level	Defect Source (Significance)
Raisins, golden	Insects and eggs	10 or more whole or equivalent insects and 35 Drosophila eggs/8 oz	Postharvest and/or processing infestation
Spinach, canned or frozen	Insects and mites	Average of 50 or more aphids, thrips, and/or mites/100 g	Preharvest infestation
		2 or more 3 mm or longer larvae and/or larval fragments of spinach worms (caterpillars) whose aggregate length exceeds 12 mm are present in 24 lb	
		Leaf miners of any size average 8 or more/100 g or leaf miners 3 mm or longer average 4 or more/100 g	
Strawberries, frozen, whole, or sliced	Mold	Average mold count of 45% or more and mold count of at least half of the subsamples is 55% or more	Postharvest and/or processing infection
	Grit	Berries taste gritty	Harvest contamination
Tomatoes, canned	Drosophila fly	Average of 10 or more fly eggs/500 g, or 5 or more fly eggs and 1 or more maggots/500 g, or 2 or more maggots/500 g	Pre- and/or postharvest and/or processing insect infestation
Tomatoes, canned with or without juice (based on drained juice)	Mold	Average mold count in 6 subsamples is 15% or more and the counts of all of the subsamples are more than 12%	Pre- and/or postharvest and/or processing infection
Tomatoes, canned, packed in tomato puree (based on drained liquid)	Mold	Average mold count in 6 subsamples is 29% or more and the counts of all of the subsamples are more than 25%	Pre- and/or postharvest and/or processing infection
Tomato juice	Drosophila fly	Average of 10 or more fly eggs/100 g, or 5 or more fly eggs and 1 or more maggots/100 g, or 2 or more maggots/100 g in a minimum of 12 subsamples	Pre- and postharvest and/or processing insect infestation
	Mold	Average mold count in 6 subsamples is 24% or more and the counts of all of the subsamples are more than 20%	Pre- and/or postharvest and/or processing infection
Tomato paste, pizza and other sauces	Drosophila fly	Average of 30 or more fly eggs/100 g, or 15 or more fly eggs and 1 or more maggots/100 g, or 2 or more maggots/100 g in a minimum of 12 subsamples	Pre- and/or postharvest and/or processing insect infestation

Tomato puree	Drosophila fly	Average of 20 or more fly eggs/100 g, or 10 or more fly eggs and 1 or more maggots/100 g, or 2 or more maggots/100 g in a minimum of 12 subsamples	Pre- and/or postharvest and/or processing insect infestation
Tomato paste, puree	Mold	Average mold count in 6 subsamples is 45% or more and the mold counts of all of the subsamples are more than 40%	Pre- and/or postharvest and/or processing infection
Pizza and other tomato sauces	Mold	Average mold count in 6 subsamples is 34% or more and the counts of all of the subsamples are more than 30%	Pre- and/or postharvest and/or processing infection
Tomato sauce, undiluted	Mold	Average mold count in 6 subsamples is 45% or more and the mold counts of all of the subsamples are more than 40%	Pre- and/or postharvest and/or processing infection
Tomato catsup	Mold	Average mold count in 6 subsamples is 55% or more	Pre- and/or postharvest and/or processing infection
Tomato powder, except spray-dried	Mold	Average mold count in 6 subsamples is 45% or more and the mold counts of all of the subsamples are more than 40%	Pre- and/or postharvest and/or processing infection
Tomato powder, spray-dried	Mold	Average mold count in 6 subsamples is 67% or more	Pre- and/or postharvest and/or processing infection
Tomato soup and tomato products	Mold	Average mold count in 6 subsamples is 45% or more and the mold counts of all of the subsamples are more than 40%	Pre- and/or postharvest and/or processing infection

SOURCE: CFSAN (1998).

REFERENCE

CFSAN (Center for Food Safety and Applied Nutrition). 1998. *The Food Defect Action Levels: Levels of Natural or Unavoidable Defects in Foods that Present No Health Hazards for Humans.* Online. U.S. Department of Agriculture. Available at http://vm.cfsan.fda.gov/~dms/dalbook.html. Accessed April 11, 2003.

Appendix E

International Microbiological Criteria

TABLE E-1 Ireland's Guidelines for the Microbiological Quality of Some Ready-to-Eat Foods at Point of Sale

		Microbiological Quality (cfu/g unless otherwise stated)			
Food Category[a]	Criterion	Satisfactory	Acceptable	Unsatisfactory	Unacceptable/ Potentially Hazardous
	Aerobic colony count				
A	30°C/48 h	$< 10^3$	10^3 to $< 10^4$	$\geq 10^4$	N/A[b]
B		$< 10^4$	10^4 to $< 10^5$	$\geq 10^5$	N/A
C		$< 10^5$	10^5 to $< 10^6$	$\geq 10^6$	N/A
D		$< 10^6$	10^6 to $< 10^7$	$\geq 10^7$	N/A
E		N/A	N/A	N/A	N/A
	Indicator organisms[c]				
A–E	*Enterobacteriaceae*	< 100	100 to $< 10^4$	$\geq 10^4$	N/A
A–E	*Escherichia coli* (total)	< 20	20 to < 100	≥ 100	N/A
A–E	*Listeria* spp. (total)	< 20	20 to < 100	≥ 100	N/A
	Pathogens				
A–E	*Salmonella* spp.	Not detected in 25 g			Detected in 25 g
A–E	*Campylobacter* spp.	Not detected in 25 g			Detected in 25 g
A–E	*E. coli* O157 and other verocytotoxin-producing *E. coli*	Not detected in 25 g			Detected in 25 g
A–E	*Vibrio cholerae*	Not detected in 25 g			Detected in 25 g
A–E	*Vibrio parahaemolyticus*[d]	< 20	20 to < 100	100 to $< 10^3$	
A–E	*L. monocytogenes*	< 20	20 to < 100	N/A	
A–E	*Staphylococcus aureus*	< 20	20 to < 100	100 to $< 10^4$	
A–E	*Clostridium perfringens*	< 20	20 to < 100	100 to $< 10^4$	
A–E	*Bacillus cereus* and other pathogenic *Bacillus* spp.	$< 10^3$	10^3 to $< 10^4$	10^4 to $< 10^6$	

[a] Category A includes beefburgers, meat pies, pork pies, sausage rolls, scotch eggs, raw pickled fish, mousse/desserts; Category B includes meat meals, poultry, cakes and pastries (without dairy cream), quiche, mayonnaise, dressings, vegetables, ice cream, ready-to-eat meals; Category C includes sliced beef, sliced pork,

sliced poultry, crustraceans, fish, cakes and pastries (with dairy cream), dried fruits and vegetables, rice; Category D includes sliced ham, mollusks and other shellfish, prepared mixed salads; Category E includes raw ham, smoked sausages, cheesecake, fermented foods, fresh fruits and vegetables, cheese, yogurt.

[b] N/A = not applicable.

[c] On occasion some strains may be pathogenic.

[d] Relevant to seafood only.

SOURCE: FSAI (2001).

TABLE E-2 International Commission on Microbiological Specifications for Foods (ICMSF) Sampling Plans and Recommended Microbiological Limits for Fruits, Vegetables, Nuts, and Yeast

							Limit per Gram	
Product	Test	Method Reference[a]	Case	Plan	n[b]	c[c]	m[d]	M[e]
Frozen fruits and vegetables (pH > 4.5)[f]	*Escherichia coli*	126/131	5	3	5	2	10^2[g]	10^3
Dried vegetables	*E. coli*	126/131	5	3	5	2	10^2[g]	10^3
Coconut (dessicated)	*Salmonella*	160[h]						
Growth not anticipated			11	2	10	0	0	—
Growth anticipated			12	2	20	0	0	—
Yeast	*Salmonella*	160[h]	12	2	20	0	0	—

[a] Refers to page number in ICMSF (1978) where methods are described. Use analytical unit sizes recommended in the methods.

[b] n = Number of samples taken.

[c] c = Maximum number of samples out of n that may exceed the value set for m.

[d] m = Analytical value that differentiates good quality from marginally acceptable quality.

[e] M = Analytical value that differentiates marginally acceptable quality from unacceptable quality.

[f] pH measured at the time of sampling. Commodities with pH 4.5 or less are not likely to represent a major hazard and criteria are not recommended.

[g] In the absence of systematic data m values are estimates.

[h] See also ISO 6579 (1981).

SOURCE: ICMSF (1986).

TABLE E-3 Canadian Standards for Fresh-Cut Produce

Food Category	Method or Equivalent	Guideline	Nature of Concern	Sampling Parameters[a]			
				n	*c*	*m*	*M*
Sprouted Seeds (e.g. alfalfa and bean sprouts)	MFHPB-19	Fecal coliforms	Sanitation	5	2	10^3	10^5
	MFHPB-19	*Escherichia coli*	Health 2[b]	5	2	10^2	10^3
	MFHPB-20	*Salmonella*	Health 2[c]	5	0	0	—

[a] *n* = Number of samples taken, *c* = maximum number of samples out of *n* that may exceed the value set for *m*, *m* = analytical value that differentiates good quality from marginally acceptable quality, *M* = analytical value that differentiates marginally acceptable quality from unacceptable quality.
[b] This becomes a Health 1 concern if verotoxin-producing strains are found.
[c] This becomes a Health 1 concern if targeted or distributed to a sensitive population, such as children less than five years of age, the elderly, or immunocompromised individuals.
SOURCE: HPFB (2003).

TABLE E-4 Australia and New Zealand Standards for Cultured Seeds and Grains

Food	Microorganism	n^a	C^b	m^c	M^d
Cultured seeds and grains (bean sprouts, etc.)	*Salmonella*/25 g	5	0	0	—

[a] n = Number of samples taken.
[b] c = Maximum number of samples out of n that may exceed the value set for m.
[c] m = Analytical value that differentiates good quality from marginally acceptable quality.
[d] M = Analytical value that differentiates marginally acceptable quality from unacceptable quality.
SOURCE: Food Standards Australia New Zealand (2003).

TABLE E-5 International Criteria for Produce

Country	Food Commodity	Other Information	Microorganisms or Metabolite
Canada	Apple juice	Unpasteurized	*Escherichia coli*
Canada	Apple juice	Unpasteurized	*E. coli* O157:H7
South Africa	Aromatic plants		Aerobic bacteria
South Africa	Aromatic plants		*Bacillus cereus*
South Africa	Aromatic plants		*Clostridium perfringens*
South Africa	Aromatic plants		Coliforms
South Africa	Aromatic plants		*E. coli*
South Africa	Aromatic plants		Molds
South Africa	Aromatic plants		*Salmonella* spp.
South Africa	Aromatic plants		*Staphylococcus aureus*
South Africa	Aromatic plants		Yeasts
Spain	Canned raw vegetables		Aerobic mesophilic microorganisms
Spain	Canned raw vegetables		*E. coli*
Spain	Canned raw vegetables		*Listeria monocytogenes*
Spain	Canned raw vegetables		*Salmonella* spp.
ICMSF[a]	Cereal products	Frozen and dried	*Salmonella* spp.
ICMSF	Cereal products	Frozen and dried	*S. aureus*
Cuba	Cereals	Ready-to-eat	Aerobic mesophilic microorganisms
Cuba	Cereals	Ready-to-eat	Molds
Cuba	Cereals	Ready-to-eat	Yeasts
ICMSF	Cereals		Molds
Spain	Cereals	Flakes	Aerobic mesophilic microorganisms
Spain	Cereals	Flakes or other expanded	*B. cereus*
Spain	Cereals	Flakes	*B. cereus*
Spain	Cereals	Flakes	*E. coli*
Spain	Cereals	Flakes	Molds
Spain	Cereals	Flakes	*Salmonella* spp.
Spain	Cereals	Flakes	Yeasts
Australia	Coconut	Dessicated	*Salmonella* spp.
ICMSF	Coconut	Desiccated, growth anticipated	*Salmonella* spp.
ICMSF	Coconut	Desiccated, growth not anticipated	*Salmonella* spp.
New Zealand	Coconut	Dried, grated	Coliforms faecal
New Zealand	Coconut	Dried, grated	Coliforms presumptive
New Zealand	Coconut	Dried, grated	*Salmonella* spp.

Numerical Values as Given in Original Publication[b] (in cfu/g or mL if not specified)	Sampling Plan as Given in Original Publication[c]	Point of Application	Legal Status
$m = 100$, $M = 1{,}000$	$n = 5$, $c = 2$	Manufacturing level	Guidelines
$m = 0$	$n = 5$, $c = 0$	Manufacturing level	Guidelines
1,000,000	Not specified	Retail	Mandatory
Not detectable in 20 g	Not specified	Retail	Mandatory
Not detectable in 20 g	Not specified	Retail	Mandatory
100	Not specified	Retail	Mandatory
Not detectable in 20 g	Not specified	Retail	Mandatory
10,000	Not specified	Retail	Mandatory
Not detectable in 20 g	Not specified	Retail	Mandatory
Not detectable in 20 g	Not specified	Retail	Mandatory
10,000	Not specified	Retail	Mandatory
$m = 1{,}000{,}000$, $M = 10{,}000{,}000$	$n = 5$, $c = 2$	Not specified	Not specified
$m = 100$, $M = 1{,}000$	$n = 5$, $c = 2$	Not specified	Not specified
Not detectable per 25 g	$n = 5$, $c = 0$	Not specified	Not specified
Not detectable per 25 g	$n = 5$, $c = 0$	Not specified	Not specified
$m = 0$	$n = 5$, $c = 0$	Port of entry	Guidelines
$m = 100$, $M = 10{,}000$	$n = 5$, $c = 0$	Port of entry	Guidelines
< 10,000	$n = 1$	Not specified	Mandatory
< 100	$n = 1$	Not specified	Mandatory
< 100	$n = 1$	Not specified	Mandatory
$m = 100$ to $10{,}000$, $M = 100{,}000$	$n = 5$, $c = 2$	Port of entry	Guidelines
10,000	Not specified	Not specified	Mandatory
< 10	$n = 1$	Retail/production	Mandatory
10	Not specified	Not specified	Mandatory
Not detectable	Not specified	Not specified	Mandatory
100	Not specified	Not specified	Mandatory
Not detectable per 25 g	Not specified	Not specified	Mandatory
100	Not specified	Not specified	Mandatory
$m = 0$ in 25 g	$n = 10$, $c = 0$	Not specified	Standards
$m = 0$	$n = 20$, $c = 0$	Port of entry	Guidelines
$m = 0$	$n = 10$, $c = 0$	Port of entry	Guidelines
$m = < 10$, $M = 10$	$n = 5$, $c = 2$	Not specified	Guidelines
$m = 100$, $M = 1{,}000$	$n = 5$, $c = 2$	Not specified	Guidelines
$m = 0$ per 25 g	$n = 5$, $c = 0$	Not specified	Guidelines

continued

TABLE E-5 Continued

Country	Food Commodity	Other Information	Microorganisms or Metabolite
Norway	Coconut	Grated	Coliforms
Norway	Coconut	Grated	*Salmonella* spp.
South Africa	Coconut	Dessicated	*Salmonella* spp.
South Africa	Coconut	Dessicated	*Shigella* spp.
South Africa	Coconut	Dessicated	*S. aureus*
Canada	Coleslaw	Ready-to-eat with shelf life > 10 days	*L. monocytogenes*
Ireland	Coleslaw		*B. cereus* and *B. subtilis* group
Ireland	Coleslaw		*Campylobacter*
Ireland	Coleslaw		*C. perfringens*
Ireland	Coleslaw		*E. coli*
Ireland	Coleslaw		*E. coli* O157 and other verotoxigenic *E. coli* (VTEC)
Ireland	Coleslaw		*L. monocytogenes*
Ireland	Coleslaw		*Listeria* spp. (not *L. monocytogenes*)

Numerical Values as Given in Original Publication[b] (in cfu/g or mL if not specified)	Sampling Plan as Given in Original Publication[c]	Point of Application	Legal Status
$m = 10$, $M = 100$	Not specified	Not standardized	Guidelines
$m = 0$, $M = 0$	Not specified	Not standardized	Guidelines
Not detectable	Not specified	Retail	Mandatory
Not detectable	Not specified	Retail	Mandatory
Not detectable	Not specified	Retail	Mandatory
Not detectable in 50 g	$n = 5$	Manufacturing level	Class 1 recall to retail level
Satisfactory: < 100, borderline: 1,000 to < 10,000, unsatisfactory: 10,000 to < 100,000, unacceptable: 100,000	Not specified	Retail	Guidelines
Satisfactory: not detected in 25 g, unacceptable: present in 25 g	Not specified	Retail	Guidelines
Satisfactory: < 10, borderline: 10 to < 100, unsatisfactory: 100 to < 10,000, unacceptable: 100,000	Not specified	Retail	Guidelines
Satisfactory: < 20, borderline: 20 to < 100, unsatisfactory: 100 to < 10,000, unacceptable/potentially hazardous: 10,000	Not specified	Retail	Guidelines
Satisfactory: not detected in 25 g, unacceptable: present in 25 g	Not specified	Retail	Guidelines
Satisfactory: not detected in 25 g, borderline: < 200 present in 25 g, unsatisfactory: 200 to < 1,000, unacceptable: 1,000	Not specified	Retail	Guidelines
Satisfactory: not detectable in 25 g, borderline: < 200 present in 25 g, unsatisfactory: 200 to < 10,000, unacceptable: 10,000	Not specified	Retail	Guidelines

continued

TABLE E-5 Continued

Country	Food Commodity	Other Information	Microorganisms or Metabolite
Ireland	Coleslaw		*Salmonella* spp.
Ireland	Coleslaw		*S. aureus*
Ireland	Coleslaw		*Vibrio parahaemolyticus*
Israel	Dates		Aerobic plate count
Israel	Dates		Coliforms
Israel	Dates		Molds
Israel	Dates		*Salmonella* spp.
Ireland	Dried fruit and vegetables		Aerobic microorganisms at 30°C
Ireland	Dried fruit and vegetables		Aerobic microorganisms at 30°C
Ireland	Dried fruit and vegetables		Aerobic microorganisms at 30°C
Ireland	Dried fruit and vegetables		*B. cereus* and *B. subtilis* group
Ireland	Dried fruit and vegetables		*Campylobacter*

Numerical Values as Given in Original Publication[b] (in cfu/g or mL if not specified)	Sampling Plan as Given in Original Publication[c]	Point of Application	Legal Status
Satisfactory: not detected in 25 g, unacceptable: present in 25 g	Not specified	Retail	Guidelines
Satisfactory: < 20, borderline: 20 to < 100, unsatisfactory 100 to < 10,000, unacceptable/potentially hazardous: 10,000	Not specified	Retail	Guidelines
Satisfactory: not detected in 25 g, borderline: < 200 present in 25 g, unsatisfactory: 200 to < 1,000, unacceptable: 1,000	Not specified	Retail	Guidelines
100,000	M = value of standard, $n = 1$, $c = 0$	Not specified	Mandatory
10	M = value of standard, $n = 1$, $c = 0$	Not specified	Mandatory
100	M = value of standard, $n = 1$, $c = 0$	Not specified	Mandatory
Not detectable in 20 g	M = value of standard, $n = 1$, $c = 0$	Not specified	Mandatory
Satisfactory: < 100,000	Not specified	Retail	Guidelines
Borderline: 100,000 to < 1,000,000	Not specified	Retail	Guidelines
Unsatisfactory: 1,000,000	Not specified	Retail	Guidelines
Satisfactory: < 100, borderline: 1,000 to < 10,000, unsatisfactory: 10,000 to < 100,000, unacceptable: 100,000	Not specified	Retail	Guidelines
Satisfactory: not detected in 25 g, unacceptable: present in 25 g	Not specified	Retail	Guidelines

continued

TABLE E-5 Continued

Country	Food Commodity	Other Information	Microorganisms or Metabolite
Ireland	Dried fruit and vegetables		*C. perfringens*
Ireland	Dried fruit and vegetables		*E. coli*
Ireland	Dried fruit and vegetables		*E. coli* O157 and other VTEC
Ireland	Dried fruit and vegetables		*L. monocytogenes*
Ireland	Dried fruit and vegetables		*Listeria* spp. (not *L. monocytogenes*)
Ireland	Dried fruit and vegetables		*Salmonella* spp
Ireland	Dried fruit and vegetables		*S. aureus*
Ireland	Dried fruit and vegetables		*V. parahaemolyticus*
Israel	Dried plums		Aerobic plate count

Numerical Values as Given in Original Publication[b] (in cfu/g or mL if not specified)	Sampling Plan as Given in Original Publication[c]	Point of Application	Legal Status
Satisfactory: < 10, borderline: 10 to < 100, unsatisfactory: 100 to < 10,000, unacceptable: 10,000	Not specified	Retail	Guidelines
Satisfactory: < 20, borderline: 20 to < 100, unsatisfactory: 100 to < 10,000, unacceptable/potentially hazardous: 10,000	Not specified	Retail	Guidelines
Satisfactory: not detected in 25 g, unacceptable present in 25 g	Not specified	Retail	Guidelines
Satisfactory: not detected in 25 g, borderline: < 200 present in 25 g, unsatisfactory: 200 to < 1,000, unacceptable: 1,000	Not specified	Retail	Guidelines
Satisfactory: not detectable in 25 g,: borderline: < 200 present in 25 g, unsatisfactory: 200 to < 10,000, unacceptable: 10,000	Not specified	Retail	Guidelines
Satisfactory: not detected in 25 g, unacceptable: present in 25 g	Not specified	Retail	Guidelines
Satisfactory: < 20, borderline: 20 to < 100, unsatisfactory: 100 to < 10,000, unacceptable/potentially hazardous: 10,000	Not specified	Retail	Guidelines
Satisfactory: not detected in 25 g, borderline: < 200 present in 25 g, unsatisfactory: 200 to < 1,000, unacceptable: 1,000	Not specified	Retail	Guidelines
100,000	M = value of standard, $n = 1$, $c = 0$	Not specified	Mandatory

continued

TABLE E-5 Continued

Country	Food Commodity	Other Information	Microorganisms or Metabolite
Israel	Dried plums		Coliforms
Israel	Dried plums		Molds
Israel	Dried plums		*Salmonella* spp.
Israel	Dried vegetables		Aerobic plate count
Israel	Dried vegetables		Coliforms
Israel	Dried vegetables		Coliforms
Israel	Dried vegetables		Molds
Israel	Dried vegetables		*Salmonella* spp.
Israel	Dried vegetables	Including onion and garlic	Coliforms
Israel	Dried vegetables	Including onion and garlic	Enterococci
Israel	Dried vegetables	Including onion and garlic	*E. coli*
Israel	Dried vegetables	Including onion and garlic	Mesophilic spore-forming bacteria
Israel	Dried vegetables	Including onion and garlic	Molds
Israel	Dried vegetables	Including onion and garlic	*Salmonella* spp.
Israel	Dried vegetables	Including onion and garlic in soya product	Yeasts
ICMSF	Frozen fruits	pH > 4.5	*E. coli*
Israel	Frozen fruits		Coliforms
Israel	Frozen fruits		Molds
Israel	Frozen fruits		*Salmonella* spp.
Spain	Frozen fruits		Aerobic mesophilic microorganisms
Spain	Frozen fruits		Anaerobic sulphite-reducing bacteria
Spain	Frozen fruits		Coliforms
Spain	Frozen fruits		*E. coli*

Numerical Values as Given in Original Publication[b] (in cfu/g or mL if not specified)	Sampling Plan as Given in Original Publication[c]	Point of Application	Legal Status
100	M = value of standard, $n = 1, c = 0$	Not specified	Mandatory
100	M = value of standard, $n = 1, c = 0$	Not specified	Mandatory
Not detectable in 20 g	M = value of standard, $n = 1, c = 0$	Not specified	Mandatory
100,000	M = value of standard, $n = 1, c = 0$	Not specified	Mandatory
1,000	M = value of standard, $n = 1, c = 0$	Not specified	Mandatory
10,000 (if *E. coli* = 0)	M = value of standard, $n = 1, c = 0$	Not specified	Mandatory
500	M = value of standard, $n = 1, c = 0$	Not specified	Mandatory
Not detectable in 20 g	M = value of standard, $n = 1, c = 0$	Not specified	Mandatory
100	M = value of standard, $n = 1, c = 0$	Not specified	Mandatory
500	M = value of standard, $n = 1, c = 0$	Not specified	Mandatory
0	M = value of standard, $n = 1, c = 0$	Not specified	Mandatory
10,000	M = value of standard, $n = 1, c = 0$	Not specified	Mandatory
10,000	M = value of standard, $n = 1, c = 0$	Not specified	Mandatory
Not detectable in 20 g	M = value of standard, $n = 1, c = 0$	Not specified	Mandatory
100	M = value of standard, $n = 1, c = 0$	Not specified	Mandatory
$m = 100$, $M = 1{,}000$	$n = 5, c = 2$	Port of entry	Guidelines
10	M = value of standard, $n = 1, c = 0$	Not specified	Mandatory
10	M = value of standard, $n = 1, c = 0$	Not specified	Mandatory
Not detectable in 20 g	M = value of standard, $n = 1, c = 0$	Not specified	Mandatory
500,000	Not specified	Not specified	Recommendation
10	Not specified	Not specified	Recommendation
100 to 300	Not specified	Not specified	Recommendation
10	Not specified	Not specified	Recommendation

continued

TABLE E-5 Continued

Country	Food Commodity	Other Information	Microorganisms or Metabolite
Spain	Frozen fruits		Molds
Spain	Frozen fruits		Psychrotrophic count
Spain	Frozen fruits		*Salmonella* spp.
Spain	Frozen fruits		*Shigella* spp.
Spain	Frozen fruits		*S. aureus*
Spain	Frozen fruits		Yeasts
Israel	Frozen vegetables		Aerobic plate count
Israel	Frozen vegetables		Coliforms
Israel	Frozen vegetables		Molds
Israel	Frozen vegetables		*Salmonella* spp.
Israel	Frozen vegetables		*Streptococcus faecalis*
Spain	Frozen vegetables		Aerobic mesophilic microorganisms
Spain	Frozen vegetables		Anaerobic sulphite-reducing bacteria
Spain	Frozen vegetables		Coliforms
Spain	Frozen vegetables		*E. coli*
Spain	Frozen vegetables		Molds
Spain	Frozen vegetables		Psychrotrophic count
Spain	Frozen vegetables		*Salmonella* spp.
Spain	Frozen vegetables		*Shigella* spp.
Spain	Frozen vegetables		*S. aureus*
Spain	Frozen vegetables		Yeasts
Israel	Fruit drink	Bases for preparation of heat-treated or preserved products	Lactic acid bacteria
Israel	Fruit drink	Bases for preparation of frozen products	Molds
Israel	Fruit drink	Bases for preparation of heat-treated or preserved products	Molds
Israel	Fruit drink	Bases for preparation of frozen products	Yeasts
Norway	Fruit ice		Aerobic microorganisms at 30°C
Norway	Fruit ice		Coliforms
Norway	Fruit ice		Molds
Norway	Fruit ice		Yeasts

Numerical Values as Given in Original Publication[b] (in cfu/g or mL if not specified)	Sampling Plan as Given in Original Publication[c]	Point of Application	Legal Status
100	Not specified	Not specified	Recommendation
500,000	Not specified	Not specified	Recommendation
Not detectable in 25 g	Not specified	Not specified	Recommendation
Not detectable in 25 g	Not specified	Not specified	Recommendation
100	Not specified	Not specified	Recommendation
100	Not specified	Not specified	Recommendation
500,000	M = value of standard, $n = 1, c = 0$	Not specified	Mandatory
500	M = value of standard, $n = 1, c = 0$	Not specified	Mandatory
100	M = value of standard, $n = 1, c = 0$	Not specified	Mandatory
Not detectable in 20 g	M = value of standard, $n = 1, c = 0$	Not specified	Mandatory
100	M = value of standard, $n = 1, c = 0$	Not specified	Mandatory
500,000	Not specified	Not specified	Recommendation
10	Not specified	Not specified	Recommendation
100 to 300	Not specified	Not specified	Recommendation
10	Not specified	Not specified	Recommendation
100	Not specified	Not specified	Recommendation
500,000	Not specified	Not specified	Recommendation
Not detectable in 25 g	Not specified	Not specified	Recommendation
Not detectable in 25 g	Not specified	Not specified	Recommendation
100	Not specified	Not specified	Recommendation
100	Not specified	Not specified	Recommendation
10	M = value of standard, $n = 1, c = 0$	Not specified	Mandatory
10	M = value of standard, $n = 1, c = 0$	Not specified	Mandatory
10	M = value of standard, $n = 1, c = 0$	Not specified	Mandatory
1,000	M = value of standard, $n = 1, c = 0$	Not specified	Mandatory
$m = 1{,}000$, $M = 10{,}000$	Not specified	Not standardized	Guidelines
$m = 0$, $M = 10$	Not specified	Not standardized	Guidelines
$m = 100$, $M = 1{,}000$	Not specified	Not standardized	Guidelines
$m = 100$, $M = 1{,}000$	Not specified	Not standardized	Guidelines

continued

TABLE E-5 Continued

Country	Food Commodity	Other Information	Microorganisms or Metabolite
Cuba	Fruit juices	Refrigerated	Coliforms
Cuba	Fruit juices	Canned	Commercially sterile
Cuba	Fruit nectars	Canned	Commercially sterile
New Zealand	Grains	Cultured	*E. coli*
New Zealand	Grains	Cultured	*Salmonella* spp.
New Zealand	Herbs		Aerobic microorganisms at 35°C
New Zealand	Herbs		*B. cereus*
New Zealand	Herbs		*C. perfringens*
New Zealand	Herbs		Coliforms faecal
New Zealand	Herbs		*Salmonella* spp.
New Zealand	Herbs		*Staphylococcus* coagulase positive
Spain	Honey		Aerobic mesophilic microorganisms
Spain	Honey		*Enterobacteriaceae*
Spain	Honey		*E. coli*
Spain	Honey		Molds
Spain	Honey		Pathogenic bacteria
Spain	Honey		Toxins, microbial
Spain	Honey		*Salmonella* spp.
Spain	Honey		*Shigella* spp.
Israel	Ketchup and tomato products		Molds
Israel	Marzipan		Molds
Spain	Marzipan		*Enterobacteriaceae*
Spain	Marzipan		*E. coli*
Spain	Marzipan		Molds
Spain	Marzipan		*Salmonella* spp.
Spain	Marzipan		*Shigella* spp.
Spain	Marzipan		*S. aureus*
Spain	Marzipan		*S. aureus* enterotoxic
Spain	Marzipan		Yeasts
Spain	Nougat		*S. aureus* enterotoxic
Norway	Nuts	Shelled, almonds etc.	*Salmonella* spp.
ICMSF	Peanut butters and other nut butters		*Salmonella* spp.
ICMSF	Peanut butters and other nut butters used in high moisture food		*Salmonella* spp.
Spain	Preserves	Salted, pasteurized	Aerobic mesophilic microorganisms

Numerical Values as Given in Original Publication[b] (in cfu/g or mL if not specified)	Sampling Plan as Given in Original Publication[c]	Point of Application	Legal Status
< 100	$n = 1$	Not specified	Mandatory
Commercially sterile	$n = 1$	Not specified	Mandatory
Commercially sterile	$n = 1$	Not specified	Mandatory
$m = 0$	$n = 5, c = 0$	Not specified	Guidelines
$m = 0$ per 25 g	$n = 5, c = 0$	Not specified	Guidelines
$m = 500{,}000$, $M = 5{,}000{,}000$	$n = 5, c = 2$	Not specified	Guidelines
$m = 1{,}000$, $M = 10{,}000$	$n = 5, c = 2$	Not specified	Guidelines
$m = 100$, $M = 1{,}000$	$n = 5, c = 2$	Not specified	Guidelines
$m = 10$, $M = 100$	$n = 5, c = 2$	Not specified	Guidelines
$m = 0$ per 25 g	$n = 5, c = 0$	Not specified	Guidelines
$m = 100$, $M = 1{,}000$	$n = 5, c = 2$	Not specified	Guidelines
10,000	Not specified	Not specified	Mandatory
Not detectable	Not specified	Not specified	Mandatory
Not detectable	Not specified	Not specified	Mandatory
100	Not specified	Not specified	Mandatory
Not detectable	Not specified	Not specified	Mandatory
Not detectable	Not specified	Not specified	Mandatory
Not detectable in 25 g	Not specified	Not specified	Mandatory
Not detectable in 25 g	Not specified	Not specified	Mandatory
Less than 25% of field containing molds	M = value of standard, $n = 1, c = 0$	Not specified	Mandatory
100	M = value of standard, $n = 1, c = 0$	Not specified	Mandatory
100	Not specified	Not specified	Mandatory
Not detectable	Not specified	Not specified	Mandatory
1,000	Not specified	Not specified	Mandatory
Not detectable in 25 g	Not specified	Not specified	Mandatory
Not detectable in 25 g	Not specified	Not specified	Mandatory
Not detectable	Not specified	Not specified	Mandatory
Not detectable	Not specified	Retail/production	Not specified
1,000	Not specified	Not specified	Mandatory
Not detectable	Not specified	Retail/production	Not specified
$m = 0$, $M = 0$	Not specified	Not standardized	Guidelines
$m = 0$	$n = 10, c = 0$	Port of entry	Guidelines
$m = 0$	$n = 20, c = 0$	Port of entry	Guidelines
10,000	Not specified	Not specified	Recommendation

continued

TABLE E-5 Continued

Country	Food Commodity	Other Information	Microorganisms or Metabolite
Spain	Preserves	Salted, nonpasteurized, with or without oil	Aerobic mesophilic microorganisms
Spain	Preserves	Salted, smoked, nonpasteurized	Aerobic mesophilic microorganisms
Spain	Preserves	Salted, pasteurized	*Clostridium* spp., sulphite reducing
Spain	Preserves	Salted, nonpasteurized, with or without oil	*Clostridium* spp., sulphite reducing
Spain	Preserves	Salted, smoked, nonpasteurized	*Clostridium* spp. sulphite reducing
Spain	Preserves	Salted, pasteurized	*Enterobacteriaceae*
Spain	Preserves	Salted, nonpasteurized, with or without oil	*Enterobacteriaceae*
Spain	Preserves	Salted, smoked, nonpasteurized	*Enterobacteriaceae*
Spain	Preserves	Salted, pasteurized	*E. coli*
Spain	Preserves	Salted, nonpasteurized, with or without oil	*E. coli*
Spain	Preserves	Salted, smoked, nonpasteurized	*E. coli*
Spain	Preserves	Salted, pasteurized	*Salmonella* spp.
Spain	Preserves	Salted, nonpasteurized, with or without oil	*Salmonella* spp.
Spain	Preserves	Salted, smoked, nonpasteurized	*Salmonella* spp .
Spain	Preserves	Salted, pasteurized	*Shigella* spp.
Spain	Preserves	Salted, nonpasteurized with or without oil	*Shigella* spp.
Spain	Preserves	Salted, smoked, nonpasteurized	*Shigella* spp.
Spain	Preserves	Salted, pasteurized	*S. aureus*
Spain	Preserves	Salted, nonpasteurized, with or without oil	*S. aureus*
Spain	Preserves	Salted, smoked, nonpasteurized	*S. aureus*

Numerical Values as Given in Original Publication[b] (in cfu/g or mL if not specified)	Sampling Plan as Given in Original Publication[c]	Point of Application	Legal Status
100,000	Not specified	Not specified	Recommendation
100,000	Not specified	Not specified	Recommendation
Not detectable	Not specified	Not specified	Recommendation
Not detectable	Not specified	Not specified	Recommendation
Not detectable	Not specified	Not specified	Recommendation
Not detectable	Not specified	Not specified	Recommendation
10	Not specified	Not specified	Recommendation
10	Not specified	Not specified	Recommendation
Not detectable	Not specified	Not specified	Recommendation
Not detectable	Not specified	Not specified	Recommendation
Not detectable	Not specified	Not specified	Recommendation
Not detectable in 25 g	Not specified	Not specified	Recommendation
Not detectable in 25 g	Not specified	Not specified	Recommendation
Not detectable in 25 g	Not specified	Not specified	Recommendation
Not detectable in 25 g	Not specified	Not specified	Recommendation
Not detectable in 25 g	Not specified	Not specified	Recommendation
Not detectable in 25 g	Not specified	Not specified	Recommendation
Not detectable	Not specified	Not specified	Recommendation
Not detectable	Not specified	Not specified	Recommendation
Not detectable	Not specified	Not specified	Recommendation

continued

TABLE E-5 Continued

Country	Food Commodity	Other Information	Microorganisms or Metabolite
Israel	Raisins		Aerobic plate count
Israel	Raisins		Coliforms
Israel	Raisins		Molds
Israel	Raisins		*Salmonella* spp.
New Zealand	Ready-to-eat	All components cooked in manufacturing process	Aerobic microorganisms at 35°C
New Zealand	Ready-to-eat	Some components not cooked in manufacturing process (e.g., sandwiches)	Aerobic microorganisms at 35°C
New Zealand	Ready-to-eat	All components cooked in manufacturing process	*B. cereus*
New Zealand	Ready-to-eat	Some components not cooked in manufacturing process (e.g., sandwiches)	*B. cereus*
New Zealand	Ready-to-eat	All components cooked in manufacturing process	*Campylobacter*
New Zealand	Ready-to-eat	Some components not cooked in manufacturing process (e.g., sandwiches)	*Campylobacter*
New Zealand	Ready-to-eat	All components cooked in manufacturing process	*C. perfringens*
New Zealand	Ready-to-eat	Some components not cooked in manufacturing process (e.g., sandwiches)	*C. perfringens*
New Zealand	Ready-to-eat	All components cooked in manufacturing process	*E. coli*
New Zealand	Ready-to-eat	Some components not cooked in manufacturing process (e.g., sandwiches)	Coliforms faecal

Numerical Values as Given in Original Publication[b] (in cfu/g or mL if not specified)	Sampling Plan as Given in Original Publication[c]	Point of Application	Legal Status
100,000	M = value of standard, $n = 1$, $c = 0$	Not specified	Mandatory
100	M = value of standard, $n = 1$, $c = 0$	Not specified	Mandatory
100	M = value of standard, $n = 1$, $c = 0$	Not specified	Mandatory
Not detectable in 20 g	M = value of standard, $n = 1$, $c = 0$	Not specified	Mandatory
m = 10,000, M = 100,000	$n = 5$, $c = 2$	Not specified	Guidelines
m = 100,000, M = 500,000	$n = 5$, $c = 2$	Not specified	Guidelines
m = 100, M = 1,000	$n = 5$, $c = 2$	Not specified	Guidelines
m =100, M = 1,000	$n = 5$, $c = 2$	Not specified	Guidelines
m = 0 per 10 g	$n = 5$, $c = 0$	Not specified	Guidelines
m = 0 per 10 g	$n = 5$, $c = 0$	Not specified	Guidelines
m = 100, M = 1,000	$n = 5$, $c = 2$	Not specified	Guidelines
m = 100, M = 1,000	$n = 5$, $c = 2$	Not specified	Guidelines
m = 0	$n = 5$, $c = 0$	Not specified	Guidelines
m = 10, M = 100	$n = 5$, $c = 2$	Not specified	Guidelines

continued

TABLE E-5 Continued

Country	Food Commodity	Other Information	Microorganisms or Metabolite
New Zealand	Ready-to-eat	All components cooked in manufacturing process	*L. monocytogenes*
New Zealand	Ready-to-eat	Some components not cooked in manufacturing process (e.g., sandwiches)	*L. monocytogenes*
New Zealand	Ready-to-eat	All components cooked in manufacturing process	*Salmonella* spp.
New Zealand	Ready-to-eat	Some components not cooked in manufacturing process (e.g., sandwiches)	*Salmonella* spp.
New Zealand	Ready-to-eat	All components cooked in manufacturing process	*Staphylococcus*, coagulase positive
New Zealand	Ready-to-eat	Some components not cooked in manufacturing process (e.g., sandwiches)	*Staphylococcus*, coagulase positive
Canada	Ready-to-eat foods	Supporting growth of *Listeria monocytogenes* with refrigerated shelf-life < 10 days and all ready-to-eat foods not supporting growth, produced under Good Manufacturing Practices (GMP)	*L. monocytogenes*
Canada	Ready-to-eat foods	Supporting growth of *L. monocytogenes* with refrigerated shelf-life < 10 days and all ready-to-eat foods not supporting growth, produced under no or inadequate GMP	*L. monocytogenes*
Ireland	Rice		Aerobic microorganisms at 30°C

Numerical Values as Given in Original Publication[b] (in cfu/g or mL if not specified)	Sampling Plan as Given in Original Publication[c]	Point of Application	Legal Status
$m = 0$ per 25 g	$n = 5, c = 0$	Not specified	Guidelines
$m = 0$ per 25 g	$n = 5, c = 0$	Not specified	Guidelines
$m = 0$ per 25 g	$n = 5, c = 0$	Not specified	Guidelines
$m = 0$ per 25 g	$n = 5, c = 0$	Not specified	Guidelines
$m = 100, M = 1{,}000$	$n = 5, c = 2$	Not specified	Guidelines
$m = 100, M = 1{,}000$	$n = 5, c = 2$	Not specified	Guidelines
< 100	$n = 5$	Manufacturing level	Allow sale
< 100	$n = 5$	Manufacturing level	Recall or stop sale
Satisfactory: < 100,000	Not specified	Retail	Guidelines

continued

TABLE E-5 Continued

Country	Food Commodity	Other Information	Microorganisms or Metabolite
Ireland	Rice		Aerobic microorganisms at 30°C
Ireland	Rice		Aerobic microorganisms at 30°C
Ireland	Rice		*B. cereus* and *B. subtilis* group
Ireland	Rice		*Campylobacter*
Ireland	Rice		*C. perfringens*
Ireland	Rice		*E. coli*
Ireland	Rice		*E. coli* O157 and other VTEC
Ireland	Rice		*L. monocytogenes*
Ireland	Rice		*Listeria* spp. (not *L. monocytogens*)
Ireland	Rice		*Salmonella* spp.

Numerical Values as Given in Original Publication[b] (in cfu/g or mL if not specified)	Sampling Plan as Given in Original Publication[c]	Point of Application	Legal Status
Borderline: 100,000 to < 1,000,000	Not specified	Retail	Guidelines
Unsatisfactory: 1,000,000	Not specified	Retail	Guidelines
Satisfactory: < 100, borderline: 1,000 to < 10,000, unsatisfactory: 10,000 to < 100,000, unacceptable: 100,000	Not specified	Retail	Guidelines
Satisfactory: not detected in 25 g, unacceptable: present in 25 g	Not specified	Retail	Guidelines
Satisfactory: < 10, borderline: 10 to < 100, unsatisfactory: 100 to < 10,000, unacceptable: 100,000	Not specified	Retail	Guidelines
Satisfactory: < 20, borderline: 20 to < 100, unsatisfactory: 100 to < 10,000, unacceptable/potentially hazardous: 10,000	Not specified	Retail	Guidelines
Satisfactory: not detected in 25 g, unacceptable: present in 25 g	Not specified	Retail	Guidelines
Satisfactory: not detected in 25 g, borderline: < 200 present in 25 g, unsatisfactory: 200 to < 1,000, unacceptable: 1,000	Not specified	Retail	Guidelines
Satisfactory: not detectable in 25 g, borderline: < 200 present in 25 g, unsatisfactory: 200 to < 10,000, unacceptable: 10,000	Not specified	Retail	Guidelines
Satisfactory: not detected in 25 g, unacceptable: present in 25 g	Not specified	Retail	Guidelines

continued

TABLE E-5 Continued

Country	Food Commodity	Other Information	Microorganisms or Metabolite
Ireland	Rice		*S. aureus*
Ireland	Rice		*V. parahaemolyticus*
Netherlands	Rice and rice products	Prepared, to be heated before sale/consumption	Aerobic microorganisms
Netherlands	Rice and rice products	Prepared, to be heated by consumer after sale	Aerobic microorganisms
Netherlands	Rice and rice products	Prepared, to be heated before sale/consumption	Pathogenic microorganisms
Netherlands	Rice and rice products	Prepared, to be heated by consumer after sale	Pathogenic microorganisms
Netherlands	Rice and rice products	Prepared, to be heated before sale/consumption	*S. aureus*
Netherlands	Rice and rice products	Prepared, to be heated by consumer after sale	*S. aureus*
Netherlands	Rice and rice products	Prepared, to be heated before sale/consumption	Toxins, microbial
Netherlands	Rice and rice products	Prepared, to be heated by consumer after sale	Toxins, microbial
Netherlands	Rice and rice products	Ready for consumption	Aerobic microorganisms
Netherlands	Rice and rice products	Ready for consumption	*Enterobacteriaceae*
Netherlands	Rice and rice products	Ready for consumption	Pathogenic microorganisms
Netherlands	Rice and rice products	Ready for consumption	*S. aureus*

Numerical Values as Given in Original Publication[b] (in cfu/g or mL if not specified)	Sampling Plan as Given in Original Publication[c]	Point of Application	Legal Status
Satisfactory: < 20, borderline: 20 to < 100, unsatisfactory: 100 to < 10,000, unacceptable/potentially hazardous: 10,000	Not specified	Retail	Guidelines
Satisfactory: not detected in 25 g, borderline: < 200 present in 25 g, unsatisfactory: 200 to < 1,000, unacceptable: 1,000	Not specified	Retail	Guidelines
< 1,000,000	Not specified	Retail	Mandatory
< 100,000	Not specified	Retail	Mandatory
Not detectable	Not specified	Retail	Mandatory
Not detectable	Not specified	Retail	Mandatory
< 500	Not specified	Retail	Mandatory
< 500	Not specified	Retail	Mandatory
Not detectable	Not specified	Retail	Mandatory
Not detectable	Not specified	Retail	Mandatory
< 10,000	Not specified	Consumption	Mandatory
Not detectable in 0.1 g	Not specified	Consumption	Mandatory
Not detectable	Not specified	Consumption	Mandatory
Not detectable in 0.1 g	Not specified	Consumption	Mandatory

continued

TABLE E-5 Continued

Country	Food Commodity	Other Information	Microorganisms or Metabolite
Netherlands	Rice and rice products	Ready for consumption	Toxins, microbial
Ireland	Salad	Mixed, prepared	Aerobic microorganisms at 30°C
Ireland	Salad	Mixed, prepared	Aerobic microorganisms at 30°C
Ireland	Salad	Mixed, prepared	Aerobic microorganisms at 30°C
Ireland	Salad	Mixed, prepared	*B. cereus* and *B. subtilis* group
Ireland	Salad	Mixed, prepared	*Campylobacter*
Ireland	Salad	Mixed, prepared	*C. perfringens*
Ireland	Salad	Mixed, prepared	*E. coli*
Ireland	Salad	Mixed, prepared	*E. coli* O157 and other VTEC
Ireland	Salad	Mixed, prepared	*L. monocytogenes*
Ireland	Salad	Mixed, prepared	*Listeria* spp. (not *L. monocytogens*)

Numerical Values as Given in Original Publication[b] (in cfu/g or mL if not specified)	Sampling Plan as Given in Original Publication[c]	Point of Application	Legal Status
Not detectable	Not specified	Consumption	Mandatory
Satisfactory: < 1,000,000	Not specified	Retail	Guidelines
Borderline: 1,000,000 to < 10,000,000	Not specified	Retail	Guidelines
Unsatisfactory: 10,000,000	Not specified	Retail	Guidelines
Satisfactory: < 100, borderline: 1,000 to < 10,000, unsatisfactory: 10,000 to < 100,000, unacceptable: 100,000	Not specified	Retail	Guidelines
Satisfactory: not detected in 25 g, unacceptable: present in 25 g	Not specified	Retail	Guidelines
Satisfactory: < 10, borderline: 10 to < 100, unsatisfactory: 100 to < 10,000, unacceptable: 100,000	Not specified	Retail	Guidelines
Satisfactory: < 20, borderline: 20 to < 100, unsatisfactory: 100 to < 10,000, unacceptable/potentially hazardous: 10,000	Not specified	Retail	Guidelines
Satisfactory: not detected in 25 g, unacceptable: present in 25 g	Not specified	Retail	Guidelines
Satisfactory: not detected in 25 g, borderline: < 200 present in 25 g, unsatisfactory: 200 to < 1,000, unacceptable: 1,000	Not specified	Retail	Guidelines
Satisfactory: not detectable in 25 g, borderline: < 200 present in 25 g, unsatisfactory: 200 to < 10,000, unacceptable: 10,000	Not specified	Retail	Guidelines

continued

TABLE E-5 Continued

Country	Food Commodity	Other Information	Microorganisms or Metabolite
Ireland	Salad	Mixed, prepared	*Salmonella* spp.
Ireland	Salad	Mixed, prepared	*S. aureus*
Ireland	Salad	Mixed, prepared	*V. parahaemolyticus*
Israel	Salad	Tehina type	Aerobic plate count
Israel	Salad	Tehina type	Coliforms
Israel	Salad	Tehina type	Molds
Israel	Salad	Tehina type	*Salmonella* spp.
Israel	Salad	Tehina type	*S. aureus*
Israel	Salad	Made from vegetable materials with chili pepper	Aerobic plate count
Israel	Salad	Made from vegetable materials with chili pepper	*Clostridium* spp.
Israel	Salad	Made from vegetable materials with chili pepper	Coliforms
Israel	Salad	Made from vegetable materials with chili pepper	Molds
Israel	Salad	Made from vegetable materials with chili pepper	*Salmonella* spp.
Israel	Salad	Made from vegetable materials with chili pepper	*S. aureus*

Numerical Values as Given in Original Publication[b] (in cfu/g or mL if not specified)	Sampling Plan as Given in Original Publication[c]	Point of Application	Legal Status
Satisfactory: not detected in 25 g, unacceptable: present in 25 g	Not specified	Retail	Guidelines
Satisfactory: < 20, borderline: 20 to < 100, unsatisfactory: 100 to < 10,000, unacceptable/potentially hazardous: 10,000	Not specified	Retail	Guidelines
Satisfactory: not detected in 25 g, borderline: < 200 present in 25 g, unsatisfactory: 200 to < 1,000, unacceptable: 1,000	Not specified	Retail	Guidelines
1,000,000	M = value of standard, $n = 1$, $c = 0$	Not specified	Mandatory
1,000	M = value of standard, $n = 1$, $c = 0$	Not specified	Mandatory
100	M = value of standard, $n = 1$, $c = 0$	Not specified	Mandatory
Not detectable in 20 g	M = value of standard, $n = 1$, $c = 0$	Not specified	Mandatory
< 50	M = value of standard, $n = 1$, $c = 0$	Not specified	Mandatory
100,000	M = value of standard, $n = 1$, $c = 0$	Not specified	Mandatory
100	M = value of standard, $n = 1$, $c = 0$	Not specified	Mandatory
100	M = value of standard, $n = 1$, $c = 0$	Not specified	Mandatory
100	M = value of standard, $n = 1$, $c = 0$	Not specified	Mandatory
Not detectable in 20 g	M = value of standard, $n = 1$, $c = 0$	Not specified	Mandatory
50	M = value of standard, $n = 1$, $c = 0$	Not specified	Mandatory

continued

TABLE E-5 Continued

Country	Food Commodity	Other Information	Microorganisms or Metabolite
Israel	Salad	Made from vegetable materials with chili pepper	*S. faecalis*
Israel	Salad	Made from vegetable materials	Aerobic plate count
Israel	Salad	Made from vegetable materials	*Clostridium* spp.
Israel	Salad	Made from vegetable materials	Coliforms
Israel	Salad	Made from vegetable materials	Molds
Israel	Salad	Made from vegetable materials	*Salmonella* spp.
Israel	Salad	Made from vegetable materials	*S. aureus*
Israel	Salad	Made from vegetable materials	*S. aureus*
New Zealand	Salad	Vegetable or fruits, excluding combination with meat	Aerobic microorganisms at 35°C
New Zealand	Salad	Vegetable or fruits, excluding combination with meat	Coliforms faecal
New Zealand	Salad	Vegetable or fruits, excluding combination with meat	*Salmonella* spp.
New Zealand	Salad	Vegetable or fruits, excluding combination with meat	*Staphylococcus,* coagulase positive
Norway	Salad	Containing mayonnaise	Aerobic microorganisms at 30°C
Norway	Salad	Containing mayonnaise	*B. cereus*
Norway	Salad	Containing mayonnaise	Coliforms
Norway	Salad	Containing mayonnaise	*L. monocytogenes*
Norway	Salad	Containing mayonnaise	*Salmonella* spp.

Numerical Values as Given in Original Publication[b] (in cfu/g or mL if not specified)	Sampling Plan as Given in Original Publication[c]	Point of Application	Legal Status
100	M = value of standard, $n = 1$, $c = 0$	Not specified	Mandatory
100,000	M = value of standard, $n = 1$, $c = 0$	Not specified	Mandatory
100	M = value of standard, $n = 1$, $c = 0$	Not specified	Mandatory
100	M = value of standard, $n = 1$, $c = 0$	Not specified	Mandatory
1,000	M = value of standard, $n = 1$, $c = 0$	Not specified	Mandatory
Not detectable in 20 g	M = value of standard, $n = 1$, $c = 0$	Not specified	Mandatory
50	M = value of standard, $n = 1$, $c = 0$	Not specified	Mandatory
100	M = value of standard, $n = 1$, $c = 0$	Not specified	Mandatory
m = 100,000, M = 1,000,000	$n = 5$, $c = 2$	Not specified	Guidelines
m = 100, M = 1,000	$n = 5$, $c = 2$	Not specified	Guidelines
m = 0 per 25 g	$n = 5$, $c = 0$	Not specified	Guidelines
m = 100, M = 1,000	$n = 5$, $c = 2$	Not specified	Guidelines
m = 50,000, M = 100,000	$n = 5$, $c = 2$	Date of production	Guidelines
m = 1,000, M = 10,000	$n = 5$, $c = 2$	Not standardized	Guidelines
m = 10, M = 100	$n = 5$, $c = 2$	Not standardized	Guidelines
Not detectable in 25 g	$n = 10$, $c = 1$	Not standardized	Guidelines
Not detectable in 25 g	$n = 10$, $c = 0$	Not standardized	Guidelines

continued

TABLE E-5 Continued

Country	Food Commodity	Other Information	Microorganisms or Metabolite
Norway	Salad	Containing mayonnaise	*S. aureus*, enterotoxic
Sweden	Salad	Containing mayonnaise	*Salmonella* spp.
Sweden	Salad	Vegetable	*Salmonella* spp.
Sweden	Salad	Containing mayonnaise	*S. aureus*
Sweden	Salad	Vegetable	*S. aureus*
Switzerland	Salad	Ready-to-eat, prepared leaf-salads without sauce	*E. coli*
Netherlands	Salad and similar		*Enterobacteriaceae*
Netherlands	Salad and similar		Molds and yeasts
Netherlands	Salad and similar		Pathogenic microorganisms
Netherlands	Salad and similar		*S. aureus*
New Zealand	Seeds	Cultured	*E. coli*
New Zealand	Seeds	Cultured	*Salmonella* spp.
France	Semi-preserves	Pasteurized	*S. aureus*
Israel	Sesame tahina	Raw material	Aerobic plate count
Israel	Sesame tahina	Raw material	Coliforms
Israel	Sesame tahina	Raw material	Mesophilic spore-forming bacteria
Israel	Sesame tahina	Raw material	Molds
Israel	Sesame tahina	Raw material	*Salmonella* spp.
Israel	Sesame tahina	Raw material	*S. aureus*
Norway	Vegetable salads	Raw, without mayonnaise	Coliforms
Cuba	Vegetables	Dried	Coliforms
Cuba	Vegetables	Dried	Molds
Cuba	Vegetables	Canned	Sterility test
Cuba	Vegetables	Dried	Yeasts
France	Vegetables	Raw, ready-to-eat	*S. aureus*
France	Vegetables	And preparations, ready-to-eat	*B. cereus*
France	Vegetables	And preparations, ready-to-eat	*C. perfringens*
France	Vegetables	Dehydrated/ lyophilized	*Salmonella* spp.

Numerical Values as Given in Original Publication[b] (in cfu/g or mL if not specified)	Sampling Plan as Given in Original Publication[c]	Point of Application	Legal Status
$m = 100$, $M = 1{,}000$	$n = 5$, $c = 2$	Not standardized	Guidelines
Not detectable in 10 g	Not specified	Retail	Mandatory
Not detectable in 10 g	Not specified	Retail	Mandatory
$m = 100$, $M = 1{,}000$	Not specified	Point of production/retail	Not specified
$m = 100$, $M = 1{,}000$	Not specified	Point of production/retail	Not specified
10	Swiss food manual	Swiss food manual	Tolerance value CFU
< 1,000	Not specified	Consumption	Mandatory
< 10,000	Not specified	Consumption	Mandatory
Not detectable	Not specified	Consumption	Mandatory
< 500	Not specified	Consumption	Mandatory
$m = 0$	$n = 5$, $c = 0$	Not specified	Guidelines
$m = 0$ per 25 g	$n = 5$, $c = 0$	Not specified	Guidelines
Not detectable in 1 g	Two class plan	Not specified	Not specified
50,000	M = value of standard, $n = 1$, $c = 0$	Not specified	Mandatory
100	M = value of standard, $n = 1$, $c = 0$	Not specified	Mandatory
100	M = value of standard, $n = 1$, $c = 0$	Not specified	Mandatory
100	M = value of standard, $n = 1$, $c = 0$	Not specified	Mandatory
Not detectable in 20 g	M = value of standard, $n = 1$, $c = 0$	Not specified	Mandatory
100	M = value of standard, $n = 1$, $c = 0$	Not specified	Mandatory
$m = 10$, $M = 100$	Not specified	Not standardized	Guidelines
< 100	$n = 1$	Not specified	Mandatory
< 100	$n = 1$	Not specified	Mandatory
Negative	$n = 1$	Not specified	Mandatory
< 100	$n = 1$	Not specified	Mandatory
$m = 100$, $M = 1{,}000$	Not specified	Not specified	Not specified
$m = 1{,}000$, $M = 10{,}000$	100 g: $n = 5$, $c = 2$	End of shelf life	Mandatory
$m = 100$, $M = 1{,}000$	100 g: $n = 5$, $c = 2$	End of shelf life	Mandatory
Not detectable in 25 g	$n = 5$, $c = 0$	Retail	Guidelines

continued

TABLE E-5 Continued

Country	Food Commodity	Other Information	Microorganisms or Metabolite
ICMSF	Vegetables	Dried	*E. coli*
ICMSF	Vegetables	Frozen, pH > 4.5	*E. coli*
Ireland	Vegetables	And vegetable meals, cooked	Aerobic microorganisms at 30°C
Ireland	Vegetables	And vegetable meals, cooked	Aerobic microorganisms at 30°C
Ireland	Vegetables	And vegetable meals, cooked	Aerobic microorganisms at 30°C
Ireland	Vegetables	And vegetable meals, cooked	*B. cereus* and *B. subtilis* group
Ireland	Vegetables	And vegetable meals, cooked	*Campylobacter*
Ireland	Vegetables	And vegetable meals, cooked	*C. perfringens*
Ireland	Vegetables	And vegetable meals, cooked	*E. coli*
Ireland	Vegetables	And vegetable meals, cooked	*E. coli* O157 and other VTEC
Ireland	Vegetables	And vegetable meals, cooked	*L. monocytogenes*
Ireland	Vegetables	And vegetable meals, cooked	*Listeria* spp. (not *L. monocytogenes*)

Numerical Values as Given in Original Publication[b] (in cfu/g or mL if not specified)	Sampling Plan as Given in Original Publication[c]	Point of Application	Legal Status
m = 100, M = 1,000	n = 5, c = 2	Port of entry	Guidelines
m = 100, M = 1,000	n = 5, c = 2	Port of entry	Guidelines
Satisfactory: < 10,000	Not specified	Retail	Guidelines
Borderline: 10,000 to < 100,000	Not specified	Retail	Guidelines
Unsatisfactory: 100,000	Not specified	Retail	Guidelines
Satisfactory: < 100, borderline: 1,000 to < 10,000, unsatisfactory: 10,000 to < 100,000, unacceptable: 100,000	Not specified	Retail	Guidelines
Satisfactory: not detected in 25 g, unacceptable: present in 25 g	Not specified	Retail	Guidelines
Satisfactory: < 10, borderline: 10 to < 100, unsatisfactory: 100 to < 10,000, unacceptable: 100,000	Not specified	Retail	Guidelines
Satisfactory: < 20, borderline: 20 to < 100, unsatisfactory: 100 to < 10,000, unacceptable/potentially hazardous: 10,000	Not specified	Retail	Guidelines
Satisfactory: not detected in 25 g, unacceptable: present in 25 g	Not specified	Retail	Guidelines
Satisfactory: not detected in 25 g, borderline: < 200 present in 25 g, unsatisfactory: 200 to < 1,000, unacceptable: 1,000	Not specified	Retail	Guidelines
Satisfactory: not detectable in 25 g, borderline: < 200 present in 25 g, unsatisfactory: 200 to < 10,000, unacceptable: 10,000	Not specified	Retail	Guidelines

continued

TABLE E-5 Continued

Country	Food Commodity	Other Information	Microorganisms or Metabolite
Ireland	Vegetables	And vegetable meals, cooked	*Salmonella* spp.
Ireland	Vegetables	And vegetable meals, cooked	*S. aureus*
Ireland	Vegetables	And vegetable meals, cooked	*V. parahaemolyticus*
Israel	Vegetables	Canned	Pathogenic bacteria
Norway	Vegetables	Fresh	*Salmonella* spp.
Spain	Vegetables		Aerobic mesophilic microorganisms
Spain	Vegetables		Coliforms
Spain	Vegetables		*E. coli*
Spain	Vegetables		Molds
Spain	Vegetables		*Salmonella* spp.
Spain	Vegetables		Yeasts
Sweden	Vegetables		*Salmonella* spp.
Israel	Vegetables and fruits	Fresh	Coliforms
Israel	Vegetables and fruits	Fresh	Coliforms faecal
Israel	Vegetables and fruits	Fresh	*E. coli*
Israel	Vegetables and fruits	Fresh	*L. monocytogenes*
Israel	Vegetables and fruits	Fresh	*Salmonella* spp.

[a] ICMSF = International Commission on Microbiological Specifications for Foods.
[b] m = analytical value that differentiates marginally acceptable quality from unacceptable quality, M = analytical value that differentiates good quality from marginally acceptable quality.
[c] n = number of samples taken, maximum number of samples out of n that may exceed the value set for m.
SOURCE: WHO (2000).

Numerical Values as Given in Original Publication[b] (in cfu/g or mL if not specified)	Sampling Plan as Given in Original Publication[c]	Point of Application	Legal Status
Satisfactory: not detected in 25 g, unacceptable: present in 25 g	Not specified	Retail	Guidelines
Satisfactory: < 20, borderline: 20 to < 100, unsatisfactory: 100 to < 10,000, unacceptable/potentially hazardous: 10,000	Not specified	Retail	Guidelines
Satisfactory: not detected in 25 g, borderline: < 200 present in 25 g, unsatisfactory: 200 to < 1,000, unacceptable: 1,000	Not specified	Retail	Guidelines
Not detectable	M = value of standard, $n = 1, c = 0$	Not specified	Mandatory
$m = 0, M = 0$	Not specified	Not standardized	Guidelines
100 to 100,000	Not specified	Not specified	Recommendation
100 to 10,000	Not specified	Not specified	Recommendation
10 to 100	Not specified	Not specified	Recommendation
10 to 10,000	Not specified	Not specified	Recommendation
Not detectable in 25 g	Not specified	Not specified	Recommendation
10 to 10,000	Not specified	Not specified	Recommendation
Not detectable in 10 g	Not specified	Retail	Mandatory
10,000	M = value of standard, $n = 1, c = 0$	Not specified	Mandatory
1,000	M = value of standard, $n = 1, c = 0$	Not specified	Mandatory
Not detectable	M = value of standard, $n = 1, c = 0$	Not specified	Mandatory
Not detectable in 25 g	M = value of standard, $n = 1, c = 0$	Not specified	Voluntary
Not detectable in 20 g	M = value of standard, $n = 1, c = 0$	Not specified	Mandatory

REFERENCES

Food Standards Australia New Zealand. 2003. *Standard 1.6.1: Microbiological Limits for Food.* Online. Available at http://www.foodstandards.gov.au/_srcfiles/Standard161_Micro_v63.pdf. Accessed April 11, 2003.

FSAI (Food Safety Authority of Ireland). 2001. *Guidelines for the Interpretation of Results of Microbiological Analysis of Some Ready-to-Eat Foods Sampled at Point of Sale.* Online. Available at http://www.fsai.ie/service-contracts/guidance_notes/gn3.pdf. Accessed April 14, 2003.

HPFB (Health Products and Food Branch). 2003. *Standards and Guidelines for the Microbiological Safety of Food: An Interpretive Summary.* Ottawa: Government of Canada. P. 12.

ICMSF (International Commission on Microbiological Specifications for Food). 1978. *Microorganisms in Foods 1. Their Significance and Methods of Enumeration,* 2nd ed. Toronto: University of Toronto Press.

ICMSF. 1986. The ICMSF sampling plans and recommended microbiological limits for vegetables, fruits, nuts and yeast 3. In: *Microorganisms in Foods 2, Sampling for Microbial Analysis: Principles and Specific Applications*, 2nd ed. Palo Alto, CA: ICMSF Blackwell Scientific Publications. Pp. 197–202.

ISO (International Organization for Standardization). 1981. *General Guidance for Detection of Salmonella. ISO 6579.* Washington, DC: ISO.

WHO (World Health Organization). 2000. *Database of Microbiological Specifications for Selected Countries (2000).* Online. Available at http://www.who.dk/foodsafety/Microbiological/20020418_8. Accessed March 7, 2003.

Appendix F

International Microbiological Criteria for Dairy Products

TABLE F-1 European Commission Overview of Microbiological Criteria for Dairy Products

			Sampling Plan[a]				
Food Category	Microorganisms	Limit	*N*	*c*	*m*	*M*	Additional Information
Raw milk intended to processing (Directive 92/46/EEC)	Plate count at 30°C	10^5 cfu/mL					Cow's milk
		5×10^5 or 1.5×10^6 cfu/mL					Buffalo's, goat's and sheep's milk
	Staphylococcus aureus		5	2	500 cfu/mL	2,000 cfu/mL	Milk for manufacturing of raw products
Raw cow's milk intended for direct human consumption (Directive 92/46/EEC)	*Salmonella*	Absence in 25 g	5	0			
	S. aureus		5	2	100/mL	500/mL	
	Plate count at 30°C	5×10^4 cfu/mL					
Pasteurised drinking milk (Directive 92/46/EEC)	Pathogenic microorganisms	Absent in 25 g	5	0			
	Coliforms		5	1	0 cfu/mL	5 cfu/mL	
	Plate count at 21°C		5	1	5×10^4 cfu/g	5×10^5 cfu/g	After incubation at 6°C for 5 days
UHT milk and sterilized milk (Directive 92/46/EEC)	Plate count at 30°C	10 cfu/0.1 mL					After incubation at 30°C for 15 days
Cheeses made from raw milk and from thermized milk (Directive 92/46/EEC)	*Listeria monocytogenes*	Absence in 1 g (hard cheeses) or in 25 g (other)	5	0			
	Salmonella	Absence in 1 g	5	0			
	S. aureus, guideline		5	2	1,000 cfu/g	10,000 cfu/g	
	Escherichia coli, guideline		5	2	10^4 cfu/g	10^5 cfu/g	

Soft cheese	*L. monocytogenes*	Absence in 25 g	5	0			
(made from	*Salmonella*	Absence in 1 g	5	0			
heat-treated milk)	*S. aureus,* guideline		5	2	100 cfu/g	1,000 cfu/g	
(Directive 92/46/EEC)	*E. coli,* guideline		5	2	100 cfu/g	1,000 cfu/g	
	Coliforms, guideline		5	2	10^4 cfu/g	10^5 cfu/g	
Fresh cheese	*L. monocytogenes*	Absence in 25 g	5	0			
(Directive 92/46/EEC)	*Salmonella*	Absence in 1 g	5	0			
	S. aureus, guideline		5	2	10 cfu/g	100 cfu/g	
Other cheese (Directive 92/4/EEC)	*L. monocytogenes*	Absence in 1 g (hard cheeses) or in 25 g (other)	5	0			
	Salmonella	Absence in 1 g	5	0			
Butter	*L. monocytogenes*	Absence in 1 g	5	0			
(Directive 92/46/EEC)	*Salmonella*	Absence in 1 g	5	0			
	Coliforms, guideline		5	2	0 cfu/g	10 cfu/g	
Powdered milk and	*Salmonella*	Absence in 1 g	5	0			
milk-based products	*L. monocytogenes*	Absence in 1 g	5	0			
(Directive 92/46/EEC)	*S. aureus,* guideline		5	2	10 cfu/g	100 cfu/g	Powdered milk
	Coliforms, guideline		5	2	0 cfu	10 cfu/g	Powdered milk-based products
Frozen milk-based	*Salmonella*	Absence in 1 g	5	0			
products	*L. monocytogenes*	Absence in 1 g	5	0			
(Directive 92/46/EEC)	*S. aureus,* guideline		5	2	10 cfu/g	100 cfu/g	
	Coliforms, guideline		5	2	10 cfu/g	100 cfu/g	
	Plate count, guideline		5	2	10^5 cfu/g	5×10^5 cfu/g	

continued

TABLE F-1 Continued

Food Category	Microorganisms	Limit	Sampling Plan[a]				Additional Information
			n	c	m	M	
Liquid milk-based products (Directive 92/46/EEC)	*Salmonella*	Absence in 1 g	5	0			
	L. monocytogenes	Absence in 1 g	5	0			

[a] n = number of samples taken, c = maximum number of samples out of n that may exceed the value set for m, m = analytical value that differentiates good quality from marginally acceptable quality, M = analytical value that differentiates marginally acceptable quality from unacceptable quality.
SOURCE: EC (2001).

TABLE F-2 Australian Microbiological Criteria for Dairy Products

Food	Microorganism	Sampling Plan[a]			
		n	c	m	M
Butter made from unpasteurised milk and/or unpasteurised milk products	*Campylobacter*/25 g	5	0	0	
	Coagulase-positive staphylococci/g	5	1	10	10^2
	Coliforms/g	5	1	10	10^2
	Escherichia coli/g	5	1	3	9
	Listeria monocytogenes/25 g	5	0	0	
	Salmonella/25 g	5	0	0	
	Standard plate count/g	5	0	5×10^5	

All cheese	*E. coli*/g	5	1	10	10^2
Soft and semi-soft cheese (moisture content > 39%) with pH > 5.0	*L. monocytogenes*/25 g	5	0	0	
	Salmonella/25 g	5	0	0	
All raw milk cheese (cheese made from milk not pasteurised or thermised)	*L. monocytogenes*/25 g	5	0	0	
	Salmonella/25 g	5	0	0	
Raw milk unripened cheeses (moisture content > 50% with pH > 5.0)	*Campylobacter*/25 g	5	0	0	
Dried milk	*Salmonella*/25 g	5	0	0	
Unpasteurised milk	*Campylobacter*/25 mL	5	0	0	10^2
	Coliforms/mL	5	1	10^2	9
	E. coli/mL	5	1	3	2.5×10^5
	L. monocytogenes/25 mL	5	0	0	
	Salmonella/25 mL	5	0	0	
	Standard plate count/mL	5	1	2.5×10^4	

[a] n = number of samples taken, c = maximum number of samples out of n that may exceed the value set for m, m = analytical value that differentiates good quality from marginally acceptable quality, M = analytical value that differentiates marginally acceptable quality from unacceptable quality.
SOURCE: ADASC (2000).

TABLE F-3 Codex Alimentarius Microbiological Criteria for Milk Products

Food Commodity	Other Information	Microorganisms or Metabolite	Numerical Values[a]	Sampling Plan[b]	Point of Application	Legal Status
Milk products	Dried	*Salmonella* spp.	$m = 0$	$n = 15$ $c = 0$	Endproducts	Guidelines
Milk products	Dried	Aerobic mesophilic bacteria	$m = 50{,}000$ $M = 200{,}000$	$n = 5$ $c = 2$	Endproducts	Guidelines
Milk products	Dried	Coliforms	$m = 10$ $M = 100$	$n = 5$ $c = 1$	Endproducts	Guidelines

[a] m = analytical value that differentiates good quality from marginally acceptable quality, M = analytical value that differentiates marginally acceptable quality from unacceptable quality.
[b] n = number of samples taken, c = maximum number of samples out of n that may exceed the value set for m.
SOURCE: CAC (1983)

REFERENCES

ADASC (Australian Dairy Authorities' Standards Committee). 2000. *Minimum Sampling Guidelines for Dairy Products.* Online. Available at http://www.dairysafe.vic.gov.au/documents/Minimum%20Sampling%20Guidelines%20for%20Dairy%20Products.pdf. Accessed May 27, 2003.

CAC (Codex Alimentarius Commission). 1983. *Recommended International Code of Hygienic Practice for Dried Milk.* CAC/RPC 31. Available at ftp://ftp.fao.org/codex/standard/en/CXP_031e.pdf. Accessed May 27, 2003.

EC (European Commission). 2001. *Overview of Microbiological Criteria for Foodstuffs in Community Legislation in Force.* Online. Available at http://europa.eu.int/comm/food/fs/sfp/mr/mr_crit_en.pdf. Accessed April 11, 2003.

Appendix G

U.S. Department of Agriculture—Agricultural Marketing Service Standards for Milk and Dairy Products

TABLE G-1 Microbiological Standards for Raw Milk for Manufacturing Purposes

Bacterial Estimate Classification	Direct Microscopic Count, Standard Plate Count, Plate Loop Count, Pectin Gel Plate Count, Petrifilm Aerobic Count, Spiral Plate Count, Hydrophobic Grid Membrane Filter Count, Impedence/Conductance Count, or Reflectance Calorimetry
Herd milk	Not over 500,000/mL
Commingled milk	Not over 1,000,000/mL

SOURCE: Dairy Programs (2002).

TABLE G-2 Updated Microbial Standards for Processed Milk Products: U.S. Department of Agriculture Agricultural Marketing Service Standards for Grades of Dairy Products

Product	Standard	Method[a]	Reference
Nonfat dry milk (spray process)			Dairy Programs, 2001c
U.S. extra grade	10,000/g	SPC	
U.S. standard grade	75,000/g	SPC	
U.S. grade not assigned	100×10^6/g	DMC	
Nonfat dry milk (roller process)			Dairy Division, 1984
U.S. extra grade	50,000	SPC	
U.S. standard grade	100,000/g	SPC	
U.S. grade not assigned	100×10^6/g	DMC	
Instant nonfat dry milk			Dairy Programs, 2001d
U.S. extra grade	10,000/g	SPC	
	10/g	Coliform	
U.S. grade not assigned	40×10^6/g	DMC	
Dry whole milk			Dairy Programs, 2001b
U.S. premium	Not applicable	SPC	
U.S. extra	10,000/g	SPC	
	10/g	Coliform	
U.S. standard	50,000	SPC	
	10/g	Coliform	
U.S. grade not assigned	100×10^6/g	DMC	
Dry buttermilk and buttermilk product			Dairy Programs, 2001a
U.S. extra	20,000/g	SPC	
U.S. standard	75,000/g	SPC	
Dry whey			Dairy Programs, 2000
U.S. extra	30,000/g	SPC	
	10/g	Coliform	
Butter	100/g	Proteolytic	Dairy Division, 2002
	20/g	Yeasts and molds	
	10/g	Coliform	
Whipped butter	50/g	Proteolytic	Dairy Division, 2002
	10/g	Yeasts and molds	
	10/g	Coliform	
Plastic and frozen cream	30,000/mL	SPC	AMS, 1975
	20/mL	Yeasts and molds	
	10/mL	Coliform	
Cottage cheese	10/g	Coliform	AMS, 1975
	100/g	Psychrotrophic	
	10/g	Yeasts and molds	

continued

TABLE G-2 Continued

Product	Standard	Method[a]	Reference
Ice cream	50,000/g	SPC	AMS, 1975
Plain	10/g	Coliform	
Frozen	20/g	Coliform	
Sherbet	50,000/g	SPC	AMS, 1975
	10/g	Coliform	
Sweetened condensed milk	1,000/g	SPC	AMS, 1975
	10/g	Coliform	
	5/g	Yeasts	
	5/g	Molds	
Edible dry casein (acid)			Dairy Division, 1968
U.S. extra grade	30,000/g	SPC	
	0/0.1g	Coliform	
U.S. standard grade	100,000/g	SPC	
	2/0.1g	Coliform	
	0/100g	Salmonella[b]	
	0/g	Staphylococci[b]	
	5,000/g	Thermophiles[b]	
	5/0.1g	Yeasts and molds[b]	
Cheddar cheese	Not available	Coliform	Dairy Division, 1956

[a] SPC = standard plate count, DMC = direct microscopic count.
[b] Optional.

TABLE G-3 Microbiological Standards for Raw Milk: U.S. Department of Agriculture Agricultural Marketing Service Standards for Grades of Dairy Products

Bacterial Estimate Classification	Direct Microscopic Count, Standard Plate Count, or Plate Loop Count
No. 1	Not over 500,000/mL
No. 2	Not over 1,000,000
Undergrade	Over 1,000,000

SOURCE: Dairy Division (2002).

REFERENCES

AMS (Agricultural Marketing Service). 1975. General specifications for approved dairy plants and standards for grades of dairy products. *Fed Regist* 40:47910–47940.

Dairy Division. 1956. *United States Standards for Grades of Cheddar Cheese*. Online. Agricultural Marketing Service (AMS), U.S. Department of Agriculture (USDA). Available at http://www.ams.usda.gov/standards/Cheddar.pdf. Accessed August 15, 2002.

Dairy Division. 1968. *United States Standards for Grades of Edible Dry Casein (Acid)*. Online. AMS, USDA. Available at http://www.ams.usda.gov/standards/Edible.pdf. Accessed August 15, 2002.

Dairy Division. 1984. *United States Standards for Grades of Nonfat Dry Milk (Roller Process)*. Online. AMS, USDA. Available at http://www.ams.usda.gov/standards/Roller.pdf. Accessed August 15, 2002.

Dairy Division. 2002. *General Specifications for Dairy Plants Approved for USDA Inspection and Grading Service*. Online. AMS, USDA. Available at http://www.ams.usda.gov/dairy/genpecs.pdf. Accessed August 15, 2002.

Dairy Programs. 2000. *United States Standard for Dry Whey*. Online. AMS, USDA. Available at http://www.ams.usda.gov/standards/dry_whey_standards_12-14-00.pdf. Accessed August 15, 2002.

Dairy Programs. 2001a. *United States Standards for Grades of Dry Buttermilk and Dry Buttermilk Product*. Online. AMS, USDA. Available at http://www.ams.usda.gov/standards/DBM_02-02-01.pdf. Accessed August 15, 2002.

Dairy Programs. 2001b. *United States Standards for Grades of Dry Whole Milk*. Online. AMS, USDA. Available at http://www.ams.usda.gov/standards/dry_whole_milk_04-13-01.pdf. Accessed August 15, 2002.

Dairy Programs. 2001c. *United States Standards for Grades of Nonfat Dry Milk (Spray Process)*. Online. AMS, USDA. Available at http://www.ams.usda.gov/standards/NDM_02-02-01.pdf. Accessed August 15, 2002.

Dairy Programs. 2001d. *United States Standards for Instant Nonfat Dry Milk*. Online. AMS, USDA. Available at http://www.ams.usda.gov/standards/INDM_02-02-01.pdf. Accessed August 15, 2002.

Dairy Programs. 2002. *Milk for Manufacturing Purposes and its Production and Processing*. Online. AMS, USDA. Available at http://www.ams.usda.gov/dairy/manufmlk.pdf. Accessed August 15, 2002.

Appendix H

Biographical Sketches of Committee and Subcommittee Members

Claude Earl Fox, M.D., M.P.H. *(Co-chair),* is a professor of public health in the Department of Population and Family Health Sciences with joint academic appointments in the Department of Medicine and the School of Nursing, Johns Hopkins Bloomberg School of Public Health, and founding director of the Johns Hopkins Urban Health Institute. He is also an adjunct associate professor of epidemiology and biostatistics at the School of Public Health, George Washington University. Earlier, Dr. Fox served as administrator, Health Resources and Service Administration, U.S. Department of Health and Human Services (HHS), and as Deputy Assistant Secretary for Health (Disease Prevention and Health Promotion) also at HHS, where he was a key player in setting Healthy People 2010 health objectives for the nation. He has been a Public Health Service regional health administrator, was a state health officer in the Alabama Department of Public Health for six years, and was a deputy health officer in Mississippi. Throughout his career, Dr. Fox has taught in the School of Public Health at the University of North Carolina, Chapel Hill, at the George Washington University, and at the University of Alabama, Birmingham. In addition to service in the public sector, Dr. Fox has been a consultant for the Public Health Foundation in Washington, D.C. He has received many awards and has been active as member, board member, or chair of numerous committees, advisory panels, and associations. He also served as president of the Association of State and Territorial Health Officials. Dr. Fox holds a B.S. and an M.D. from the University of Mississippi and an M.P.H. from the University of North Carolina, Chapel Hill, is board certified in preventive medicine and public health, and is licensed to practice medicine in Delaware, Maryland, and Mississippi.

Cameron R. Hackney, Ph.D. *(Co-chair),* is dean of the Davis College of Agriculture, Forestry and Consumer Sciences and director of the West Virginia Experiment Station, West Virginia University in Morgantown. Previously, Dr. Hackney held positions as department head and professor in the Department of Food Science and Technology, Virginia Polytechnic Institute and State University, Blacksburg, and superintendent of the Virginia Seafood Research and Extension Center in Hampton. His academic background is in food science, and he has taught undergraduate and graduate courses in food microbiology, food toxicology, and dairy processing, and was an extension project leader for food science and technology at the Virginia Polytechnic and State University from 1992 to 1997. He has edited two books on seafood safety and has published or presented over 250 scientific papers and presentations. In addition, he has given over 200 presentations as part of extension workshops. Dr. Hackney was a member of the Institute of Medicine Committee on Evaluation of the Safety of Fishery Products (1988–1990) that produced the report, *Seafood Safety*. He has served on numerous national and state committees, including the Microbiology Committee of the Interstate Shellfish Sanitation Conference (1984–1991), the Methods Committee of the National Indicator Study (1991), and the National Indicator Study's Microbiology Committee (1987–1992), which he chaired. He has helped organize over 75 national and international workshops, and has international experience as a consultant. Dr. Hackney holds a B.S. in animal science and an M.S. in agricultural microbiology from West Virginia University, and a Ph.D. in food science from North Carolina State University. He is past chair of the Council of Food Science Administrators and chair of the Northeast Experiment Station Directors. He is a fellow of the International Association for Food Protection and is a member of the Institute of Food Technologists and the Atlantic Fisheries Technology Society.

Kathryn J. Boor, Ph.D., is an associate professor of food processing microbiology in the Department of Food Science at Cornell University, Ithaca, New York. Her research interests include dairy microbiology and product safety, bacterial transmission in food processing systems (dairy and seafood), bacterial food safety, food processing microbiology, product shelf-life extension, and food biotechnology. Dr. Boor is a member of the American Association for the Advancement of Science, the American Society for Microbiology, the American Dairy Science Association, the Institute of Food Technologists, the International Association for Food Protection, and The Dairy Practices Council. She is currently on the board of directors for the American Dairy Science Association. She is also the scientific advisor for the New York State Cheese Manufacturers' Association. She has received many honors, including most recently the 2000 U.S. Department of Agriculture Honor Award for her work with the Listeria Outbreak Working Group. Dr. Boor holds a B.S. in food science from Cornell University, an M.S. in food science from the University of Wisconsin, and a Ph.D. in microbiology from the University of California at Davis.

Elizabeth Boyle, Ph.D., is a professor in the Department of Animal Sciences and Industry at Kansas State University in Manhattan. Her area of expertise is in meat processing, safety, and quality. She works mainly in extension to enhance the quality and safety of meat products and to provide scientific and technical assistance to meat processors and trade associations. She also teaches Hazard Analysis and Critical Control Point (HACCP) workshops nationally as a certified lead HACCP instructor and teaches undergraduate and graduate courses in HACCP and advanced HACCP. Her research interests focus on the impact of HACCP on small and very small meat and poultry processing facilities, and meat safety and quality. She has received several awards, has published numerous scientific and extension publications and abstracts, and has made presentations at many professional and industrial meetings. She is a member of the Institute of Food Technologists, the American Meat Science Association, the Council for Agricultural Science and Technology, and the Kansas Meat Processors Association. Dr. Boyle holds a B.S. in wildlife biology from the University of Minnesota, an M.S. in food science and human nutrition and a Ph.D. in meat science and technology from Colorado State University.

Marsha N. Cohen, J.D., is a professor of law at Hastings College of the Law, University of California, San Francisco. Professor Cohen's publications and lectures focus on pharmacy law, food law, and consumer protection issues. She participated in the Institute of Medicine's 1998 Committee to Ensure Safe Food from Production to Consumption and served as a member of the Institute of Medicine's Food Forum. Earlier, she was a member of the Food and Drug Administration's Food Advisory Committee, the California State Board of Pharmacy, and other national and state committees. Prior to her position at Hastings, Professor Cohen was a staff attorney for the Washington, D.C., office of Consumers Union. Professor Cohen obtained a B.A. from Smith College and a J.D. from Harvard Law School. She is a member of the Bar in California and the District of Columbia.

James S. Dickson, Ph.D. (*Chair, Subcommittee on Meat and Poultry*), is a professor and chair of the Microbiology Department at Iowa State University in Ames. His academic background is in food science and microbiology. Dr. Dickson is a recognized scientist in the area of microbiology of foods of animal origin in relation to pathogens, their etiology, detection and isolation methods, and decontamination interventions. He is also interested in predictive microbiology. Dr. Dickson is a certified HACCP instructor and has chaired subcommittees of the International HACCP Alliance. He has authored over 60 scientific papers and five book chapters and has received several awards. He is a fellow of the American Academy of Microbiology and a member of the American Society for Microbiology and the Institute of Food Technologists. He was the 2001–2002 president of the International Association for Food Protection. Dr. Dickson holds a B.S. in microbiology from Clemson University, an M.S. in dairy science from the University of Georgia, and a Ph.D. in food science and technology from the University of Nebraska.

Darrell W. Donahue, Ph.D., is an associate professor and coordinator of Biological Engineering in the Department of Chemical and Biological Engineering at the University of Maine in Orono. Previously he was the director of information systems and a visiting assistant professor at North Carolina State University. He also has industrial experience working as a process engineer and a process engineering consultant for two major food companies. Currently, his research interests include engineering support for quality assurance systems and design and evaluation of biological sensors for food processing applications. Dr. Donahue is involved in many professional societies, including the Institute of Food Technologists, the American Society of Agricultural Engineers, the Institute for Operations Research and Management Science, and the American Society of Quality. He has been a reviewer and editor of many journals and proposals. Dr. Donahue holds a B.S. in zoology and chemistry, an M.S. in biological and agricultural engineering and mathematics, and a Ph.D. in engineering and operations research, all from North Carolina State University.

Jeffrey M. Farber, Ph.D., is the director of the Bureau of Microbial Hazards in the Health Products and Food Branch, Food Directorate, Health Canada; as such, he is an employee of the Canadian government. Earlier, he was research scientist and scientific advisor with that unit for many years. Dr. Farber is an internationally recognized food microbiologist and a member and treasurer of the International Commission on the Microbiological Safety of Foods, which has proposed a description of the role of food safety objectives as a basis for setting food process control criteria (performance standards) within a HACCP system. He is a member of the International Association for Food Protection and holds a Ph.D. in microbiology.

Robert Gravani, Ph.D. (*Chair, Subcommittee on Produce and Related Products, Seafood, and Dairy Products*), is a professor of food science at Cornell University, Ithaca, New York. His fields of expertise are food microbiology; food safety and sanitation in the food processing, food service, and retail food industries; food regulations; and consumer food safety information. His work, mainly in extension/outreach, currently emphasizes the development of Good Agricultural Practices to reduce microbial risks in fruits and vegetables. He is also involved in providing scientific and technical assistance to constituents and trade associations in all areas of food safety and sanitation, including basic food microbiology, food regulations, good manufacturing practices, prerequisite programs, and the HACCP system. He coteaches a popular course on food choices and issues. Dr. Gravani's research has focused on the use of natural microbial growth inhibitors in foods and on consumer and retail workers' knowledge of food safety. He is a past member of the National Advisory Committee on Microbiological Safety of Foods and serves currently on the Accreditation Review Committee of the International HACCP Alliance. Dr. Gravani has published numerous scientific papers and abstracts. He is a fellow of the Institute of Food Technologists, a member of the American Society for Microbiology, the International Association for Food Protection, the Association of Food and Drug Officials, the National Restaurant Association, and the Council for Agricultural Science and Technology. He also belongs to various honor societies and has received multiple awards for excellence in teaching and extension activities. Dr. Gravani holds a B.S. in food science from Rutgers University, and an M.S. and a Ph.D. in food science from Cornell University.

Richard L. Guerrant, M.D., is the Thomas H. Hunter Professor of International Medicine, and director of the Center for Global Health at the University of Virginia School of Medicine. He was trained in internal medicine and infectious diseases at the Harvard Service of Boston City Hospital, Johns Hopkins, the National Institutes of Health, and the University of Virginia. Dr. Guerrant's research interests focus on the recognition, diagnosis, pathogenesis, and treatment of enteric diseases. An important area of his research has focused on pathogenesis of foodborne disease agents. His current work involves investigating the role of key mediators in inflammatory parasitic infections (e.g., from *Cryptosporidium*) and diarrheas due to microbial adhesion or toxins (i.e., enteroaggregative *Escherichia coli*). He has done extensive fieldwork defining the magnitude of diarrheal diseases and their nutritional impact in rural and urban communities, including studies in northeastern Brazil, the Congo, and Bangladesh, and he started the Division of Geographic and International Medicine with Kellogg and Rockefeller support in 1978. Dr. Guerrant is the author of more than 400 scientific and clinical articles, reviews, and numerous major textbook chapters, and editor of 7 books, and is on the editorial board of the *Reviews of Infectious Diseases*. Among his most recent awards are the Henderson Award, the IDSA Abbott Award, the ACCA Award, and the Smadel and Abbot Award. Dr. Guerrant holds a B.S. from Davidson College and an M.D. from the University of Virginia School of Medicine.

Linda J. Harris, Ph.D., is a cooperative extension specialist in the Department of Food Science and Technology at the University of California at Davis. Her current research interests focus on microbial safety and spoilage issues related to fresh and processed fruits and vegetables. Her extension programs cover microbial food safety of meat, dairy products, and fruits and vegetables for producers, processors, retailers, and consumers. Dr. Harris is a member of the American Society for Microbiology, International Association for Food Protection, Institute of Food Technologists, and International Fresh-cut Fruit and Vegetable Association. She has served on the editorial board of *Applied and Environmental Microbiology* and the *Journal of Food Protection* and is a past member of the Institute of Food Technologists/Food and Drug Administration Task Force on the Microbiological Safety of Fresh and Fresh-cut Fruits and Vegetables. Dr. Harris holds a B.S. in food science and an M.S. in food microbiology from the University of Alberta and a Ph.D. in microbiology from North Carolina State University.

Craig W. Hedberg, Ph.D., is an associate professor in the Division of Environmental and Occupational Health in the School of Public Health at the University of Minnesota. Previously he held positions as a supervisor of the Foodborne, Vectorborne, and Zoonotic Diseases Unit and the Surveillance and Disease Investigations Unit at the Minnesota Department of Health (MDH), and as communicable disease epidemiologist at Hennepin County Community Health Department and MDH. His current research interests include food-borne disease surveillance and the use of epidemiological methods in outbreak investigation and disease control. Dr. Hedberg has received many honors, including the Charles C. Shepard Science Award from the Centers for Disease Control and Prevention in 1991 and a Commissioner's Special Citation (Schwans outbreak) from the Food and Drug Administration in 1995. He is a member of many professional associations, including the International Association for Food Protection, and has been appointed or elected to many boards, including the Minnesota Environmental Health Association and School of Public Health Policy Council. He also serves as an editor of *Epidemiology and Infection* and is a reviewer for many journals. Dr. Hedberg holds a B.S. in biology from the University of Connecticut and an M.S. in environmental health and a Ph.D. in epidemiology from the University of Minnesota.

Neal H. Hooker, Ph.D., is an assistant professor in the Department of Agricultural, Environmental, and Development Economics at Ohio State University. His research and extension interests include agribusiness management and marketing, food safety and economics, E-agribusiness, policy, and international trade. He is a member of the American Agricultural Economical Association, the International Food and Agribusiness Management Association, the Food Distribution Research Society, and the International Fresh-cut Produce Association. Dr. Hooker holds a B.S. in economics from the University of Essex, an M.A. in economics from the University of British Columbia, and a Ph.D. in resource economics from the University of Massachusetts.

John A. Marcy, Ph.D., is an extension food scientist with The Center for Excellence in Poultry Science at the University of Arkansas in Fayetteville. His academic training is in food science, food microbiology, and statistics. Dr. Marcy's expertise in poultry processing, HACCP methodology and plans, and U.S. Department of Agriculture regulations is well recognized by the poultry industry. Although his work is mainly in extension, he also conducts research on poultry processing and quality factors, meat microbiology, and food safety. He has received awards for establishing food service training partnerships in several states. He has authored several scientific papers and three book chapters, and has taught HACCP at many workshops nationally and internationally as a Certified Lead HACCP Instructor. He is a member of the Institute of Food Technologists, the International Association for Food Protection, the Conference for Food Protection, the National Environmental Health Association, the Society for the Advancement of Foodservice Research, the Poultry Science Association, and several honor societies. Dr. Marcy holds a B.S. in food technology and science from the University of Tennessee and an M.S. and a Ph.D. in food technology from Iowa State University.

W. Steven Otwell, Ph.D., is a professor and Florida Sea Grant Seafood Specialist in the Aquatic Food Products Lab of the University of Florida. His research interests address all aspects of seafood product quality and safety from production through processing to retail and food services. He currently serves as a national coordinator for the Seafood HACCP Alliance for Education and Training, the executive director of the Seafood Science and Technology Society of the Americas, a fellow for the Institute of Food Technologists, and the director of the Annual Shrimp School. He serves on the editorial staff of the *Journal of Aquatic Food Product Technology*. Dr. Otwell is developing generic HACCP models for smoked fish and primary shrimp processing. He holds a B.S. in biology from Virginia Military Institute, an M.S. in marine science from the University of Virginia, and a Ph.D. in food science from North Carolina State University.

Jim E. Riviere, D.V.M, Ph.D., is Distinguished Professor of Pharmacology and director of the Center for Chemical Toxicology Research and Pharmacokinetics at the College of Veterinary Medicine, North Carolina State University, Raleigh. He has conducted extensive research into the fate and effects of veterinary drug residues, including antibiotics, and many toxic substances in food animals and their presence in foods derived from animals. The focus of his research is mathematical modeling of drug and chemicals disposition and comparative pharmacokinetics and prediction of drug residues in food animals. He teaches courses in pharmacokinetics and drug delivery. He is a member of the Food and Drug Administration Science Board, co-founder and co-director of the global Food Animal Residue Avoidance Databank, now an official program of the Food and Agriculture Organization of the United Nations, and a former member of the U.S. Pharmacopoeia's General Committee on Revision. Dr. Riviere has been the recipient of many awards and is a fellow of the Academy of Toxicological Sciences. He is a member of the American Association for the Advancement of Science, the American Association of Pharmaceutical Sciences, the American Academy of Veterinary Pharmacology and Therapeutics, the American Veterinary Medical Association, and the Society of Toxicology. He has written six books and more than 150 original scientific papers and many book chapters and reviews. Dr. Riviere holds a B.S. in biology and an M.S. in endocrinology from Boston College and a Ph.D. in pharmacology and a D.V.M. from Purdue University.

Donald W. Schaffner, Ph.D., is an extension specialist and professor in the Department of Food Science at Rutgers University in New Jersey. His research interests include quantitative risk assessment and predictive modeling. Dr. Schaffner has authored more than 100 peer-reviewed publications, book chapters, and abstracts. He has educated thousands of food industry professionals through numerous short courses and workshops in the United States and more than a dozen countries around the world. He recently chaired two World Health Organization/Food and Agriculture Organization expert workshops on the development of exposure assessment and risk characterization guidelines for microbiological hazards in food. He has also served on several Institute of Food Technologists Expert Panels for a variety of food safety-related topics. Dr. Schaffner is active in several scientific associations including the International Association for Food Protection, the Institute of Food Technologists, the Society for Risk Analysis, and the American Society for Microbiology. He holds a B.S. in food science from Cornell University and an M.S. and a Ph.D. in food science and technology from the University of Georgia.

John G. Surak, Ph.D., is a professor of food science and coordinator of International Programs for the College of Agriculture, Forestry, and Life Sciences at Clemson University, Clemson, South Carolina. Dr. Surak has academic training in food science and in veterinary science (pathology and toxicology) and works primarily in extension services. His work focuses on the development of quality management systems for food safety and emphasizes statistical process control for the food industry. Dr. Surak teaches the statistical process control part of the HACCP Implementation Model Program to Food Safety and Inspection Service inspectors and to industry participants of the pilot study. He is also a consultant to the U.S. Department of Agriculture's Agricultural Marketing Service on purchasing specifications for meat and poultry for the School Lunch Program and to the Grain Inspection Packers and Stockyard Administration on assessment of their quality assurance programs. He has conducted economic analyses of HACCP regulations. He has received many awards and has written more than 100 publications. Dr. Surak is a member of the American Society for Quality Control and the Institute of Food Technologists and is a fellow of both societies. He holds a B.S. and an M.S. in food science and a Ph.D. in food science and veterinary science, all from the University of Wisconsin.

Donn R. Ward, Ph.D., is a professor (extension specialist) and associate head of the Department of Food Science at North Carolina State University in Raleigh. As an extension specialist in seafood technology, his research interests include HACCP education and the development and implementation of HACCP systems in the food processing industry associated with aquatic food products. He is currently a member of the Institute of Food Technologists, the International Association for Food Protection, and the Association of Food and Drug Officials, and the honor societies Gamma Sigma Delta, Phi Sigma, and Phi Tau Sigma. Dr. Ward is currently a co-chair of the National Sanitation Foundation International's Food Safety and Quality Advisory Council. He has served on various committees of the Institute of Food Technologists, the Tropical and Subtropical Fisheries Technological Conference of the Americas, and various editorial boards. Dr. Ward holds a B.S. in biology and an M.S. in food science from Virginia Polytechnic Institute and State University and a Ph.D. in food science and technology from Texas A&M University.

Terri Wenger, Ph.D., is the chief of the Grading, Labeling, and Evaluation Section in the Division of Food Safety of the Wisconsin Department of Agriculture, Trade, and Consumer Protection. She is responsible for statewide program and policy development and day-to-day direction in food product standards and labeling; cheese, butter, and egg grading and egg processor inspection and licensing; and laboratory evaluation. She received the departmental Exceptional Performance Award in 1994. Dr. Wenger is a member of many professional organizations, including the Association of Food and Drug Officials, the North Central Association of Food and Drug Officials, the Institute of Food Technologists, and the American Diabetes Association. She is a certified professional food manager, has a restaurant manager certification (Wisconsin), and is certified in family and consumer sciences. Dr. Wenger holds a B.S. in home economics and a Ph.D. in nutritional sciences with a minor in food science from the University of Wisconsin.

Index

A

B

C

D

E

F

G

H

I

J

L

M

N

S

T

U

V

W

Y

Z